BLACK WOMEN'S REPRODUCTIVE HEALTH & SEXUALITY
~A HOLISTIC PUBLIC HEALTH APPROACH~

For access to digital chapters,
visit the APHA Press bookstore (www.apha.org).

BLACK WOMEN'S REPRODUCTIVE HEALTH & SEXUALITY
~A HOLISTIC PUBLIC HEALTH APPROACH~

REGINA DAVIS MOSS, PhD, MPH
~EDITOR~

APHA PRESS
AN IMPRINT OF AMERICAN PUBLIC HEALTH ASSOCIATION

American Public Health Association
800 I Street, NW
Washington, DC 20001-3710
www.apha.org

© 2023 by the American Public Health Association

All rights reserved. No part of this publication may be reproduced, stored in a retrieval system, or transmitted in any form or by any means, electronic, mechanical, photocopying, recording, scanning, or otherwise, except as permitted under Sections 107 and 108 of the 1976 United States Copyright Act, without either the prior written permission of the Publisher or authorization through payment of the appropriate per-copy fee to the Copyright Clearance Center [222 Rosewood Drive, Danvers, MA 01923, (978) 750-8400, fax (978) 646-8600, www.copyright.com]. Requests to the Publisher for permission should be addressed to the Permissions Department, American Public Health Association, 800 I Street, NW, Washington, DC 20001-3710; fax (202) 777-2531.

DISCLAIMER: Any discussion of medical or legal issues in this publication is being provided for informational purposes only. Nothing in this publication is intended to constitute medical or legal advice, and it should not be construed as such. This book is not intended to be and should not be used as a substitute for specific medical or legal advice, since medical and legal opinions may only be given in response to inquiries regarding specific factual situations. If medical or legal advice is desired by the reader of this book, a medical doctor or attorney should be consulted. The use of trade names and commercial sources in this book does not imply endorsement by the American Public Health Association. The views expressed in the publications of the American Public Health Association are those of the contributors and do not necessarily reflect the views of the American Public Health Association, or its staff, advisory panels, officers, or members of the Association's Executive Board. While the publisher and contributors have used their best efforts in preparing this book, they make no representations with respect to the accuracy or completeness of the content. The findings and conclusions in this book are those of the contributors and do not necessarily represent the official positions of the institutions with which they are affiliated.

Georges C. Benjamin, MD, MACP, Executive Director

Printed and bound in the United States of America
Book Production Editor: Maya Ribault
Typesetting: The Charlesworth Group
Cover Design: Alan Giarcanella
Printing and Binding: Sheridan Books

About the Cover: "Mother" was created by Black artist Alan Giarcanella in honor of his mother who was being treated for breast cancer. The piece is a figurative exploration of the strong Black woman as the original mother of humanity and her ascension over oppression. The subject's skin tone is a rich black, conveying the intentionality of the book. The abstract figures cradling her face—a woman's back symbolizing sensuality, and pregnant silhouette signifying life, rebirth, and fertility—infuse the beauty of the womb, sex positivity, and maternity. The subtle purple on her eyelids is an homage to royalty, freedom, Alice Walker, and Black feminism. Her hair, which morphs into a golden glow of African textiles, represents resistance against western beauty ideals and her return to her throne as Mother Goddess.

Library of Congress Cataloging-in-Publication Data

Names: Davis Moss, Regina, editor. | American Public Health Association, issuing body.
Title: Black women's reproductive health and sexuality : a holistic public health approach / [edited by] Regina Davis Moss.
Description: Washington, DC : American Public Health Association, 2023. | Includes bibliographical references and index. | Summary: "Intended as a resource for public health professionals and others committed to improving the reproductive and sexual health outcomes for Black women in America, this book takes a holistic look at the many facets of the reproductive health and sexuality of Black women by providing the readers with a life course perspective as well as a historical context"-- Provided by publisher.
Identifiers: LCCN 2023012827 (print) | LCCN 2023012828 (ebook) | ISBN 9780875533407 (paperback) | ISBN 9780875533414 (adobe pdf)
Subjects: MESH: Reproductive Health | Women's Health | Black or African American | Sexual Health | Systemic Racism | Social Determinants of Health | Health Inequities | United States
Classification: LCC RG136.2 (print) | LCC RG136.2 (ebook) | NLM WA 309 AA1 | DDC 613.9/408996073--dc23/eng/20230615
LC record available at https://lccn.loc.gov/2023012827
LC ebook record available at https://lccn.loc.gov/2023012828

I dedicate this book to my mother, Delphynne Jones Davis, and the long legacy of strong, smart, and trailblazing women in my family. My mother's kindness, compassion, gentle spirit, and beautiful smile is truly missed.

I also dedicate the book to my family and friends; they have been among my strongest and most unwavering supporters. Thank you for all the unconditional love you offered me as I curated and wrote.

Contents

Foreword xiii
Gail Elizabeth Wyatt, PhD, MA

Preface xvii
Regina Davis Moss, PhD, MPH

I. REBORN NOT REFORMED: REIMAGINING RESEARCH ON BLACK WOMEN'S REPRODUCTIVE HEALTH AND SEXUALITY

1. The Exploitation of Black Women's Bodies in the United States: 3
   A Historical Perspective of a Modern Problem
   *Nicole L. Harris, MA, Haywood L. Brown, MD, and
   Maria J. Small, MD, MPH*

2. The Legal Subjugation of Black Women and the Fight for 15
   Reproductive Justice
   Akayla Galloway, JD

3. Black Women's Reproductive Health and Sexuality: A Literature 27
   Review Within the Context of US Society
   Stacey C. Penny, MSW, MPH

4. Determinants of Chronic Stress and the Impact on Black Women's 45
   Maternal and Reproductive Outcomes
   *Blessing Chidiuto Lawrence, MPH, Rauta Aver Yakubu, MPH, MHA,
   Anna Kheyfets, Candace Stewart, MPH, Shubhecchha Dhaurali,
   Keri Carvalho, PhD, MS, Siwaar Abouhala,
   Kobi V. Ajayi, PhD, MPH, MBA, Marwah Kiani,
   and Ndidiamaka Amutah-Onukagha, PhD, MPH*

5. Disrupting the System to Provide the Care Black Women Deserve: 61
   An Imperative for a Holistic Evidence-Based Systems Approach
   Christy M. Gamble, JD, DrPH, MPH, and Osub Ahmed, MPH

Appendix I: From the Archives 71

II. REEMBODIMENT OF THE SELF: DISPELLING MYTHS IN MEDIA AND SOCIETY

6. Reframing Historical Narratives, Images, and Beliefs About the Sexuality of Black Women 75
   Regina Davis Moss, PhD, MPH

7. Black Feminist Digital Erotic Resistance as a Harm-Reduction Strategy to Positively Impact the Sexual Health Behaviors of Black Women 87
   Shawna G. Shipley-Gates, MA, MPH

8. Black Women's Experiences With Infertility: Messages About Reproductive Health on the *Being Mary Jane* Television Show 97
   DaKysha Moore, PhD, MHS, MS, and Elijah O. Onsomu, PhD, MHS, MS

Appendix II: From the Archives 105

III. REVOLUTIONIZING JUSTICE, ACTIVISM, AND POLICY: CREATING MOVEMENTS OF TRUE LIBERATION

9. Using Justice-Oriented Frameworks to Understand Black Women's Reproductive Health 109
   Dawn Godbolt, PhD, MS, and Hena Wadhwa, PhD, MS, MA

10. #MeToo: Changing the Narrative for Black Women Experiencing Sexual Violence, Intimate Partner Violence, and Sexual Aggression 121
    Camille A. Clare, MD, MPH, and Torie Comeaux Plowden, MD, MPH

11. The Liberation Health Framework as a Strategy to Advance Birth Control Access 135
    Kimberly A. Baker, DrPH, MPH, and Kenya Johnson, PhD, MSW

12. The Black Maternal Health Momnibus Act: A Labor of Love Led by Black Women 145
    Jamila K. Taylor, PhD, MPA

Appendix III: From the Archives 157

IV. RE-CENTERING HEALTH AND WELL-BEING: SETTING THE STANDARD FOR HOLISTIC SOLUTIONS

13. A Holistic Public Health Solution Approach to Reducing Maternal Mortality — 161
Wendy C. Wilcox, MD, MPH, MBA, Maria J. Small, MD, MPH, and Sascha James-Conterelli, DNP

14. Perinatal Safety, Midwifery Model Care, and Public Health: Delivering Optimal Outcomes at the Intersection — 179
Jennie Joseph, LM, Claudia Tillman, PhD, MA, Kendra Ippel, MS, Aurora Sullivan, MPH, and Deanna J. Wathington, MD, MPH

15. Community-Based Doulas: A Critical Part of the Paradigm Shift to Create Birth Equity — 193
Kanika A. Harris, PhD, MPH, Mother Mother Binahkaye Joy, and Zainab Sulaiman, MSc

16. We Are Not a Monolith: Nativity, Racial Discrimination, and Maternal/Infant Health Across the Black Diaspora — 203
Yanica F. Faustin, PhD, MPH, Kristin Z. Black, PhD, MPH, and Jon M. Hussey, PhD, MPH

17. Reclaiming Black Breast Power: Breastfeeding and Chestfeeding Among Black Birthing Persons — 215
Camille A. Clare, MD, MPH, and Nekisha Killings, MPH

18. Fertility, Infertility, and Family-Building Considerations Among Black Women — 227
Jerrine R. Morris, MD, MPH, Tia Jackson-Bey, MD, MPH, and Torie Comeaux Plowden, MD, MPH

19. Changing Our Perception of the Change: The Impact of Chronic Stress on Menopausal Black Women — 247
Lesley L. Green-Rennis, EdD, MPH, Lisa Grace-Leitch, EdD, MPH, MA, and Gloria Shine McNamara, PhD, MS

20. Sexual Agency, Behaviors, and Decision-Making Throughout the Life Span — 263
Torie Comeaux Plowden, MD, MPH, and Camille A. Clare, MD, MPH

21.	Creating Hope and Ending Stigma: A Holistic Approach to HIV/AIDS *Ashleigh LoVette, PhD, MA, Brenice Duroseau, MSN, Angela Wangari Walter, PhD, MPH, MSW, and Kamila A. Alexander, PhD, MPH, RN*	275
22.	Don't You Forget About Us: Sexuality and the Sexual and Reproductive Health of Black LGBTQ+ Women *Daphne Scott-Henderson, MS, RN*	291
23.	Wellness for Black Adolescent Girls and Young Women *Ndidiamaka Amutah-Onukagha, PhD, MPH, Vanessa Nicholson, DrPH, MPH, Telesha B. Zabie, MD, MBA, Lorraine J. Lacroix-Williamson, MPH, Elizabeth Bolarinwa, Aishwarya Amarnath, Michelle S. Jerry, Ruth Vigue, MS, and Yoann Sophie Antoine, MPH*	301
24.	How Much Longer? Exploring the State of Comprehensive Sexual and Reproductive Health Education for Black Girls in the United States *Aja Clark, MPH, Phoebe Wescott, MPH, and Joia Crear-Perry, MD*	311
25.	Sex Positivity and Culturally Affirming Sexuality Education *Ashley Townes, PhD, MPH, and Shemeka Thorpe, PhD*	325
26.	A Lifespan Approach to Black Women's Mental Health and Sexuality: Kellye's Story *Kisha B. Holden, PhD, MSCR, Sharon Rachel, MA, MPH, Rhonda Reid, MD, Allyson S. Belton, MPH, and Folashade Omole, MD*	335
27.	Well-Educated: Culturally Centered Sexual Wellness With and by Sex Educators *Davondra I. Brown, MEd, and Tiffany L. Reddick, MEd, LPC*	347
28.	Perinatal Health Care With Sexual Abuse Survivors in Mind: Trauma-Responsive Care as a Reproductive Justice Strategy *Inas K. Mahdi, MPH*	359
29.	An Approach to Applying an Intersectional Lens to Research on Black Women's Reproductive and Sexual Health *Maranda C. Ward, EdD, MPH, Bailey Moore, and Anna Barickman*	367

30.	Designing New Futures: Essential Wrap-Around Services for Reproductive Justice–Informed Scholars *Joia Crear-Perry, MD, Asha Hassan, MPH, Tonni Oberly, MPH, Jaleah Rutledge, MA, Daphne Scott-Henderson, MS, RN, Daniel Suárez-Baquero, PhD, MSN, RN, Najjuwah Walden, MSW, and Monica R. McLemore, PhD, MPH, RN*	379
31.	We're at a Turning Point: How Investments in Black Women–Focused Organizations and Leaders in Philanthropy Are Impacting Black Women's Reproductive Health and Sexuality *Regina Davis Moss, PhD, MPH*	393

Appendix IV: From the Archives   407

Afterword   409
Linda Goler Blount, MPH

Contributors   413

Index   427

Foreword

America is a representative democracy and the wealthiest country in the world but continues to lag far behind global leaders in its inclusiveness, regardless of gender, sexual orientation, ethnicity, and background. However, the wealth of this nation has depended on the exercise of power and a form of population control that has assigned limited opportunities to many groups, not least among them Black women.

Historical stereotypes about Black women's sexuality have been used as a rationale for their mistreatment as subhumans, the exploitation of their reproductive abilities, and their exposure to capricious sexual violation for more than 400 years as enslaved and oppressed people. While they have been the child bearers, caretakers of the vulnerable, and centers of family life and culture, the value of these roles has been met with marginal levels of health care, navigating health literacy in the face of medical mistrust, and limited opportunities for meaningful and sustained employment. Health and mental health problems often go undiagnosed, are misdiagnosed, or are punished with incarceration rather than treatment. Homeless rates among Black women and their children are higher today than ever. Generational poverty and vulnerability to violence continue to plague families and communities, and harsh sentences are given to women who fight back to protect themselves and their families.

These realities of existence are further intensified by voter suppression and an effort to once again deny not only Black women, but all women, the right to control their own bodies and sexuality. The patterns of devaluation and mistreatment are cyclic. And the stakes are getting higher to control segments of America so that white supremacy can reign.

It is clear to many that the structure of American democracy and opportunities for all is not working if it requires the subjugation of Black women. We need to reexamine the misinformation and myths that shape what we perceive about Black women and adopt a more comprehensive approach that requires the integration of intersectionality in theories and practice. We can join the effort to disempower those who lie and deny with *Black Women's Reproductive Health and Sexuality: A Holistic Public Health Approach.*

The assumption might be that the quality of life for the most vulnerable has little chance of improving because of structural racism that has fostered the creation of social, economic, educational, and financial barriers to a full life. This book defies that thinking in four interconnected sections and with the assemblage of noted authors.

Section I begins with the historical context of enslavement in America and its effects on the exploitation and regulation of Black women's bodies and fertility and continues with a discussion of the determinants of chronic stress and overall health, including the effects of racism on reproduction. A biological perspective provides a sober view of the physical toll that Black women's bodies continue to take, as evidenced in high rates of maternal mortality and poor health outcomes. Black women often have to survive and try to keep their families together without the full understanding of all the options available to women. A systems approach is recommended to better address health inequities by including the environments and conditions in which Black women are born and adopting a holistic and multilayered view of health in community-based settings.

In Section II, a bio-behavioral approach begins to re-create the narrative of Black women by dispelling myths and stereotypes and encouraging self-defining, sexually affirming messages and portrayals.

Section III addresses sexual violence and its impact on well-being, how Black women fight against sexual oppression and injustice by creating their own movements and frameworks, and the long legacy of Black women-led activism. The growing attention to well-established health disparities and the maternal health crises at federal, state, and local levels have sparked reproductive justice, social change, and public policy efforts that ensure equitable patient-centered care for all.

In Section IV, innovative models, Black-led practices, and responsive care and training are described. The need to include lesbian, gay, bisexual, transgender, queer or questioning, and intersex (LGBTQI) issues within trauma-informed perspectives is also discussed.

Both qualitative and quantitative methods are utilized beginning with a unidimensional view of reproductive health and sexuality using women's voices, to broader approaches addressing mental health, biological conditions, and societal norms.

Black Women's Reproductive Health and Sexuality: A Holistic Public Health Approach takes the reader beyond a description of who is more likely to be vulnerable to public health crises in America. It answers that question with why and how disparate patterns of health care and mental health delivery as well as the training of professionals to provide services to the vulnerable have become well entrenched in the American health care system. Ensuring that current practices, some of which are built on principles of structural racism, are challenged and replaced by more holistic models of care is the task for today. Current approaches to public health have been used for far too long in our universities, clinics, and public health organizations.

This book provides a wealth of information and prescriptions for change that redefine health for Black women whose contributions have been overlooked and resilience long misunderstood. The cultural context of their beliefs and values has been mimicked but rarely understood. This holistic approach to reproductive health and sexuality provides the reader with a comprehensive view of what is needed in policy, practice, research, training, mentorship, and philanthropy to better enlighten and promote Black women's health within the context of their power, intelligence, and will to survive and thrive in this society.

Gail Elizabeth Wyatt, PhD, MA

Preface

Black women's reproductive health and sexuality is a complex concept, which encompasses physical, mental, and social well-being. Research and practice that effectively address the diverse and intersectional causes disproportionately harming Black women require multisectoral, multilevel, and interdisciplinary collaborations emanating from a systems paradigm.

Very few efforts at the academic level have specifically explored the nuanced health outcomes that Black women face. Research related to Black women's reproductive health interventions have often focused on adverse risks and outcomes without considering the many social and institutional factors that contribute to ongoing disparities. Sex-positive data about US Black women and their sexuality is also underrepresented in sexuality education.

Black Women's Reproductive Health and Sexuality: A Holistic Public Health Approach transcends these disparate methods by integrating intersectionality into theory and practice and by presenting the field of Black women's reproductive health and sexuality alongside its history and future. This book utilizes a health equity lens as well as qualitative and quantitative approaches to advance the development, implementation, and evaluation of holistic approaches that bolster innovation in supporting Black women, girls, and gender-expansive individuals. The book is divided into four interconnected sections focused on a (1) historical review of the subjugation of Black women's bodies, fertility, and sexuality; (2) society and culture; (3) social justice, activism, and policy; and (4) health and well-being. Each of these sections provide a critical analysis of the unique health concerns of Black women as well as their contributions as thought leaders and catalysts for systems transformation in the United States.

WHY THIS BOOK?

Black women in the United States, irrespective of socioeconomic status, education, and geographic region, are fighting against horrifying rates of maternal mortality and morbidity, infant mortality, breast cancer, sexual and intimate partner violence, environmental exposures, and other issues. While well meaning, we often focus only on partitioned treatments or individual health behaviors and then judge the effectiveness of those interventions by the failures of the very same systems and cultural norms that gave birth to the health outcomes to begin with. This should not be the only approach. There is an urgent demand to better understand and consider all the factors that influence a Black woman's ability to realize her full reproductive and sexual self. What's missing from Black women's care? Their own centered voice, a validation of lived experience, and the freedom to choose and be informed. Without these, there is a gaping silence. And in that silence lies the real horror.

A liberation mindset calls for a long memory to contextualize contemporary systemic outcomes. Dorothy Roberts, Kimberlé Williams Crenshaw, Patricia Hill Collins, Loretta Ross, Byllye Avery, Toni M. Bond, Linda Villarosa, Alice Walker, Nikki Giovanni, Paula J. Giddings, Maya Angelou, Toni Morrison, Mara Brock Akil, and many others have provided foundations for sociocultural learning and understanding of Black women's daily lives. These Black women understood all too well that contributing critical analysis to the body of literature and legitimizing lived experiences were tools to fight against gender and racial retrenchment. This book includes contributions from researchers, public health practitioners, health providers, community leaders, advocates, policymakers, funders, and other sectors engaged in Black women's maternal and reproductive health. They have allowed for the centering of that work in ways that other peer-reviewed manuscripts, praxes, and moments have not.

There are many other reasons I sought to create this book, but perhaps the main ones can be summarized as follows: to locate the entrenched practices and assumptions that have impacted Black women's reproductive health and sexuality, to illuminate the contours of intersectionality, to celebrate and honor Black women's intellectual production, and to impact the full spectrum of reproductive health, rights, and justice for Black women in the public policy arena. This book was conceived as a comprehensive compendium of research, policy, and practice in which each chapter was designed to stand alone yet belong together. Its unity of purpose and its structure—the way the chapters build upon each other—form a coherent narrative. Nothing is inconsequential.

This book reflects a lifetime of WHYs. It represents a journey of trying to create a more equitable and inclusive future in which all our human and life needs are met, of trying to equip Black women and girls to walk in confidence in a world that can make them feel invisible, of synthesizing not only what I gleaned as a public health professional but also through the first-hand experiences I endured and witnessed, which gave me the necessary expertise to conceive this collection.

The information presented throughout the book is not intended to be exhaustive. Instead, what is offered are necessary considerations that impel the systemic examination, the cultural affirmation, the person-centered quality care, the investments in programs and community-informed practices, and the diversification of the workforce that has long been called for. As we work to advance the health, safety, and well-being of Black women, girls, and gender-expansive people, there is one thing we're clear on: Now more than ever, we need to employ multifaceted and holistic solutions, and we cannot leave any aspect of this approach behind. This is something that we CAN do. It is up to us.

ACKNOWLEDGMENTS

I wish to thank the entire publications teams who worked on this book, with special thanks to Maya Ribault for her invaluable support during the production process. I would also like to thank Michelle Quirk who read and gave helpful suggestions on the final manuscript, as well as the anonymous peer reviewers provided by APHA Press.

Regina Davis Moss, PhD, MPH

I. REBORN NOT REFORMED: REIMAGINING RESEARCH ON BLACK WOMEN'S REPRODUCTIVE HEALTH AND SEXUALITY

1

The Exploitation of Black Women's Bodies in the United States: A Historical Perspective of a Modern Problem

Nicole L. Harris, MA, Haywood L. Brown, MD, and Maria J. Small, MD, MPH

For more than a century, Black women have shouldered the burden of the maternal mortality crisis in the United States, with current rates nearly 2.5 times that of the total population, and there is no sign of this trend reversing (Centers for Disease Control and Prevention [CDC] n.d.-a; Declercq and Zephryin 2020). Intuitively, this longstanding disparity would prompt increased attention and care from health care providers, but many Black women report the opposite: their concerns, pain, and discomfort are routinely dismissed, ignored, or weaponized against them during prenatal care, labor, and delivery, creating an environment bereft of warmth, respect, and dignity (McLemore et al. 2018; Vedam et al. 2019).

In this chapter, we make the case that the fields of medicine and public health thrived because of the original sin of slavery and that the practices and ideologies used to justify its existence have rippled through time, resulting in the modern problem of Black maternal mortality we see today. We posit that to understand Black women's reproductive health and sexuality, it is critical that we situate it in its greater context. We must start at the beginning.

SLAVERY (1619–1865)

Historians often engage in the erasure of Black women's trauma, exploitation, and pain by centering forced labor as the only true harm of slavery when the reality is that sexual coercion and abuse were fundamental features of their bondage (Bridgewater 2001). In fact, when the first Africans arrived in the United States in 1619, women and girls had already survived and witnessed unspeakable acts of sexual violence at the hands of their captors aboard the slave ships (Bridgewater 2001). They were stripped naked, fondled, and placed on auction blocks, where their fecundity meant premium prices for buyers and maximum profits for slave owners (Bridgewater 2001). Furthermore, women were coerced to reproduce through a system of rewards and punishments that could mean more privileges and food for their family or physical abuse and separation from their children, subject to their compliance (Bridgewater 2001). It was not until the end of the transatlantic slave trade in 1808 that the weight of the American agricultural economy was placed on Black women's and girls' capacity to replenish and grow the population of slaves, and, consequently, the practice of sexual coercion, assault, and forced reproduction was brought to scale.

Forced Reproduction for Profit

Virginia was one of several states that embarked upon the task of supplying the United States with slaves by leveraging techniques learned through animal husbandry (Bridgewater 2001; Brown et al. 2021). Brown et al. (2021) describe young women and men being stripped down, corralled into a barn, and forced to remain overnight with the mandate to procreate—sometimes resulting in dozens of children. However, extreme duress, lack of nutrition, disease, and other factors left some slaves unable to have children, which was often met with brutality and ostracism by owners unable to collect a return on their investment (Bridgewater 2001). This economic loss was then passed down to future buyers, with damning consequences for girls and women when their infertility was discovered (Bridgewater 2001). Children were also sold on the auction block due to "status of the mother laws"—first introduced by Virginia in 1662—which established that "the offspring follow the condition of the mother, no matter the father" (Bridgewater 2001; Brown et al. 2021). These laws cemented Black women's status and that of their children as the property of their enslaver, with no legal rights or recourse to protect themselves or their children from physical assault, rape, or separation (Bridgewater 2001; Brown et al. 2021).

Profiting From Pain

Doctors were paid handsomely to ensure that the slave economy thrived by helping insurance companies determine the fitness of each slave for the purposes of underwriting policy coverage, assisting owners in determining their market value before auction, or providing routine medical services (Owens and Fett 2019). J. Marion Sims, perhaps the most well-known "women's health" physician of the time, built a career off the experimentation and exploitation of enslaved women, earning him riches, renown, and, later, a position as the president of the American Medical Association (Nelson 2007).

Sims had no initial interest in surgical gynecology but saw an opening to develop new surgical techniques that would help him achieve recognition within the nascent field of medicine (Axelsen 1985). Sims had more than 10 slaves under his care; his most well-known were Anarcha, Lucy, and Betsy, who suffered from a vesico-vaginal fistula or a childbirth-related tear in the vaginal wall, which created a hole between the bladder and vagina and caused urinary incontinence (Axelsen 1985). For four years, Sims performed countless surgeries on these women without the benefit of anesthesia, and after approximately 30 operations on Anarcha alone, successfully repaired the vesico-vaginal fistula (Brown et al. 2021; Savit 1982). After perfecting the fistula repair surgery on slaves, Sims sought business from wealthy white women with the same condition, assuring them that his method was rigorously tested and effective (Axelsen 1985; Nelson 2007). None, however, were able to complete his surgery without anesthesia, which fed the mythos he propagated of Black women having a much higher pain threshold, making them ideal subjects for experimentation (Axelsen 1985; Nelson 2007).

The deep ties between medicine and slavery go beyond the machinations of Sims, the "Father of Gynecology." Medical schools profited from the exploitation of slave men and women, using their cadavers as training material for dissection and surgery (Kenny 2015; Owens and Fett 2019). Some were even located near slave-trading stocks and used their unfettered access to slaves as a recruitment tool to boost student enrollment (Nuriddin, Mooney, and White 2020; Savit 1982). The Medical College of Georgia, for example, was well known for its hiring of "resurrectionists," who exhumed the gravesites of newly deceased slaves for medical research and student training (Nuriddin, Mooney, and White 2020).

Black women and girls are estimated to have grown the slave population from one million to three million, which created generational wealth for slave owners, bolstered the careers of physicians, and made academic medicine the economic engine it is today (Bray and McLemore 2021; Kenny 2015). This was not by accident. To build America, a Black woman's reproduction had to be fundamentally severed from her humanity and instead tied to economics—a trend that will carry through time and serve as a root cause of modern-day perinatal health disparities.

JIM CROW (1877–1968)

The Black Codes of Reconstruction, which restricted freed people's decisions of when and where they could work, gave way to Jim Crow laws, which segregated them from the rest of society and cemented white supremacy as the primary doctrine of the country (Prather et al. 2018). Jim Crow permeated every element of life, particularly in the South, leaving freed people to be seen, to be treated, and to live as second-class citizens. These dynamics left Black women and girls especially vulnerable to the machinations of racist policymakers and the rising eugenics movement, without the political capital to intervene.

Eugenics Movement

The eugenics movement operated under the premise that people designated as undesirable—women of color, those experiencing mental illness or disability, the incarcerated, and the impoverished—should be restricted in their ability to reproduce due to inferior genes that would create a population rife with low intelligence, criminality, and infirmity (Blake 1995). This ideology became prominent after the freeing of slaves but reached its zenith during Jim Crow when the national political discourse on race intensified, and public sentiment shifted on the value of Black women's reproduction (Nelson 2007). No longer able to profit from the offspring of enslaved women, a growing population of Black people was viewed as a fundamental threat to the financial security and culture of white supremacy in the United States, prompting policymakers to both devise and financially support attempts to curb Black women's reproduction (Nelson 2007).

Margaret Sanger and Eugenics

Margaret Sanger is an iconic figure who is considered the founder of the modern birth control revolution in the United States, having helped to develop the first birth control pill, Enovid, and having started what is now the Planned Parenthood Federation of America (Brown et al. 2021). Sanger lobbied for and was successful in bringing government-subsidized clinics to low-income Black and Latinx neighborhoods, a move largely well received, albeit with some detractors concerned about the potential for "genocide" (Brown et al. 2021; Nelson 2007; Roberts 1997). In the end, Sanger *was* a product of her time, holding simultaneously the belief that no woman should have to bear the burden of unwanted pregnancy and the eugenicist notion that not every woman was worthy of childbirth (Nelson 2007; Roberts 1997).

Beyond these contradictory views, Sanger's legacy is complicated by the work she spurred. The makers of other birth control pills routinely deployed their product first in Black communities, with little safety testing, or within Puerto Rico, for human trials (Brown et al. 2021; Feagin and Bennefield 2014). Some contraceptives had significantly high levels of hormones, resulting in hypertension and an elevated risk for stroke among Black women, while others, namely the intrauterine device (IUD), brought about infections that caused several deaths (Feagin and Bennefield 2014). As in the case of slavery, the experimentation and exploitation of Black women—this time to stop their reproduction—presented a tangible benefit for white women, who throughout history were seen as delicate and worthy of being shielded from harm (Feagin and Bennefield 2014; Nelson 2007). Once tested on Black and Brown women and girls, contraceptives were distributed to white communities.

The eugenicist movement was not just an American aberration: its presence was felt globally, and its rhetoric both propagated and propped itself upon a vast body of pseudoscience that sought to find biological, intellectual, social, and physical differences among races, which served as justification for Black women's exploitation. Sarah Baartman, dubbed the "Hottentot Venus," was a slave in South Africa, known for her full figure, who was sold by her owners to be shown in human displays (Briggs 2000). Either stripped naked or wearing stereotypical tribal garb, Sarah's exposition was the culmination of centuries of racist and gendered stereotypes that reduced her to a bestial caricature whose figure was a source of entertainment, awe, and disdain (Briggs 2000; Henderson 2014). In the end, she died young and in the custody of her captor, who dissected her postmortem and sold her brain, skeleton, and genitals to the Paris Museum of Mankind for a profit (Henderson 2014). She remained an exhibit until 1982 and was not buried in her homeland until 2002 (Henderson 2014).

The Short Life of the Sheppard-Towner Act of 1921

The Sheppard-Towner Act of 1921 lasted until 1929 and was the nation's first attempt to improve the health of both mothers and babies (Baker 2021). Physicians and nurses traveled across the country delivering health care, health education, and lactation support within homes, churches, schools, and community centers—efforts that are credited with reducing infant deaths by up to 20% (Baker 2021). The program was not without its flaws: it was complicit in the segregation of health care systems in the South and upended the Black midwifery tradition by replacing them with white nurses (Baker 2021; Brown et al. 2021). The American Medical Association, the premier professional organization for physicians, was instrumental in the discontinuation of the Sheppard-Towner Act, which allowed physicians with no previous training in reproductive health care or pediatrics to open family clinics for profit (Baker 2021; Bray and McLemore 2021).

CIVIL RIGHTS ERA (1954–1968)

The Civil Rights Act of 1964 prohibited race-based discrimination and mandated the desegregation of public spaces and federally funded facilities—although segregated hospital wings persisted, resulting in dual systems of care (Brown et al. 2021; Prather et al. 2018). Coinciding with what should have been a seismic shift in American life, most medical schools began to implement oath-taking, or a pledge among students and staff to operate ethically in their practice of medicine (Gamble et al. 2019). Thus, it is surprising that in the backdrop of an era meant for their liberation, two of the most oft-cited abuses of Black people in medical research were ongoing: the Tuskegee Syphilis Study and the theft of Henrietta Lacks's cervical cancer cells.

In 1932, the US Public Health Service and the Tuskegee Institute launched the "Tuskegee Study of Untreated Syphilis in the Negro Male" with the purpose of understanding how syphilis progresses and impacts the brain and body if untreated, hypothesizing that white and Black men experience the disease differently (CDC n.d.-c; Feagin and Bennefield 2014). The study ceased in 1972 after being exposed by the Associated Press and deemed unethical by a federal review panel, citing participants not receiving treatment despite the widespread availability of penicillin (CDC n.d.-c). Today, the Tuskegee Syphilis Study, as it is now known, is taught to researchers across the

United States as a mandatory element of ethics courses and training. Less attention, however, has been paid to the impact of Black men's exploitation on the health of their partners and infants, several of whom contracted or were born with syphilis due to the men's lack of treatment (Gamble 1997; Prather et al. 2018).

In 1951, Henrietta Lacks was treated at the Johns Hopkins Hospital for cancer and had samples of blood drawn without her consent (Feagin and Bennefield 2014; Nuriddin, Mooney, and White 2020). After her death, George Gey, a clinical researcher at Johns Hopkins University, noted that while others' cells died, Lacks's doubled, prompting him to clone them for his own research on immortal cell lines, unbeknownst to her family until the 1970s (Feagin and Bennefield 2014). HeLa cells, as they are now referred to, have spurred countless scientific advancements and insights, some of which led to the development of an effective polio vaccine (Feagin and Bennefield 2014). Billion-dollar immunology and cancer research industries were built on Lacks's exploitation and the taking of her cells, but, to this day, her family has yet to receive recompense (Feagin and Bennefield 2014; Nuriddin, Mooney, and White 2020).

POST-CIVIL RIGHTS ERA (1968–PRESENT)

Despite the historic legal successes of the Civil Rights Movement, the abuses of Black women, in the form of forced sterilizations and hysterectomies, continued but under the guise of less-invasive and unrelated treatment, as punishment for alleged misdoings or in exchange for a social safety net (Blake 1995; Prather et al. 2018). Many physicians who supported eugenic sterilization would use "the event of childbirth or nongynecological surgeries, like appendectomies, to perform a tubal ligation" (Cahn 2007, p. 174). Other women were denied routine medical or obstetric care if they did not consent to a subsequent sterilization procedure or a long-term birth control method (Prather et al. 2018; Taylor 2020). The federal government's complicity in attempts to reduce Black women's reproduction was an open secret. In fact, President Richard Nixon signed the Title X program under the Public Health Service Act into law with the hopes that a more robust, fully funded family planning regime would curb pregnancies and reduce the burden on the welfare system (Brown et al. 2021).

Un-ringing the Bell

Simultaneous to these harms were the federal government's attempts to undo them. After the shuttering of the Tuskegee Syphilis Study, the National Research Act of 1974 was passed, requiring voluntary informed consent and the use of institutional review boards for all federally funded projects (CDC n.d.-d). In 2010, the Patient Protection and Affordable Care Act was signed into law with the intention of closing the gap in health outcomes in the United States by expanding Medicaid coverage to millions of the previously uninsured and ensuring that essential services are covered (Brown et al. 2021). Medicaid expansion, however, is voluntary, and most states that have opted out of such efforts are in the Southeast, where a large proportion of Black people in the United States reside, allowing disparities in perinatal health, access to care, and health outcomes to persist (Brown et al. 2021; Lee, Dodge, and Terrault 2022).

PROMISING APPROACHES TO ADDRESSING HISTORICAL HARMS

In 2019, the United States faced a crisis with the emergence of the COVID-19 pandemic that upended our way of life and disproportionately sickened and killed Black men and women. We also grappled with the permanence of racism within longstanding institutions, which prompted CDC and hundreds of municipalities to declare racism as a threat to public health, and leaders across states, cities, and professional organizations to pledge to dismantle racism within their respective spheres of influence, despite their own racist pasts (American Public Health Association n.d.; CDC n.d.-b). With this newfound interest and momentum, how should we proceed?

- Pass the Black Maternal Momnibus Act of 2021 (Momnibus): Twelve bills comprise the Momnibus that range from expanding Medicaid coverage from 60 days to one year postpartum to ensuring that Black mothers and infants are protected from the deleterious effects of climate change (US House of Representatives n.d.). These key investments have been vetted by more than 250 advocacy organizations and more than 100 members of Congress and have the power to close the disparity gap and put the United States on a path to Black maternal and infant health equity (US House of Representatives n.d.).
- Adopt a respectful maternity care (RMC) model: To undo harms, past and present, widespread adoption of RMC is required. The World Health Organization (2018) defines RMC as "care organized for and provided to all women in a manner that maintains their dignity, privacy and confidentiality, ensures freedom from harm and mistreatment, and enables informed choice and continuous support during labour and childbirth…" The Green et al. (2021) RMC framework, developed using the feedback of Black women and community stakeholders, enables health care providers and facilities to identify and address threats to respectful, holistic, person-centered maternity care. In addition, the Association of Women's Health Obstetric and Neonatal Nurses (2022) provides RMC clinical guidelines and an implementation framework to help providers improve care and potentially reduce maternal health disparities.
- Make reproductive justice integral to research and practice: SisterSong (n.d.) proposes that to address the impact of intersecting forms of oppression in the reproductive lives of the most vulnerable, we must center those populations and assess the complex

systems that exert power over them. To do this work and to address the role of racism, sexism, and classism on perinatal health, both public health and medicine have to (1) listen to Black women and center their experiences and expressed wishes; (2) share in decision-making with Black women and recognize them as the experts of their bodies and health; (3) engage in work that is of *mutual* benefit and profits their community; and (4) create a pathway for Black people to be in positions of power to tackle issues that most impact them.

- Cease race-based medicine: Although centuries of eugenics-inspired pseudoscience have been thoroughly debunked, medicine still uses race-adjusted treatment algorithms that center white people as the biological standard from which Black, Indigenous, and people of color (BIPOC) vary (Cerdeña, Plaisime, and Tsai 2020). Cerdeña, Plaisime, and Tsai (2020) note that using race, instead of symptom presentation, as a guide in treatment decisions has the potential to deepen disparities by increasing the odds of medical error, causing BIPOC to present with more severe illness before treatment is indicated, and delaying access to social services that require a medical diagnosis or designation of disability. Instead, Cerdeña, Plaisime, and Tsai (2020) recommend a race-conscious approach to medicine in which treatment planning includes the consideration of structural racism, *not* race, to contextualize symptom presentation, patients' health behaviors, and their health outcomes.
- Add informed refusals/declinations to study protocols: Researchers such as Benjamin (2016) and Darcell et al. (2010) implore us to see refusals/declinations to participate in clinical and public health research not as antiscience or an inevitable consequence of abuses long ago (e.g., the Tuskegee Syphilis Study) but as a form of resistance and protection from the present-day danger presented by fields that exploit BIPOC. Researchers should make space within their study protocols to collect informed refusals/declinations, in addition to informed consent, to understand patterns of why the Black community is disinterested in participating and to use those insights to devise better, more mutually beneficial studies *alongside* them.

CONCLUSION

To achieve equity in Black women's reproductive, maternal, and sexual health, we must disabuse ourselves of the notion that racism is dead and, instead, recognize that the historical abuses of slavery have rippled through time to shape the modern-day practice of medicine and research in the United States. *Today*, half of medical students believe that Black people have a higher threshold for pain and thicker skin than their white counterparts, echoing rhetoric from J. Marion Sims and other physicians of his time (Hoffman et al. 2016). *Today*, Black girls are viewed as more grown up, more sexual, less innocent, and less deserving of protection than their white peers, harkening back to slave owners' sexualization and adultification of enslaved children to justify their sexual assault (Epstein, Blake, and Gonzalez 2017). Finally, *today*, when Black newborns are cared for by a Black neonatologist, Black–white disparities in survival rates are reduced by as much as 50%, regardless of how complex the childbirth was (Greenwood et al. 2020). It is clear: racism is alive and well and will continue to thrive in the darkness of indifference. It is up to us as policymakers, researchers, clinicians, students, and laypeople alike to work alongside Black women and girls to dismantle sexist and racist systems of oppression that have exploited and profited from their pain since the days of slavery.

REFERENCES

American Public Health Association. Analysis: declarations of racism as a public health crisis. Available at: https://www.apha.org/-/media/Files/PDF/topics/racism/Racism_Declarations_Analysis.ashx

Association of Women's Health Obstetric and Neonatal Nurses. Respectful maternity care framework and evidence-based clinical practice guideline. *J Obstet Gynecol Neonatal Nurs.* 2022;51(2):e3–e54. https://doi.org/10.1016/j.jogn.2022.01.001

Axelsen DE. Women as victims of medical experimentation: J. Marion Sims' surgery on slave women, 1845–1850. *Sage.* 1985;2(2):10–13.

Baker JP. When women and children made the policy agenda—the Sheppard–Towner Act, 100 years later. *N Engl J Med.* 2021;385(20):1827–1829. https://doi.org/10.1056/NEJMp2031669

Benjamin R. Informed refusal: toward a justice-based bioethics. *Sci Tech Hum Values.* 2016;41(6): 967–990. https://doi.org/10.1177/0162243916656059

Blake M. Welfare and coerced contraception: morality implications of state sponsored reproductive control. *Univ Louisv J Fam Law.* 1995;34(2):311–344.

Bray SRM, McLemore MR. Demolishing the myth of the default human that is killing Black mothers. *Front Public Health.* 2021;9:675788. https://doi.org/10.3389/fpubh.2021.675788

Bridgewater PD. Un/re/dis covering slave breeding in Thirteenth Amendment jurisprudence. *Wash Lee Race Ethnic Anc Law J.* 2001;7:11. Available at: https://scholarlycommons.law.wlu.edu/crsj/vol7/iss1/4

Briggs L. The race of hysteria: "overcivilization" and the "savage" woman in late nineteenth-century obstetrics and gynecology. *Am Q.* 2000;52(2):246–273. https://doi.org/10.1353/aq.2000.0013

Brown HL, Small MJ, Clare CA, Hill WC. Black women health inequity: the origin of perinatal health disparity. *J Natl Med Assoc.* 2021;113(1):105–113. https://doi.org/10.1016/j.jnma.2020.11.008

Cahn SK. *Sexual Reckonings: Southern Girls in a Troubling Age.* Cambridge, MA: Harvard University Press; 2007.

Centers for Disease Control and Prevention. Pregnancy Mortality Surveillance System. n.d.-a. Available at: https://www.cdc.gov/reproductivehealth/maternal-mortality/pregnancy-mortality-surveillance-system.htm

Centers for Disease Control and Prevention. Racism and health. n.d.-b. Available at: https://www.cdc.gov/minorityhealth/racism-disparities/index.html

Centers for Disease Control and Prevention. The Syphilis Study at Tuskegee timeline. n.d.-c. Available at: https://www.cdc.gov/tuskegee/timeline.htm

Centers for Disease Control and Prevention. The US Public Health Service Syphilis Study at Tuskegee. n.d.-d. Available at: https://www.cdc.gov/tuskegee/after.htm

Cerdeña JP, Plaisime MV, Tsai J. From race-based to race-conscious medicine: how anti-racist uprisings call us to act. *Lancet.* 2020;396(10257):1125–1128. https://doi.org/10.1016/s0140-6736(20)32076-6

Declercq E, Zephryin L. Maternal mortality in the United States: a primer. Commonwealth Fund. 2020. Available at: https://www.commonwealthfund.org/sites/default/files/2020-12/Declercq_maternal_mortality_primer_db.pdf

Epstein R, Blake JJ, González T. Girlhood interrupted: the erasure of Black girls' childhood. *Social Science Research Network.* June 27, 2017. http://dx.doi.org/10.2139/ssrn.3000695

Feagin J, Bennefield Z. Systemic racism and US health care. *Soc Sci Med.* 2014;103:7–14. https://doi.org/10.1016/j.socscimed.2013.09.006

Gamble N, Holler B, Thomson S, Murata S, Stahnisch FW, Russell G. Is the writing on the wall for current medical oaths? A brief historical review of oath taking at medical schools. *Med Sci Educ.* 2019;29(2):603–607. https://doi.org/10.1007/s40670-019-00704-6

Gamble VN. The Tuskegee syphilis study and women's health. *J Am Med Womens Assoc (1972).* 1997;52(4):195–196.

Green CL, Perez SL, Walker A, et al. The cycle to respectful care: a qualitative approach to the creation of an actionable framework to address maternal outcome disparities. *Int J Environ Res Public Health.* 2021;18(9):4933. https://doi.org/10.3390/ijerph18094933

Greenwood BN, Hardeman RR, Huang L, Sojourner A. Physician–patient racial concordance and disparities in birthing mortality for newborns. *Proc Natl Acad Sci U S A.* 2020;117(35):21194–21200. https://doi.org/10.1073/pnas.1913405117

Henderson CE. AKA: Sarah Baartman, the Hottentot Venus, and Black women's identity. *Womens Stud.* 2014;43(7):946–959. https://doi.org/10.1080/00497878.2014.938191

Hoffman KM, Trawalter S, Axt JR Oliver MN. Racial bias in pain assessment and treatment recommendations, and false beliefs about biological differences between Blacks and whites. *Proc Natl Acad Sci U S A.* 2016;113(16):4296–4301. https://doi.org/10.1073/pnas.1516047113

Kenny SC. Power, opportunism, racism: human experiments under American slavery. *Endeavour.* 2015;39(1):10–20. https://doi.org/10.1016/j.endeavour.2015.02.002

Lee BP, Dodge JL, Terrault NA. Medicaid expansion and variability in mortality in the USA: a national, observational cohort study. *Lancet Public Health.* 2022;7(1):e48–e55. https://doi.org/10.1016/s2468-2667(21)00252-8

McLemore MR, Altman MR, Cooper N, Williams S, Rand L, Franck L. Health care experiences of pregnant, birthing and postnatal women of color at risk for preterm birth. *Soc Sci Med.* 2018;201:127–135. https://doi.org/10.1016/j.socscimed.2018.02.013

Nelson CA. American husbandry: legal norms impacting the production of (re)productivity. *Yale J Law Feminism.* 2007;19(1):1–48.

Nuriddin A, Mooney G, White AIR. Reckoning with histories of medical racism and violence in the USA. *Lancet.* 2020;396(10256):949–951. https://doi.org/10.1016/s0140-6736(20)32032-8

Owens DC, Fett SM. Black maternal and infant health: historical legacies of slavery. *Am J Public Health.* 2019:109(10):1342–1345. https://doi.org/10.2105/ajph.2019.305243

Prather C, Fuller TR, Jeffries WLT, et al. Racism, African American women, and their sexual and reproductive health: a review of historical and contemporary evidence and implications for health equity. *Health Equity.* 2018;2(1):249–259. https://doi.org/10.1089/heq.2017.0045

Roberts D. *Killing the Black Body: Race, Reproduction, and the Meaning of Liberty.* New York, NY: Penguin Random House LLC; 1997.

Savit TL. The use of Blacks for medical experimentation and demonstration in the old South. *J South Hist.* 1982;48(3):331–348.

Scharff DP, Mathews KJ, Jackson P, Hoffsuemmer J, Martin E, Edwards D. More than Tuskegee: understanding mistrust about research participation. *J Health Care Poor Underserved.* 2010;21(3):879–897. https://doi.org/10.1353/hpu.0.0323

SisterSong. Reproductive justice. Available at: https://www.sistersong.net/reproductive-justice

Taylor JK. Structural racism and maternal health among Black women. *J Law Med Ethics.* 2020;48(3):506–517. https://doi.org/10.1177/1073110520958875

US House of Representatives. Black Maternal Health Momnibus Act of 2021. Available at: https://blackmaternalhealthcaucus-underwood.house.gov/Momnibus

Vedam S, Stoll K, Taiwo TK, et al. The Giving Voice to Mothers Study: inequity and mistreatment during pregnancy and childbirth in the United States. *Reprod Health.* 2019;16(1):77. https://doi.org/10.1186/s12978-019-0729-2

World Health Organization. WHO recommendations: intrapartum care for a positive childbirth experience. 2018.

2

The Legal Subjugation of Black Women and the Fight for Reproductive Justice

Akayla Galloway, JD

I am a Black Feminist. I mean I recognize that my power as well as my primary oppressions come as a result of my blackness as well as my womaness and therefore my struggles on both of these fronts are inseparable.

–Audre Lorde (1985)

There is a long history of the regulation of Black birthing persons' fertility, along with a narrative depicting Black women as unfit to have children. Black women, girls, femmes, and gender-expansive folx have seemingly been erased in the mainstream, whitewashed version of reproductive health and rights. The reproductive justice framework was birthed from the womb of Black women, stemming from lack of control over our bodies and the ongoing struggle to reclaim our autonomy. Chronicling the reproductive violations of US Black women from slavery until now—including instances of rape, state-sanctioned violence, inadequate health care, and the silencing of our political voice and power—this chapter examines the strict measures employed to control Black women's childbearing and fertility. The main objectives are to (1) catalog the historical violations of Black women's autonomy and (2) discuss Black women's needs as they pertain to the ongoing struggle to obtain true liberation.

The term "Black women" used throughout this chapter is defined as women-identified persons who also identify as Black and, as a result of racial inequities and gender-based discrimination, are a target of a rare form of oppression. As not all people who have the ability to become pregnant and give birth self-identify as women, the violation of rights and unmet health needs of gender-nonconforming persons and transgender men are also discussed.

BLACK WOMEN, RAPE, AND THE LACK OF LIBERTY

Oftentimes, when the story of Black women is told, it starts after the slave ships docked in America. However, our story and the story of our victimization is one that begins long before we arrived. Before we were kidnapped from our land, we were free. We were wives, daughters, sisters, and mothers living in kingdoms and villages, each with its own language and culture (Hallam 2022). The transatlantic slave trade was a devastating experience. We were forced to live under terrible conditions and subject to control that extended to every aspect of our sexuality and biology. For slavery to be looked at as anything other than subjugation and oppression, owners had to develop and maintain a doctrine that treated slave mother and child as property, which allowed every tool of property law to protect and be supported by the legal system (Pokorak 2006).

Black women were denied their personal liberties, and many suffered sexual or reproductive harm simply because of their race and gender identity. These historical experiences include rape, state-sanctioned violence, forced sterilization, health care disenfranchisement, and others that still manifest today through birth injustices such as infant and maternal mortality.

Throughout slavery, Black women's sexual and reproductive health was exploited and industrialized to create and continuously replenish a working class. To meet the demands of human labor, the legal systems of slavery had to control slave women's reproduction, which negated any suggestion that a Black woman could be violated as an autonomous person (Pokorak 2006). Among the most egregious forms of discrimination perpetrated by the institution of slavery was the criminal law response to Black sexuality. For the majority of this nation's history, raping a Black woman was simply not a crime. In the very few places where the law did not bar rape prosecutions either explicitly or procedurally, prejudices and practices kept prosecutions a rare, if extant, occurrence (Pokorak 2006). This resulted in the legitimization of the rape of Black women and them subsequently being forced to bear children without protestation. Now, when we look at the modern landscape of the complete overhaul of abortion protections and near total evisceration of access, Black pregnant people are again being forced to carry pregnancies, an assault on their reproductive liberties.

For the enslaved Black women, white men's control over their bodies also came in the acts of sexual violence against enslaved men. Because Black men were viewed as social threats and had few criminal justice protections, mobs of white men publicly lynched and/or castrated them in efforts to assert their dominance (Prather et al. 2018). In addition to disrupting relationships between enslaved women and their male partners and challenging enslaved men's ability to protect and support enslaved Black women, such occurrences restricted their opportunities to reproduce with a partner of their choosing (Prather et al. 2018).

Childbearing during slavery was often intrinsically related to an economic system. The lack of criminality, combined with the 1662 statutory classification of the child of a white man and a slave woman as a "slave," created an economic incentive for owners to rape their slaves (Roberts 1997). Research estimates that almost 60% of Black women aged 15 to 30 years who were enslaved were sexually assaulted by slave owners and other white men (Prather et al. 2018). Some enslaved women attempted to avoid being sexually exploited for these purposes and aborted their pregnancies as an act of resistance (Prather et al. 2018).

STATE-SANCTIONED SEXUAL VIOLENCE

Policy has historically been designed to control and ultimately police the lives of Black people. The US government has aided in the continuous exploitation and abuse of Black people, especially women, girls, femmes, and gender-expansive folx.

The Hyde Amendment and its impact on low-income Black folx continues to be a barrier to access to abortion care. However, it is predated by punitive prison and welfare policies enacted to dictate Black women's ability to even get pregnant or have children. Eugenics is a science that tries to improve the human race by controlling which people become parents (Wilson 2023). The United States established eugenics boards whose primary function was to review candidates for sterilization.

COMPULSORY STERILIZATION

Sterilizations were often conducted without the informed consent of Black women. In the cases where consent was given, it was often with coercion and without the full knowledge that the procedures were not reversible (Schoen 2005). Coercion constitutes sexual battery because the consent obtained is not freely given. Teaching hospitals often routinely performed hysterectomies on poor Black women. These operations were so common in Mississippi, they became known as "Mississippi appendectomies" (Kugler 2014). Many state governments, even those with passed sterilization laws, documented as much sterilization as they could as therapeutic to avoid the procedural safeguards of sterilization laws: "State governments…misrepresented the number of mandated sterilizations they performed by labeling a significant number of them 'therapeutic' rather than 'eugenic'" (Cahn 2007, p. 173).

State policies often did not create a safe environment for Black folx to birth or parent children free of the policing of their households and wombs. Many, particularly those living in poverty, were illiterate and tricked by public assistance officials into getting their children and/or themselves sterilized. Under coercion or threats of revocation of benefits unless they cooperated, many Black women agreed to procedures. Frequently, private doctors took sterilization into their own hands, pressuring Black women to agree before they would be accepted as patients. At various times during the 20th century, 32 states ran federally funded programs that allowed for the compulsory sterilization of those the government deemed unfit to procreate (Ko 2016).

It is peculiar that the US government can mandate and fund the sterilization of nonconsenting persons but today cannot find the funds to expand health care to cover the reproductive needs of its citizens. The United States used sterilization as a weapon to discriminate against and control the fertility of anyone with an "undesirable" trait: Black women, migrants, the disabled, the mentally ill, the poor, those who were unmarried, and those deemed sexually promiscuous or wayward. In some cases, they were deceived into believing that the procedure was merely temporary. The intentionally ambiguous language that misled sterilization patients still is apparent today; tubal ligation is often called "tube tying," misleading a person to think that the tubes can be untied.

In the early 1990s, the Food and Drug Administration (FDA) approved Norplant and Depo-Provera for use as contraceptives. However, Black women were some of the first test subjects for the birth control drugs between 1967 to 1978 before they were approved—again stripping Black women of their humanity and reducing them to guinea pigs. Contemporaneously, legislators were proposing policies that would mandate those on public assistance to be on birth control, and a new narrative of Black women as "welfare queens" emerged.

Placing the blame of having to rely on public assistance on the very person the system is designed to bankrupt is another tool used to try to portray Black childbearing as a defective reproduction process. It reinforces the scapegoating of Black mothers dating back to slavery days and the notion that Black women are irresponsible and incapable of controlling their sexuality without state regulation. Blaming also encourages the policing of Black people and seeks to establish additional ways to punish them, even if no crime has been committed.

This coercion and abuse of authority is no different from when Indigenous women were sterilized by the federally run Indian Health Service (Gillespie 2000). Health care is provided by a government that murdered their forefathers, stole their land, and continues to be an oppressive presence. Even today, Indigenous peoples' reproductive health services are provided by the Indian Health Service.

One should not have to relinquish their bodily autonomy to receive assistance. Black women deserve to be trusted to choose whatever birth control or family planning method they use. Black women should be able to make their own reproductive choices free from government entanglement, regardless of if they live above or below the federal poverty level or are dealing with economic instability or insecurity.

The Relf sisters—Katie, 16; Mary Alice, 14; and Minnie, 12—were given Depo-Provera injections without consent before its approval by the FDA. Months after the girls had already been receiving the shots, their mother was finally asked to sign a consent form. Mrs. Relf, who could neither read nor write, signed the form with an "X." Told only that they would receive "some shots" and not provided with any details regarding the procedure, she unknowingly authorized the tubal ligation of her two youngest children (Gillespie 2000). The Southern Poverty Law Center filed a case on their behalf that brought the prevalence of sterilization abuse to light. As a result of the Relf case, the concept of reproductive freedom evolved to include freedom to reproduce as well as freedom from unwanted pregnancies.

INCARCERATION AND INHUMANE MEDICAL PRACTICES

Many Black and migrant women experience state-sanctioned violence in our detention and prison systems, having to undergo forced sterilization, being coerced into having abortions, or being separated from their children. Birthing people who experience incarceration are often stripped of their autonomy when they are taken into custody. This includes their right to make decisions related to their health and their Eighth Amendment right to be free from cruel and unusual punishment.

Nearly 4% of women are pregnant when they enter the carceral system (Marushack 2004). Incarcerated birthing people are often routinely shackled during pregnancy and childbirth. These barbaric practices of our subjugation during slavery are embedded into the US carceral system and are regarded as inhumane, unnecessary, and unsafe medical practices. Restraining pregnant persons at any time increases their potential for an accidental trip or fall. It also poses a significant risk of serious harm to the fetus, including the potential for loss of pregnancy. During labor, delivery, and postpartum recovery, shackling can interfere with the medical staff's ability to conduct emergency procedures (e.g., cesarean delivery). Shackling also restricts the ability of a person to move during labor, leaving the birthing person unable to make necessary shifts and positions to help them manage the pains of childbirth (Amnesty International 2011). Shackling during labor can lead to bruising as a result of leg and abdomen restraints and cause severe cuts on the ankles due to the straining during childbirth (American College of Obstetricians and Gynecologists 2011). Using restraints after delivery has also been found to prevent some people from effectively healing and chest- or breastfeeding (Amnesty International 2011).

When Black women and gender-nonconforming people give birth while incarcerated, they are often immediately separated from their child and denied the opportunity to hold their newborn, breastfeed, or spend quality time with their infant (Marushack 2004). Separating children from their parents at birth robs them of their lineage and passes trauma directly to their child.

Many transgender and gender-expansive folx experience state-sanctioned violence while incarcerated, especially when they are denied gender-affirming care that impacts their reproductive and sexual health. Gender-affirming care is a model of care that affirms the gender identity of a person as they navigate expressing, defining, and understanding their gender and gender identity, free of any shame or disrespect (Matouk and Wald 2022). Too often, experiences of sexual violence and unreliable gender-affirming care in prison are reported. Many prisons refuse to house transgender folx consistent with their gender and refuse to provide medically necessary health care.

The Trump administration's rollback in protections for those seeking gender-affirming care further marginalizes Black transgender and gender-nonconforming folx, who already encounter stigmatized health care (Forestiere 2020). Legislative anti-queer attacks send the message that lesbian, gay, bisexual, transgender, queer or questioning, intersex, asexual, and other gender minority (LGBTQIA+) folx do not matter and that their abuse is somehow justified under the laws of the United States. Violence against Black transgender women has been referred to as "a pandemic within a pandemic" (Forestiere 2020). In 2020, 28 states had hate crime laws that did not include protections for transgender people (Forestiere 2020). The jails and prisons in the United States are not safe for Black women, transgender men, and their families.

POVERTY AND UNEQUAL HEALTH CARE

In the mainstream pro-choice movement, there is an emphasis on choice, as if choice is all that is needed. However, when a person lacks or has limited resources, it is yet another barrier to care. The social determinants of health associated with institutionalized and interpersonal racism, including poverty, shape access to health care and interactions with medical professionals (Prather 2018). Lack of access to quality health care services and opportunities make Black women more vulnerable to not having control of their fertility.

During the Civil Rights Era, unequal reproductive health care continued, particularly among Black women living in poverty. In 1972, 9 of 15 women, mostly young, Black, and poor, were grievously wounded by abortions induced by insertion of the super coil, a relatively new and untested method. The super coil was a device intended to terminate pregnancies that caused uncontrollable bleeding and, in some cases, led to hysterectomies, abdominal pain, and anemia. In addition, many poor Black women underwent unnecessary hysterectomies as practice for medical students at select teaching hospitals. Today, Black women continue to undergo more hysterectomies than their counterparts due to conditions (e.g., uterine fibroids) that are potentially treatable by less-aggressive procedures, a perpetuation of the eugenics movement. The frequency of hysterectomies among Black women with low education has also amplified concerns about the frequency with which this procedure is used (Prather 2018).

Although long-acting reversible contraceptives (i.e., implants) are now recommended as an effective contraception option for many women, including adolescents, regardless of race and ethnicity, debates about reproductive justice and the use of these contraceptives among Black women persist. Black women report experiences of racial discrimination when seeking family planning services and are more likely than white women to be advised to restrict childbearing. Likewise, Black women of low socioeconomic status (SES) are more likely than white women of low SES to be recommended by their health care provider for intrauterine contraception (Prather 2018)

In the United States, women of color are more likely to live in poverty than men across almost all races and ethnicities (Bleiweis et al. 2020). Our economic system continues to maintain inequities between the rich and the poor while simultaneously cutting funding for social programs like Medicare and Social Security. Many people who lack economic security are un- or underinsured and rely on public funds to access reproductive care.

Medicaid covers a substantial number of births in the United States; however, there are gaps in care. In some states, Medicaid patients only receive care coverage for 60 days postpartum. A few states fund abortion services, and most do not, which means that if a person does not have private insurance, they must pay out of their own pocket. Abortion access includes the ability to pay for the procedure, transportation to and from the appointment, and employers that allow time off for appointments. Many grassroots organizations have taken up initiatives to help those in need through abortion funds. As of 2023, more than a dozen states have enacted abortion bans and/or made them unavailable, which has caused many to have to travel to great lengths to receive abortion care. Those who are unable or incapable of traveling are forced to continue their pregnancies. According to The Turnaway Study (Advancing New Standards in Reproductive Health 2022), women who are forced to have unplanned, unintended, and mistimed pregnancies are more likely to be impoverished and experience financial hardship for years following the pregnancy and birth—thus, keeping pregnant persons in a cycle of poverty.

Most important, Black women have a three to four times higher risk of pregnancy-related death compared with women of other races (Hoyert 2022). Black women also have increased risk for infant mortality. This increased risk of mortality suggests that Black women are less likely to receive quality prenatal care and other preventive services (e.g., preconception health counseling, quality care for pre-existing medical conditions such as hypertension; Tucker et al. 2007). Black women need comprehensive health care that allows them to assess their needs and craft a care plan that meets or exceeds those needs. Poverty should not be a determining factor for which reproductive options are available.

DENIAL OF BLACK WOMEN'S VICTIMHOOD

Media stereotypes of Black women as lustful beings deny Black women victimhood and are born of representations that emerged in the past. Myths of Black women as hypersexual serve to justify their sexual assault and continue to inform public opinion that upholds the racialized gender oppression and misogynoir that Black women face. Young Black girls are often considered "fast," a word that suggests budding promiscuity, aiding in their adultification and aging them to a point where their victimization is justified. The adultification of Black girls and theme of them being responsible for their own victimization was exemplified in the Robert Kelly (R. Kelly) sex trafficking and racketeering case. R. Kelly is a celebrated R&B singer and had a history of sexually assaulting young girls since the 1990s. However, most of the narrative surrounding the cancellation of the artist was about how the girls "wanted" a relationship and how it was their fault for engaging with him. R. Kelly was able to use his wealth and power to coerce and abuse young girls, predominantly underage Black girls. These same girls are held responsible for their own abuse despite R. Kelly's history and reputation.

The American justice system has done an insufficient job of protecting Black women from sexual violence. Black women, girls, femmes, and gender-expansive folx are seldom granted the opportunity to be seen as victims. Black women continue to suffer from tactics they adopted to survive a subjugated world during and after slavery. That social structure, by its very design, imposed a code of silence upon Black women that has enabled and protected those who have abused them for decades (Broussard 2013). Despite this, Black women have always demanded justice and that their voices be heard.

BLACK WOMEN AND THE BODY POLITIC

Black women have always played an active role in the American political process. Even during the institution of slavery, they fought for their freedom and to be treated as respected human beings. Black women fought for the rights to their children and to protect their families. They fought for their rights of citizenship, even when they were denied protection under the nation's laws.

The right to vote is arguably the defining characteristic of one's citizenship. By this standard, Black folx were not able to establish full citizenship until the passage of the Voting Rights Act of 1965 (Bailey 2020). In 1920, the passage of the 19th Amendment gave white women the right to vote, but racist restrictions like poll taxes and literacy tests continued to deprive Black women of the same right (Brown 2018). The fight for the right to vote was tied to other injustices Black people were experiencing, including Jim Crow laws and racial violence. While white female suffragists gathered and advocated for the right of white women to vote, Black women were excluded (Brown 2018). The National American Woman Suffrage Association even prevented Black women from attending their conventions. Black women often had to march separately from white women in suffrage parades (Bailey 2020).

White suffragists ignored the plight of Black women and were frankly unwilling to consider the various needs of Black women's families and communities. Despite being left out of the mainstream demand for suffrage, Black women continued advocating for the right to vote (Jones 2020). However, Black women in the 19th century did not have the choice to focus on just one issue. They were fighting for rights and freedom on multiple fronts.

When Black women are excluded from the mainstream, we create our own movements to fight back and focus on the issues that affect us. Black women's social justice movements have always included the duality of our experiences with both racism and sexism. We come from a long legacy of activism and grassroots organizing to make sure that we have a more equitable society.

Black women are some of the most politically engaged, yet our interests are still not reflected in legislation (Jones 2020). Today, various tactics are still used to discourage and undermine our voter engagement and collective political power.

Not having our voices centered in political spaces has had harsh implications for Black women's reproductive health. The most recent example was that of *Dobbs v. Jackson,* the case that ultimately removed pregnant people's right to control their own reproduction. This, however, was far from the first attack on Black women's rights and accessibility. Many Black feminists refer to *Roe v. Wade* as the "floor" as far as reproductive protections for Black women are concerned. Pro-choice movements focus on having a choice, not the limited or nonexistent access to abortion care nor the harms that happen inside marginalized communities. Politics are being weaponized through pro-choice movements (Strongman 2022). Interestingly, the states attacking abortion access seem to be the states that are causing the most egregious harm to voting rights.

In the summer of 1994, a group of Black women convened to discuss the specific needs of women of color and poor women that were unaddressed by the larger women's rights movement. The mainstream women's rights and pro-choice movements were largely focused on the reproductive rights of white women and failed to account for the intersectional impact of one's race, gender, class, disability, immigration, or incarceration status (SisterSong n.d.). Neglecting to make the connection between these intertwined and inseparable concepts meant the advocacy goals of reproductive justice could not be met by the pro-choice movement because they failed to acknowledge and respond to the needs of all folx (Williams 2019). Reproductive justice stems from Black women's struggle for control over their bodies and a more than century-long battle to obtain bodily autonomy.

CONCLUSION

There are deep-rooted historical systems of oppression that are still reflected in the ongoing oppression of Black women, femmes, girls, and gender-expansive folx. These structural oppressions under systems of racism, sexism, capitalism, homophobia, and transphobia are products of state-sanctioned violence. White heteronormativity is the standard in the United States and is so embedded in the country's fabric that it is often difficult to disentangle. Failing to recognize or name the historical experiences and legal measures used to regulate Black women's bodily autonomy allows these systems to continue. We must be mindful of how the historical impact of state-sanctioned violence and medical racism links past events to present sexual and reproductive health outcomes.

To believe in reproductive justice is to believe in the value of Black lives and the power of collectivism. It is to believe in liberty for Black women.

We Remember.[1]

---

[1] See African American Women Are for Reproductive Freedom: We Remember (1989).

REFERENCES

Advancing New Standards in Reproductive Health. The Turnaway Study. August 31, 2022. Available at: https://www.ansirh.org/research/ongoing/turnaway-study

African American Women Are for Reproductive Freedom: We Remember. 1989. On file with National Council of Negro Women Inc, Washington, DC.

American College of Obstetricians and Gynecologists. Health care for pregnant and postpartum incarcerated women and adolescent females. *Obstet Gynecol.* 2011;118(5):1198–1202. https://doi.org/10.1097/AOG.0b013e31823b17e3

Amnesty International. "Not part of my sentence": violations of the human rights of women in custody. 2011. Available at: https://www.amnestyusa.org/reports/usa-not-part-of-my-sentence-violations-of-the-human-rights-of-women-in-custody

Bailey M. Between two worlds: Black women and the fight for voting rights. National Park Service. October 9, 2020. Available at: https://www.nps.gov/articles/black-women-and-the-fight-for-voting-rights.htm

Bleiweis R, Boesch D, Gaines AC. The basic facts about women in poverty. Center for American Progress. August 3, 2020. Available at: https://www.americanprogress.org/article/basic-facts-women-poverty

Brown TL. Celebrate women's suffrage, but don't whitewash the movement's racism. American Civil Liberties Union. August 24, 2018. Available at: https://www.aclu.org/blog/womens-rights/celebrate-womens-suffrage-dont-whitewash-movements-racism

Broussard PA. Black women's post-slavery silence syndrome: a twenty-first century remnant of slavery, Jim Crow, and systemic racism—who will tell her stories? *J Gender Race Just.* 2013;16:373.

Cahn SK. *Sexual Reckonings: Southern Girls in a Troubling Age.* Cambridge, MA: Harvard University Press; 2007.

Forestiere A. America's war on Black trans women. *Harvard Civil Rights-Civil Liberties Law Review.* September 23, 2020. Available at: https://harvardcrcl.org/americas-war-on-black-trans-women

Gillespie K. Defining reproductive freedom for women "living under a microscope": Relf v. Weinberger and the involuntary sterilization of poor women of color. Digital Georgetown. January 2000. Available at: https://repository.library.georgetown.edu/handle/10822/1051142

Hallam J. Slavery and the making of America. The slave experience: men, women & gender. PBS. 2022. Available at: https://www.thirteen.org/wnet/slavery/experience/gender/history2.html

Hoyert DL. Maternal mortality rates in the United States, 2020. NCHS Health E-Stats. 2022. https://dx.doi.org/10.15620/cdc:113967

Hyde Amendment, Pub L 117-103, Div H, §§506–507.

Jones MS. *Vanguard: How Black Women Broke Barriers, Won the Vote, and Insisted on Equality for All.* New York, NY: Basic Books; 2020.

Ko L. Unwanted sterilization and eugenics programs in the United States. PBS. January 19, 2016. Available at: https://www.pbs.org/independentlens/blog/unwanted-sterilization-and-eugenics-programs-in-the-united-states

Kugler S. Day 17: Mississippi appendectomies and reproductive justice. MSNBC. March 27, 2014. Available at: https://www.msnbc.com/msnbc/day-17-mississippi-appendectomies-msna293361

Lorde A. *I Am Your Sister: Black Women Organizing Across Sexualities*. New York, NY: Kitchen Table, Women of Color Press; 1985.

Marushack LM. Medical problems of prisoners. Bureau of Justice Statistics. 2004. Available at: https://www.bjs.gov/content/pub/html/mpp/mpp.cfm

Matouk KM, Wald M. Gender-affirming care saves lives. Columbia University Department of Psychiatry. March 30, 2022. Available at: https://www.columbiapsychiatry.org/news/gender-affirming-care-saves-lives

Pokorak JJ. Rape as a badge of slavery: the legal history of, and remedies for, prosecutorial race-of-victim charging disparities. *Nev Law J*. 2006;7(1): Article 2. https://scholars.law.unlv.edu/nlj/vol7/iss1/2

Prather C, Fuller TR, Jeffries WL, et al. Racism, African American women, and their sexual and reproductive health: a review of historical and contemporary evidence and implications for health equity. *Health Equity*. 2018;2(1):249–259. https://doi.org/10.1089/heq.2017.0045

Roberts DE. *Killing the Black Body: Race, Reproduction, and the Meaning of Liberty*. New York, NY: Pantheon Books; 1997.

SisterSong. Reproductive justice. Available at: https://www.sistersong.net/reproductive-justice

Schoen J. *Choice and Coercion: Birth Control, Sterilization, and Abortion in Public Health and Welfare*. Chapel Hill, NC: University of North Carolina Press; 2005.

Strongman SE. Despite antiabortion campaigns, Black feminists support abortion rights. *Washington Post*. June 29, 2022. Available at: https://www.washingtonpost.com/outlook/2022/06/29/despite-anti-abortion-campaigns-black-feminists-support-abortion-rights

Tucker MJ, Berg CJ, Callaghan WM, et al. The Black-white disparity in pregnancy-related mortality from 5 conditions: differences in prevalence and case fatality rates. *Am J Public Health*. 2007;97(2):247–251. https://doi.org/10.2105/AJPH.2005.072975

Williams V. Why Black women issued a public demand for "reproductive justice" 25 years ago. *Washington Post*. August 17, 2019. Available at: https://www.washingtonpost.com/nation/2019/08/16/reproductive-justice-how-women-color-asserted-their-voice-abortion-rights-movement

Wilson PK. Eugenics. In: *Encyclopedia Britannica*. January 6, 2023. Available at: https://www.britannica.com/science/eugenics-genetics

3

Black Women's Reproductive Health and Sexuality: A Literature Review Within the Context of US Society

Stacey C. Penny, MSW, MPH

In 2018, the Guttmacher Institute updated its definition of sexual and reproductive health to be more comprehensive and holistic: "a state of physical, emotional, mental and social well-being in relation to all aspects of sexuality and reproduction, not merely the absence of disease, dysfunction or infirmity" (Starrs et al. 2018). As a country, the United States is far from embracing this definition when caring for the health of Black women. Decades of systemic and structural inequities have severely impacted the overall health and mental well-being of Black women, creating significant racial and health disparities. As a result, Black women are at a considerably higher risk for chronic health conditions and pregnancy complications, delayed access to care, toxic stress, and death, regardless of education and income level (Thompson et al. 2022).

This chapter provides an overview of the current state of Black women's reproductive and sexual health in the United States, including the complex environmental and systems-level factors that drive their health outcomes. Using a life course perspective, this literature review highlights the harmful exposures and factors Black women experience throughout their lifetime that may explain racial inequalities and health disparities (Salinas-Miranda et al. 2017). To truly understand how Black women are faring today, it is imperative to acknowledge and discuss the history of racism, discrimination, and reproductive oppression as contributors.

THE ROLE OF RACISM IN REPRODUCTIVE AND SEXUAL HEALTH

On the heels of the Black Lives Matter protests and at the height of a global health pandemic that unearthed systemic inequities, the Centers for Disease Control and Prevention (CDC) called out racism as a serious threat to public health in the United States (Wamsley 2021). Researchers have found that the agonizing history of structural and individual racism has led to a high level of distrust in the health care system and delays in accessing timely medical care (Collier and Molina 2020). Wariness of providers stems from painful and violent historical narratives of gynecological and obstetric practices performed on Black women dating back to slavery (Cooper Owens 2017; Davis 2019b; Roberts 1997). The impact of these incidences on the reproductive and sexual health (RSH) of women of color is increasingly being explored to explain large gaps in health outcomes and profound inequities.

There is overwhelming evidence that Black women's RSH has been long jeopardized. Beginning with the unfathomable exploitation of their bodies during slavery, throughout the Jim Crow and Civil Rights eras, and post-Civil Rights Era, Black women were recipients of inhumane and poor-quality health care and the victims of unnecessary gynecological procedures such as forced hysterectomies and sterilization (Roberts 1997). Lauded in American history as groundbreaking, the often-unethical medical experimentation paved the way for future physicians to continue pursuing "medical success" at the cost of Black women's lives and well-being (Cooper Owens 2017; Prather et al. 2018). A form of obstetric racism,[1] false perceptions that Black women are able to endure high thresholds of pain unfortunately still exist among some health care providers, medical professionals, and residents in training (Hoffman et al. 2016; Davis 2019b). Systemic drivers like these and others have continued to devalue the bodies of Black women and significantly contribute to the intergenerational, gendered, racialized trauma experienced by Black women (Barlow and Jones 2018).

CHRONIC HEALTH CONDITIONS

Although there have been improvements in Black women's health within the last century, they remain at increased risk for chronic disease, with obesity rates at 56% among those aged 20 years and older and with nearly 60% of Black women aged 20 years and older having hypertension or taking high-blood-pressure medication (National Center for Health Statistics [NCHS] 2022). When compared to non-Hispanic white women, Black women also have a higher prevalence of risk factors related to cardiovascular disease, including diabetes (Virani et al. 2020).

Navigating chronic health issues before, during, and after pregnancy has been demonstrated to have an impact on a woman's health, especially among Black women who experience more risk factors compared to white women. Black women are at a higher risk for gestational diabetes, preeclampsia, and cardiovascular issues, which can also lead to a high-risk pregnancy and maternal morbidity and mortality (Eunice Kennedy Shriver National Institute for Child Health and Human Development 2020). In a 2021 study that examined racial and health disparities in chronic conditions among women, Black

---

[1] Defined by Dana Ain Davis as, but not limited to, "critical lapses in diagnosis; being neglectful, dismissive, or disrespectful; causing pain; and engaging in medical abuse through coercion to perform procedures or performing procedures without consent." (Davis 2019a)

women with gestational diabetes were not only disproportionately affected but were also 2.5 times more likely to suffer from chronic health conditions compared to other racial/ethnic groups (Bazargan-Hejazi et al. 2021).

In addition, place matters when considering risk factors that disproportionately impact the health of Black women. Social determinants of health such as neighborhood, housing, and environment play a role in chronic illnesses such as asthma and high blood pressure (Cockerham et al. 2017). Redlining has segregated neighborhoods by race, resulting in Black people being cyclically barred from living in safe and healthy communities. Black women, who are more likely to live in polluted neighborhoods, are therefore most likely to experience deteriorated respiratory health (American Lung Association 2020). An association between exposure to high doses of ground-level ozone and preterm birth has been found, noting that Black women had the highest levels of preterm birth (Bekkar et al. 2020). A lack of clean air, healthy housing structures, and walkable neighborhoods may explain why, when compared to whites, Blacks are 40% more than likely to have asthma, and Black women are nearly 60% more likely to have high blood pressure (Office of Minority Health 2021a; 2021b).

Beyond chronic unhealthy exposures in the built environment, enduring adversity throughout life can eventually take a toll on an individual's physical and mental well-being. For Black women who are already facing physiological and psychological stress because of pregnancy, systemic racism and discrimination can have a significant effect on their pregnancy and birth outcomes. Exposure to cumulative adverse experiences and marginalization across the lifespan has been coined as "weathering" to explain the early health deterioration among Black people (Geronimus 1992). This "wear and tear" on the body stems from chronic, prolonged, or persistent stress or stressful life conditions and has been found to negatively impact a woman's overall reproductive health (O'Campo et al. 2016). The intense level of stress on the body causes Black women to appear biologically older, potentially making them more susceptible to a multitude of general health and RSH complications (Geronimus 1992). Chronic conditions including diabetes, obesity, hypertension, and heart disease are also exacerbated by weathering (Chinn et al. 2021).

The prevalence of chronic disease among Black women is concerning, especially when research has demonstrated that many chronic diseases are preventable by dismantling a health care delivery system and policies that are steeped in structural racism and bias.

PRECONCEPTION, REPRODUCTIVE, AND SEXUAL HEALTH CARE

Preconception care (PCC) should be provided for all women capable of becoming pregnant to identify and address preconception health (PCH) risks for adverse perinatal outcomes. CDC defines PCC as interventions that aim to identify and modify biomedical, behavioral, and social risks to a woman's health or pregnancy outcome through prevention and management by emphasizing factors that must be acted on before conception or early in pregnancy to have maximal impact. (CDC 2006)

PCH and PCC involve addressing a range of RSH issues such as sexually transmitted infections (STIs), specific chronic health conditions (e.g., diabetes), exposure to toxins, family planning, and preventive interventions (e.g., screening; Jack et al. 2015). It is particularly important for Black women given national persistent health outcomes and health care disparities.

Sexually Transmitted Infections

Black women are significantly more likely to contract an STI than white women (CDC 2020). As a result, chronic reproductive health issues such as infertility and cervical cancer are exacerbated.

Infertility

Despite the 6.7 million women of childbearing age who struggle with getting pregnant, infertility is not widely discussed (NCHS 2021). Although studies have shown that Black women aged 33 to 44 years are twice as likely to experience infertility in comparison to white women (Eichelberger et al. 2018), Black women often suffer with infertility in silence. With an estimated four million new infections in the United States in 2018 and 1.5 million new cases in 2020, chlamydia is one of the most common and most preventable causes of infertility (CDC 2022). In 2020, US Black women had the highest rate of reported cases of chlamydia (1,270/100,000) and faced the greatest disparity with a rate that was 5.3 times that of white women (CDC 2022). The updated CDC sexually transmitted infection guidelines and increased access to STI screenings may explain the higher chlamydia rates (Patel et al. 2016), but the lack of quality RSH counseling provided to Black women (Frederiksen et al. 2021) may perpetuate a continuous and vicious cycle of adverse health outcomes.

Uterine fibroids (fibroids) are often misdiagnosed (Bellamy 2022) as an STI and disproportionately affect more than 80% of Black women (Eltoukhi et al. 2014). Another contributor to infertility, these benign tumors are the leading cause of hysterectomies, with Black women 2.4 more times likely to undergo surgery (Stewart et al. 2013). Fibroids are an aspect of reproductive health that is rarely talked about, despite the problems they cause with pregnancy and delivery such as the increased likelihood of a caesarean delivery, preterm delivery, and postpartum hemorrhage (Al-Hendy et al. 2017)—all of which are adverse pregnancy outcomes that Black women experience at higher rates (CDC Division of Reproductive Health 2022). There is limited evidence that explains the biologic cause or onset of fibroids or why Black women have larger or more numerous tumors and develop them earlier in life (Baird et al. 2020). However, their existence is a painful and stressful burden that impacts Black women's overall health and well-being.

Cancer

In a systematic review of Black women's perspectives and experiences of cervical cancer screenings, researchers found that, compared to white women, Black women are 41% more likely to develop cervical cancer and 75% more likely to die from the disease (Christy et al. 2021). Despite having the highest rate (79%) of Papanicolaou (Pap) testing among all women (Frederiksen et al. 2021), Black women may be delaying care after being diagnosed with a chronic or potentially fatal condition.

The number of cases of cancer of the uterus, also called endometrial cancer, is on the rise, with the greatest increase among Black women. Black women are nearly twice as likely as white women to die of endometrial cancer, even though the disease is actually slightly more common in white women than in Black women (Doll, Winn, and Goff 2017; Henley et al. 2018). Black women are less likely to be diagnosed early in the course of the illness, and their survival rates are worse no matter when they are diagnosed and what subtype of the cancer they have.

A panel of experts conducted an evidence review and found racial and ethnic disparities in the care given to Black and Hispanic women with uterine cancer (Whetstone et al. 2022; Mukerji et al. 2018). Black women were less likely than white women to undergo hysterectomy, less likely to have their lymph nodes properly biopsied to see if the cancer had spread, and less likely to receive chemotherapy, even for a more threatening cancer. Research also shows inadequate screening methods, such as some tools to measure endometrial thickness—a possible sign of endometrial cancer—miss almost five times more cases of endometrial cancer in Black women than white women (Doll, Winn, and Goff 2017).

ACCESS TO REPRODUCTIVE AND SEXUAL HEALTH CARE AND SERVICES

Through the expansion of Medicaid eligibility and increased affordability of private insurance, the Affordable Care Act (ACA) has provided many women with increased access to RSH counseling and screenings (US Department of Health and Human Services 2022). The ACA also mandated private insurers to cover all 18 US Food and Drug Administration-approved contraceptive options (Howell, Pinckney, and White 2020). However, social determinants of health, such as poverty, geographic access, and lack of transportation, greatly impact a woman's ability to access these resources and services (Etheredge 2020).

Systemic racism and discrimination, as well as adverse interactions with providers, also significantly contribute to the level of care women receive (Frederiksen et al. 2021). Black women have indicated that they are less likely to receive high-quality, patient-led care during which they are respected, their concerns and preferences are heard around birth control methods, and they are given enough information to make decisions about their birth control choices (Frederiksen et al. 2021). There is evidence that clinicians are more verbally dominant and less patient-centered with Black patients (Johnson et al. 2004). These negative experiences continue to threaten Black women's right to receive holistic, equitable care. Ensuring equitable access to quality family planning services and resources, STI screenings, and gynecological visits is critical to reducing adverse pregnancy outcomes (Atrash et al. 2006).

Nearly half of all pregnancies in the United States are unintended. The rate of intended pregnancy for Black women is double that of white women (Sawhill and Guyot 2019). Systemic barriers to RSH counseling and care may explain why Black women are approximately four times more likely to have an induced abortion compared to their white counterparts (Jatlaoui et al. 2019). Lack of access to quality contraceptive services, affordability, and real-life challenges to effective contraceptive use over long periods of time, as well as feeling unsupported during pregnancy, leaves a woman with few reproductive health choices (Frederiksen et al. 2021). The US Supreme Court's ruling overturning *Roe v. Wade* further threatens these choices.

The 1973 landmark ruling of the *Roe v. Wade* case provided women with the constitutional right to make choices about their bodies along with personal liberties around family and contraception (Center for Reproductive Rights n.d.). However, the fight over body autonomy experienced by Black women has been historically and drastically different than that of white women. Centuries of enslavement violated not only their human rights but also their reproductive rights (Prather et al. 2018). The continuance of hegemonic forces in this country further limits and denies Black women their RSH choices through racialized science and medicine (Cooper Owens and Fett 2019), capitalism, and coerced sterilization (Stern 2020). The ramifications of these historical events remain woven into the fabric of our US health care system and greatly contribute to Black women feeling unheard, unseen, and marginalized when seeking varying levels of care (Sakala et al. 2018; Frederiksen et al. 2021).

By handing RSH autonomy over to the states, the Supreme Court's verdict is an added layer of pain, fear, and burden experienced by Black women who already lack access to abortion care. Coined the "coming of the new Jane Crow era" by Michele Goodwin (Goodwin 2021, p. 509), Black and Brown women will bear the brunt of the negative RSH outcomes and consequences of the restriction and criminalization of abortion. Given that the abortion rate is highest among Black women (Kortsmit 2021), they will face even more financial hardships and risks of health complications (Artiga et al. 2022). With the higher rates of adolescent pregnancy (Martin et al. 2021) and maternal mortality and morbidity (Hoyert 2022; MacDorman et al. 2021) among girls and Black women with high-risk pregnancies, existing disparities in maternal and infant health may increase as it becomes more difficult to access safe and life-saving abortions. Moreover, if states become more aggressive in prosecuting women who get abortions or obtaining data on reproductive habits, the crackdown will fall heaviest on Black women who are most likely to seek care.

With more than 30% of US Black women in the head of household role (Tamir et al. 2021), we must also consider that, as they face limitations in their RSH choices, other aspects of their lives may also be severely impacted. Having autonomy over contraception choices has enabled Black women to pursue educational, professional, and financial goals without the worry of an unintended pregnancy (Maxwell 2012). However, the denial of abortions creates long-term economic hardship and instability, including increased poverty and financial debt (Miller et al. 2020). The Black-white wealth gap places Black female breadwinners and their families at greater risk (Moss et al. 2020) whether they make the decision to travel out of state seeking an abortion or to continue the pregnancy. With a high percentage of Black women being denied or lacking access to paid leave (Milli, Frye, and Buchanan 2022), as sole earners, they are more susceptible to postpartum depression, pregnancy-related complications, and loss of health insurance (Cosse and Hernandez 2018). As a consequence, Black women are forced to make a choice between their health and a paycheck. The denial of RSH autonomy also exacerbates costs related to transportation and childcare—thus further placing undue economic burden on Black families (Artiga et al. 2022).

PERINATAL AND POSTPARTUM HEALTH

Maternal Mortality and Morbidity

From the *Harvard Public Health Magazine* to the *New York Times*, media outlets have helped to elevate the Black maternal mortality crisis in this country. This critical public health issue has been prioritized by the Biden administration and other policymakers through proposed legislation like the Black Maternal Health Momnibus Act of 2021. These policies propose a shift in our existing health care system and address multiple drivers that influence care and treatment within US hospitals and birthing facilities. Philanthropic entities such as Merck for Mothers have also invested millions of dollars into programs and initiatives to identify solutions and create strategies to mitigate complex factors that play a role in maternal health outcomes (Merck for Mothers 2021). Despite these efforts, Black women continue to die at startling rates in one of the wealthiest, most developed countries.

Maternal death rates are often seen as a country's indicator of development and quality of health care. Defined as the death of a woman during pregnancy or within one year of the end of pregnancy (National Research Council 2000), this rate can be seen as the barometer on how well the mothers are doing in a nation. Unfortunately, the United States is not faring well with its mothers and is the only developed country whose maternal mortality rates are increasing at an alarming pace. With an overall increase of pregnancy-related deaths by 40% from 2020 to 2021, Black women continued to die at significantly higher rates than white and Hispanic women, with 66.9 deaths per 100,000 live births compared to 26.6 and 28, respectively (Hoyert 2023). Researchers have suggested that inequitable health care models combined with racial disparities, social determinants of health, and a lack of access to adequate and timely care are the cause for these increasingly higher rates (Lopez, Hart, and Katz 2021). Sadly, these factors are not new because Black mothers have been dying at a rate that is three to four times higher than their white counterparts since 1950.

In addition, researchers in Washington State found that Black women had 2.1 times higher rates of severe morbidity compared with white women from seven states when they conducted a population-based case-control study linking birth certificate and hospital discharge data (Gray et al. 2012). Regardless of protective factors such as educational attainment, prenatal care, and socioeconomic status, the excessive disparities gap between Black and white maternal morbidity outcomes continues to widen (CDC 2022).

Across all income levels, Black infants have much worse health than their non-Hispanic white counterparts. Strikingly, the low birth weight and preterm birth rates for infants of Black women in the top of the income distribution have been found to be around 1.5 times higher than those for infants of white women in the bottom of the distribution. Similarly, infant mortality for Black infants in the top of the income distribution was approximately 23% higher than the rate of deaths per 1,000 births among white infants in the bottom of the income bracket (Kennedy-Moulton et al. 2023). Black women with advanced education degrees—doctors, lawyers, and those with master's degrees in business administration—are more likely to lose infants than white women who have not graduated from high school (Carpenter 2017). This evidence implies that policies seeking to achieve racial health equity cannot succeed if they only target economic markers of disadvantage (Kennedy-Moulton et al. 2023).

Maternal Mental Health

The "strong Black woman" or "superwoman" phrase has been historically used in Black communities to describe women because of their strength, resilience, and ability to endure adversity, especially racism (Woods-Giscombé 2010). Personifying such characteristics has been necessary for survival, as Black people in general have had to overcome tremendous hardships in their lifetimes. While some researchers have found that displaying this level of strength and resilience has some positive benefits for Black women (American Heart Association 2020), maintaining the superwoman status may be a double-edged sword. With a large percentage of Black women leading households, the burden of financial and familial responsibilities places them at risk for chronic stress as well as poor physical and mental health (Chatterjee and Davis 2017). Some Black women may also feel the need to uphold the superwoman phenomena and exhibit strength and perseverance to cope during pregnancy and motherhood (Gary et al. 2020). As described earlier, the persistence of multiple stress-related factors and coping mechanisms expose Black women to an increased allostatic load and weathering. Mood disorders can also arise that greatly impact birth and pregnancy outcomes.

According to a recent report by the Maternal Mental Health Leadership Alliance (MMHLA), approximately 40% of Black people who gave birth experienced maternal mental health conditions (MMHLA 2021). In addition, the report found that Black women were twice as likely to suffer from depression than white women (MMHLA 2021) and that they were also often undertreated (Martin and Montagne 2017). Untreated perinatal depression and anxiety are associated with pregnancy complications and adverse outcomes during the perinatal period, including impaired lactation and infanticide. Mothers who experience depression or anxiety and lack of social support may find it challenging to build a secure attachment, leading to an insecure attachment (Woolhouse et al. 2015).

The stigma that is often tied to mental illness in the Black community further complicates a woman's decision to seek help or suffer through the pain (Ward, Clark, and Heidrich 2009). Therefore, it is not a surprise that Black women are also half as likely to access mental health treatment (MMHLA 2021). By ignoring the need for mental health care, Black women face several conditions including obsessive-compulsive disorder, depression, posttraumatic stress disorder, anxiety disorders, bipolar illness, and substance use disorders (MMHLA 2021).

Limited access to resources, lack of universal screening and mental health education, lack of culturally congruent providers, and fractured health care systems limit the ways Black mothers and birthing people often seek and receive health services (Crear-Perry et al. 2021; Howell and Zeitlin 2018). Maternal mental health symptoms and issues among Black women are often overlooked and underaddressed.

There is growing evidence of the relationship between poor health outcomes and Black women feeling dismissed and ignored during health visits. In 2018, the New York State Department of Health (NYSDOH) held a series of listening sessions with women of color who revealed that they felt providers did not listen to them and that the care they received was impacted by judgment and racism (NYSDOH 2019). Evident throughout this chapter, persistent bias, implicit forms of structural racism, and false beliefs of how Black women feel pain and discomfort have led to Black women feeling invisible to health care providers and throughout the health care system.

THE ROLE OF COMMUNITY PARTNERSHIPS AND COLLABORATIONS

Improving the care continuum for Black women's RSH and closing the racial gap in pregnancy and birth outcomes requires strategic, multisectoral, and diverse (e.g., background, thought, practice) partnerships. This complex and massive public health issue cannot be effectively addressed when organizations, health systems and providers, communities, and government agencies work in silos (McCoy-Thompson 1994). Collaboration is key to creating the level of systems change that is needed to impact Black women's reproductive and sexual health in the United States.

Federal programs such as Healthy Start have demonstrated great success over the last three decades by including and leveraging the voices and lived experiences of families through its Community Action Network and engaging other community-based entities to improve US infant mortality rates (Bradley et al. 2017; Berry 2010). State Perinatal Quality Collaboratives, composed of multidisciplinary networks, have contributed to significant improvements in perinatal care such as reductions of morbidity from hemorrhage and hypertension because of data-driven quality improvement methods and practices used by birthing facility partners (Mason et al. 2022). Furthermore, public-private partnerships to address implicit bias among health care providers and systemic bias at the organizational level, such as those formed between Blue Cross Blue Shield companies and the March of Dimes, are extremely critical to making measurable impact on the RSH inequities facing Black women (Keck 2022).

CONCLUSION

The most disrespected person in America is the Black woman. The most unprotected person in America is the Black woman. The most neglected person in America is the Black woman.

–Malcolm X (1962)

Many Black women, and social and reproductive justice advocates, would agree that these words of Malcolm X continue to ring true today—especially when comparing Black women's health outcomes to those of white women. When we consider what is happening to Black women that is not happening to other women, it is important to remember this country's tragic and painful history with Black people. The United States is steeped in centuries of structural racism and discrimination, broken systems, and antiquated beliefs that have significantly contributed to the excessive health disparities experienced by Black women. Knowing the drivers that act at multiple levels and perpetuate the life-threatening RSH outcomes that Black women face may bring us one step closer to identifying adaptive strategies and solutions that improve their lives.

REFERENCES

Al-Hendy A, Myers ER, Stewart E. Uterine fibroids: burden and unmet medical need. *Semin Reprod Med.* 2017;35(6):473–80. https://doi.org/ 10.1055/s-0037-1607264

American Heart Association. Being an African American "superwoman" might come with a price. February 11, 2020. Available at: https://www.heart.org/en/news/2020/02/11/being-an-african-american-superwoman-might-come-with-a-price

American Lung Association. Disparities in the impact of air pollution. 2020. Available at: https://www.lung.org/clean-air/outdoors/who-is-at-risk/disparities

Artiga S, Hill L, Ranji U, Gomez I. What are the implications of the overturning of Roe v. Wade for racial disparities? Kaiser Family Foundation. *Racial Equity and Healthy Policy.* July 15, 2022. Available at: https://www.kff.org/racial-equity-and-health-policy/issue-brief/what-are-the-implications-of-the-overturning-of-roe-v-wade-for-racial-disparities

Atrash HK, Johnson K, Adams M, et al. Preconception care for improving perinatal outcomes: the time to act. *Matern Child Health J.* 2006;10(suppl 1):S3–S11. https://doi.org/10.1007/s10995-006-0100-4

Baird DD, Patchel SA, Saldana TM, et al. Uterine fibroid incidence and growth in an ultrasound-based, prospective study of young African Americans. *Am J Obstet Gynecol.* 2020;223(3):402.e1–402.e18. https://doi.org/10.1016/j.ajog.2020.02.016

Barlow JN, Jones TC. Reclaiming health for Black women and girls: a conversation with Dr. Jameta Nicole Barlow. *J Crit Thought Praxis.* 2018;7(2):64–65.

Bazargan-Hejazi S, Ruiz M, Ullah S, et al. Racial and ethnic disparities in chronic health conditions among women with a history of gestational diabetes mellitus. *Health Promot Perspect.* 2021:11(1):54–59. https://doi.org/10.34172/hpp.2021.08

Bekkar B, Pacheco S, Basu R, DeNicola N. Association of air pollution and heat exposure with preterm birth, low birth weight, and stillbirth in the US. *JAMA Netw Open.* 2020;3(6):e208243. https://doi.org/10.1001/jamanetworkopen.2020.8243

Bellamy C. Black women start to talk about uterine fibroids, a condition many get but few speak about. March 2022. NBC News. Available at: https://www.nbcnews.com/news/nbcblk/black-women-start-talk-uterine-fibroids-condition-many-get-speak-rcna20478

Berry E, Brady C, Cunningham SD, et al. Federal Healthy Start Initiative: a national network for effective home visitation and family support services. National Healthy Start Association. August 2010.

Bradley K, Chibber KS, Cozier N, Meulen PV, Ayres-Griffin C. Building Healthy Start grantees' capacity to achieve collective impact: lessons from the field. *Matern Child Health J.* 2017;21(suppl 1):32–39. https://doi.org/10.1007/s10995-017-2373-1

Carpenter Z. What's killing America's Black infants? Racism is fueling a national health crisis. *The Nation.* February 17, 2017. Available at: https://www.thenation.com/article/archive/whats-killing-americas-black-infants

Center for Reproductive Rights. Roe v. Wade, the landmark US Supreme Court ruling recognizing the right to abortion. Available at: https://reproductiverights.org/roe-v-wade

Centers for Disease Control and Prevention. Health disparities in HIV/AIDS, viral hepatitis, STDs, and TB: African Americans/Blacks. September 14, 2020. Available at: https://www.cdc.gov/nchhstp/healthdisparities/africanamericans.html

Centers for Disease Control and Prevention. Recommendations for improving preconception health and health care—United States: a report of the CC/ATSDR Preconception Care Workgroup and the Select Panel on Preconception Care. *MMWR Recomm Rep.* 2006;55(RR-6): 1–23.

Centers for Disease Control and Prevention, Division of Reproductive Health, National Center for Chronic Disease Prevention and Health Promotion. Racial/ethnic disparities in pregnancy related death—United States, 2007-2016. April 2022. Available at: https://www.cdc.gov/reproductivehealth/maternal-mortality/disparities-pregnancy-related-deaths/infographic.html

Centers for Disease Control and Prevention, Division of STD Prevention, National Center for HIV, Viral Hepatitis, STD, and TB Prevention. STDs and infertility, STD surveillance April-May 2022. Available at: https://www.cdc.gov/std/infertility/default.htm

Chatterjee R, Davis R. How racism may cause Black mothers to suffer the deaths of their infants. National Public Radio. December 20, 2017. Available at: https://www.npr.org/sections/health-shots/2017/12/20/570777510/how-racism-may-cause-black-mothers-to-suffer-the-death-of-their-infants

Chinn JJ, Martin IK, Redmond N. Health equity among Black women in the United States. *J Womens Health (Larchmt).* 2021;30(2):212–219. http://doi.org/10.1089/jwh.2020.8868

Christy K, Kandasamy S, Majid U, Farrah K, Vanstone M. Understanding Black women's perspectives and experiences of cervical cancer screening: a systematic review and qualitative metasynthesis. *J Health Care Poor Underserved.* 2021;32(4):1675–1697. https://doi.org/10.1353/hpu.2021.0159

Cockerham WC, Hamby BW, Oates GR. The social determinants of chronic disease. *Am J Prev Med.* 2017;52(1 suppl 1):S5–S12. https://doi.org/10.1016/j.amepre.2016.09.010

Collier AY, Molina RL. Maternal mortality in the United States: updates on trends, causes, and solutions. *Neoreviews.* 2019;20(10):e561–e574. https://doi.org/10.1542/neo.20-10-e561

Cooper Owens D. *Medical Bondage: Race, Gender, and the Origins of American Gynecology.* Athens, GA: The University of Georgia Press; 2017.

Cooper Owens D, Fett SM. Black maternal and infant health: historical legacies of slavery. *Am J Public Health.* 2019;109(10):1342–1345. https://doi.org/10.2105/AJPH.2019.305243

Cosse R, Hernandez E. America's workplaces are destroying Black maternal health. The Center for Law and Social Policy. February 27, 2018. Available at: https://www.clasp.org/blog/americas-workplaces-are-destroying-black-maternal-health

Crear-Perry J, Correa-de-Araujo R, Lewis Johnson T, McLemore MR, Neilson E, Wallace M. Social and structural determinants of health inequities in maternal health. *J Womens Health (Larchmt).* 2021;30(2):230–235. https://doi.org/10.1089/jwh.2020.8882

Davis DA. Obstetric racism: the racial politics of pregnancy, labor, and birthing. *Med Anthropol.* 2019a;38(7):560–573. https://doi.org/10.1080/01459740.2018.1549389

Davis DA. *Reproductive Injustice: Racism, Pregnancy, and Premature Birth (Anthropologies of American Medicine: Culture, Power and Practice).* New York, NY: New York University Press; 2019b.

Doll KM, Winn AN, Goff BA. Untangling the Black-white mortality gap in endometrial cancer: a cohort simulation. *Am J Obstet Gynecol.* 2017;216(3):324–325. https://doi.org/10.1016/j.ajog.2016.12.023.

Eichelberger KY, Doll K, Ekpo GE, Zerden ML. Black lives matter: claiming a space for evidence-based outrage in obstetrics and gynecology. *Am J Public Health.* 2016;106(10):1771–1772. https://doi.org/10.2105/AJPH.2016.303313

Eltoukhi HM, Modi MN, Weston M, Armstrong AY, Stewart EA. The health disparities of uterine fibroid tumors for African American women: a public health issue. *Am J Obstet Gynecol.* 2014;210(3):194–199. https://doi.org/10.1016/j.ajog.2013.08.008

Etheredge S. Why the social determinants of health (SDOH) is a women's health issue. Planned Parenthood. January 2020. Available at: https://ppfa.medium.com/why-the-social-determinants-of-health-sdoh-is-a-womens-health-issue-14b8d392972a

Eunice Kennedy Shriver National Institute for Child Health and Human Development. What factors increase the risk of maternal morbidity and mortality? May 14, 2020. Available at: https://www.nichd.nih.gov/health/topics/maternal-morbidity-mortality/conditioninfo/factors

Frederiksen B, Ranji U, Salganicoff A, Long M. Women's sexual and reproductive health services: key findings from the 2020 KFF Women's Health Survey. Kaiser Family Foundation. 2021. Available at: https://www.kff.org/womens-health-policy/issue-brief/womens-sexual-and-reproductive-health-services-key-findings-from-the-2020-kff-womens-health-survey

Gary JC, Dormire SL, Norman J, Harvey IS. The lived experience of pregnancy as a Black woman in America: a descriptive phenomenological case study. *Online J Interprofessional Health Promot.* 2020;2(1):3. Available at: https://repository.ulm.edu/ojihp/vol2/iss1/3

Geronimus AT. The weathering hypothesis and the health of African-American women and infants: evidence and speculations. *Ethn Dis.* 1992;2(3):207–221.

Goodwin M. Pregnancy and the New Jane Crow. *Connecticut Law Review.* 2021:509. Available at: https://opencommons.uconn.edu/law_review/509

Gray KE, Wallace ER, Nelson KR, Reed SD, Schiff MA. Population-based study of risk factors for severe maternal morbidity. *Paediatr Perinat Epidemiol.* 2012;26(6):506–514. https://doi.org/10.1111/ppe.12011

Henley SJ, Miller JW, Dowling NF, Benard VB, Richardson LC. Uterine cancer incidence and mortality—United States, 1999–2016. *MMWR Morb Mortal Wkly Rep.* 2018;67:1333–1338. https://doi.org/10.15585/mmwr.mm6748a1

Hoffman KM, Trawalter S, Axt JR, Oliver MN. Racial bias in pain assessment and treatment recommendations, and false beliefs about biological differences between Blacks and whites. *Proc Natl Acad Sci U S A.* 2016;113(16):4296–4301. https://doi.org/10.1073/pnas.1516047113

Howell E, Zeitlin J. Improving hospital quality to reduce disparities in severe maternal morbidity and mortality. *Semin Perinatol.* 2017;41(5):266–272. https://doi.org/10.1053/j.semperi.2017.04.00

Howell M, Pinckney J, White L. Contraception equity for Black women. In our own voice: National Black Women's Reproductive Justice Agenda. 2020. Available at: http://blackrj.org/wp-content/uploads/2020/04/6217-IOOV_ContraceptiveEquity.pdf

Hoyert DL. Maternal mortality rates in the United States, 2021. NCHS Health E-Stats. 2023. https://dx.doi.org/10.15620/cdc:124678

Jack B, Bickmore T, Hempstead M, et al. Reducing preconception risks among African American women with conversational agent technology. *J Am Board Fam Med.* 2015;28(4):441–451. https://doi.org/10.3122/jabfm.2015.04.140327

Jatlaoui TC, Eckhaus L, Mandel MG, et al. Abortion surveillance—United States, 2016. *MMWR Surveill Summ.* 2019;68(11):1–41. https://doi.org/10.15585/mmwr.ss6811a1

Johnson RL, Roter D, Powe NR, Cooper LA. Patient race/ethnicity and patient–physician communication during medical visits. *Am J Public Health.* 2004;94(12):2084–2090. https://doi.org/10.2105/ajph.94.12.2084

Keck K. Taking action to reduce maternal health disparities. Blue Cross Blue Shield. April 8, 2022. Available at: https://www.bcbs.com/the-health-of-america/healthequity/taking-action-to-reduce-maternal-health-disparities

Kennedy-Moulton K, Miller S, Persson P, Rossin-Slater M, Wherry L, Aldana G. Maternal and infant health inequality: new evidence from linked administrative data. NBER Working Paper No. 30693. National Bureau of Economic Research. November 2022. Available at: https://www.nber.org/system/files/working_papers/w30693/w30693.pdf

Kortsmit K, Mandel MG, Reeves JA, et al. Abortion surveillance—United States, 2019 [erratum: *MMWR Morb Mortal Wkly Rep.* 2022;71:1247]. *MMWR Surveill Summ.* 2021;70(SS-9):1–29. https://www.cdc.gov/mmwr/volumes/70/ss/ss7009a1.htm

Lopez L, Hart LH, Katz MH. Racial and ethnic health disparities related to COVID-19. *JAMA.* 2021;325(8):719–720. https://doi.org/10.1001/jama.2020.26443

MacDorman MF, Thoma M, Declcerq E, Howell EA. Racial and ethnic disparities in maternal mortality in the United States using enhanced vital records, 2016–2017. *Am J Public Health.* 2021;111(9):1673–1681. https://doi.org/10.2105/AJPH.2021.306375

Martin JA, Hamilton BE, Osterman MJK, Driscoll AK. Births: final data for 2019. *Natl Vital Stat Rep.* 2021;70(2). https://dx.doi.org/10.15620/cdc:100472

Martin N, Montagne R. Lost mothers: maternal care and preventable deaths, nothing protects Black women from dying in pregnancy and childbirth. *Propublica.* December 7, 2017. Available at: https://www.propublica.org/article/nothing-protects-black-women-from-dying-in-pregnancy-and-childbirth

Mason CL, Collier CH, Penny SC. Perinatal quality collaboratives and birth equity. *Curr Opin Anaesthesiol.* 2022;35(3):299–305. https://doi.org/10.1097/ACO.0000000000001143

Maternal Mental Health Leadership Alliance. Fact sheet: maternal mental health: Black women and birthing people. November 2021. Available at: https://static1.squarespace.com/static/637b72cb2e3c555fa412eaf0/t/63da5d28d1a1dd20ff42bba7/1675255082829/Fact-Sheet-MMHLA-Black-Women-Birthing-People.pdf

Maxwell Z. Women as breadwinners? Nothing new for Black folks. *Ebony.* April 4, 2012. Available at: https://www.ebony.com/women-as-breadwinners-nothing-new-for-the-black-community

McCoy-Thompson M. The Healthy Start Initiative: a community-driven approach to infant mortality reduction—vol. I, consortia development. Arlington, VA: National Center for Education in Maternal and Child Health; 1994.

Merck for Mothers. Safer Childbirth Cities Initiative. June 2021. Available at: https://www.merckformothers.com/docs/safer_childbirth_mfm.pdf

Miller S, Wherry LR, Foster DG. The economic consequences of being denied an abortion. NBER Working Paper No. 26662. National Bureau of Economic Research. January 2020.

Milli J, Frye J, Buchanan MJ. Black women need access to paid family and medical leave. The Center for American Progress. March 4, 2022. Available at: https://www.americanprogress.org/article/black-women-need-access-to-paid-family-and-medical-leave

Moss E, McIntosh K, Edleberg W, Broady K. The Black-white wealth gap left Black households more vulnerable. Brookings. December 8, 2020. Available at: https://www.brookings.edu/blog/up-front/2020/12/08/the-black-white-wealth-gap-left-black-households-more-vulnerable

Mukerji B, Baptiste C, Chen L, et al. Racial disparities in young women with endometrial cancer. *Gynecol Oncol.* 2018;148(3):527–534. https://doi.org/10.1016/j.ygyno.2017.12.032

National Center for Health Statistics. Health of Black or African American non-Hispanic population. 2022. Available at: https://www.cdc.gov/nchs/fastats/black-health.htm

National Center for Health Statistics. Key statistics from the National Survey of Family Growth - I listing. Infertility. 2021. Available at: https://www.cdc.gov/nchs/nsfg/key_statistics/i.htm#infertility

National Research Council Committee on Population; Reed HE, Koblinsky MA, Mosley WH, eds. Appendix A, definitions. In: *The Consequences of Maternal Morbidity and Maternal Mortality: Report of a Workshop.* Washington, DC: National Academies Press; 2000. Available at: https://www.ncbi.nlm.nih.gov/books/NBK225430

New York State Department of Health, New York State Taskforce on Maternal Mortality and Disparate Racial Outcomes. Recommendations to the governor to reduce maternal mortality and racial disparities. March 2019. Available at: https://www.health.ny.gov/community/adults/women/task_force_maternal_mortality/docs/maternal_mortality_report.pdf

O'Campo P, Schetter CD, Guardino CM, et al. Explaining racial and ethnic inequalities in postpartum allostatic load: results from a multisite study of low to middle income women. *SSM Popul Health.* 2016;2:850–858. https://doi.org/10.1016/j.ssmph.2016.10.014

Office of Minority Health, US Department of Health and Human Services. Asthma and African Americans. 2021a. Available at: https://minorityhealth.hhs.gov/omh/browse.aspx?lvl=4&lvlid=15

Office of Minority Health, US Department of Health and Human Services. Heart disease and African Americans. 2021b. Available at: https://minorityhealth.hhs.gov/omh/browse.aspx?lvl=4&lvlid=19

Office on Women's Health, US Department of Health and Human Services. Uterine fibroids. February 19, 2021. Available at: https://www.womenshealth.gov/a-z-topics/uterine-fibroids

Patel CG, Chesson HW, Tao G. Racial differences in receipt of chlamydia testing among Medicaid-insured women in 2013. *Sex Transm Dis.* 2016;43(3):147–151. https://doi.org/10.1097/OLQ.0000000000000405

Prather C, Fuller TR, Jeffries WL 4th, et al. Racism, African American women, and their sexual and reproductive health: a review of historical and contemporary evidence and implications for health equity. *Health Equity.* 2018;2(1):249–259. https://doi.org/10.1089/heq.2017.0045

Roberts D. *Killing the Black Body: Race, Reproduction and the Meaning of Liberty.* New York, NY: Pantheon Books; 1997.

Sakala C, Declercq ER, Turon JM, Corry MP. Listening to mothers in California: a population-based survey of women's childbearing experiences, full survey. National Partnership for Women and Families. 2018. Available at: https://www.chcf.org/wp-content/uploads/2018/09/Listening-MothersCAFullSurveyReport2018.pdf

Salinas-Miranda AA, King LM, Salihu HM, et al. Exploring the life course perspective in maternal and child health through community-based participatory focus groups: social risks assessment. *J Health Dispar Res Pract.* 2017;10(1):143–166.

Sawhill I, Guyot K. Preventing unplanned pregnancy: lessons from the states. Brookings. June 24, 2019. Available at: https://www.brookings.edu/research/preventing-unplanned-pregnancy-lessons-from-the-states

Starrs, AM, Ezeh AC, Barker G, et al. Accelerate progress—sexual and reproductive health and rights for all: report of the Guttmacher–Lancet Commission. *Lancet* 2018;391(10140):2642–2692. https://doi.org/10.1016/S0140-6736(18)30293-9

Stern A. Forced sterilization policies in the US targeted minorities and those with disabilities—and lasted into the 21st century. Michigan Institute for Healthcare Policy and Innovation. September 23, 2020. Available at: https://ihpi.umich.edu/news/forced-sterilization-policies-us-targeted-minorities-and-those-disabilities-and-lasted-21st#:~:text=Preliminary%20analysis%20shows%20that%20from,the%20rate%20of%20white%20men

Stewart EA, Nicholson WK, Bradley L, Borah BJ. The burden of uterine fibroids for African-American women: results of a national survey. *J Womens Health Larchmt.* 2013;22(10):807–816. https://doi.org/10.1089/jwh.2013.4334

Tamir C, Budiman A, Noe-Bustamante L, Mora L. Facts about the Black population. Pew Research Center. March 25, 2021. Available at: https://www.pewresearch.org/social-trends/fact-sheet/facts-about-the-us-black-population

Thompson TM, Young YY, Bass T, et al. Racism runs through it: examining the sexual and reproductive health experience of Black women in the South. *Health Aff (Millwood).* 2022;41(2):195–202. https://doi.org/10.1377/hlthaff.2021.01422

US Department of Health and Human Services. HRSA updates the Affordable Care Act Preventive Health Care Guidelines to improve care for women and children. January 12, 2022. Available at: https://www.hiv.gov/blog/hrsa-updates-affordable-care-act-preventive-health-care-guidelines-improve-care-women-and

Virani SS, Alonso A, Benjamin EJ, et al. Heart disease and stroke statistics—2020 update: a report from the American Heart Association. *Circulation.* 2020;141(9):e139–e596. https://doi.org/10.1161/CIR.0000000000000757

Wamsley L. CDC director declares racism a "serious public health threat." National Public Radio. April 2021. Available at: https://www.npr.org/2021/04/08/985524494/cdc-director-declares-racism-a-serious-public-health-threat

Ward EC, Clark L, Heidrich S. African American women's beliefs, coping behaviors, and barriers to seeking mental health services. *Qual Health Res.* 2009;19(11):1589–1601. https://doi.org/10.1177/1049732309350686

Whetstone S, Burke W, Sheth SS, et al. Health disparities in uterine cancer: report from the Uterine Cancer Evidence Review Conference. *Obstet Gynecol.* 2022;139(4):645–659. https://doi.org/10.1097/AOG.0000000000004710

Woods-Giscombé CL. Superwoman schema: African American women's views on stress, strength, and health. *Qual Health Res.* 2010;20(5):668–683. https://doi.org/10.1177/1049732310361892

Woolhouse H, Gartland D, Mensah F, Brown S. Maternal depression from early pregnancy to 4 years postpartum in a prospective pregnancy cohort study: implications for primary health care. *BJOG.* 2015;122(3):312–321. https://doi.org/10.1111/1471-0528.12837

X Malcolm. The most disrespected person in America, is the Black woman. May 22, 1962. Available at: https://speakola.com/political/malcolm-x-speech-to-black-women-1962

4

Determinants of Chronic Stress and the Impact on Black Women's Maternal and Reproductive Outcomes

Blessing Chidiuto Lawrence, MPH, Rauta Aver Yakubu, MPH, MHA, Anna Kheyfets, Candace Stewart, MPH, Shubhecchha Dhaurali, Keri Carvalho, PhD, MS, Siwaar Abouhala, Kobi V. Ajayi, PhD, MPH, MBA, Marwah Kiani, and Ndidiamaka Amutah-Onukagha, PhD, MPH

The United States has the highest maternal mortality rate amongst developed countries (Tikkanen et al. 2020). Despite advancements in technology and health care (Chinn et al. 2020), significant racial disparities persist in maternal mortality rates, with US Black women disproportionately affected.

Several hypotheses around the causes for the Black-white racial disparities have been proposed, such as access to health insurance, socioeconomic status, and neighborhood conditions. Yet, a study comparing risk factors based on differing medical insurance status (public vs. private) found no association of higher mortality among Black or Hispanic women with public insurance (Howell et al. 2020a).

Racial disparities persist regardless of protective factors. Black women with college degrees are significantly more likely to die of a pregnancy-related cause than white, Hispanic, and Asian women without high-school diplomas, and more than five times more likely compared with white women with college degrees (Centers for Disease Control and Prevention [CDC] 2019; Chappel et al. 2020).

Factors exacerbating these disparities include an increased likelihood for Black and Hispanic women to deliver at hospitals with worse outcomes for maternal morbidity and mortality and limited quality of resources at hospitals in racially segregated zip codes (Howell et al. 2020b; Janevic et al. 2020). While hospital quality and residential segregation can partially explain the racial disparities in maternal outcomes, they themselves are symptoms of systemic and structural racism, which refers to the totality of ways in which societal systems reinforce discriminatory beliefs, values, and distribution of resources through laws, policies, entrenched practices, and established attitudes that produce and perpetuate widespread unfair treatment and oppression of people of color (Bailey et al. 2017; Bonilla-Silva 1997; Feagin et al. 2018). These systems and structures expose people of color to health-harming conditions that impose and sustain barriers to opportunities that promote health and well-being.

The Black-white gap in outcomes has not been fully explained by existing medical and health literature. This is in part a result of the lack of systematic data collection to analyze the impact of structural and interpersonal racism on health outcomes of Black people (Davis 2019; Janevic et al. 2020), particularly Black women. This chapter explains how the persistent racial differences in maternal and reproductive health outcomes can be attributed to the chronic stress of exposure to racism, depicts systemic and structural determinants, and presents recommendations for addressing them.

CHRONIC STRESS

Stress is defined as any effect that threatens homeostasis, a regulation of body processes and functions (Schneiderman et al. 2005; Selye 1956). Not all stress is bad, as acute stress, or the short-term (fight-or-flight) stress response, can be a survival mechanism that enhances protection and performance under conditions involving challenge or threat (Schneiderman et al. 2005). However, prolonged and unremitting exposure to stress, **chronic stress**, has been shown to have harmful effects on health. Chronic stress results from biological, sociological, environmental, and economic factors and significantly impacts physiological and psychological changes that predispose individuals to adverse health outcomes (Kogler et al. 2015; Schneiderman et al. 2005). Still, the detrimental effects of stress on maternal and reproductive health among Black women are often understated and trivialized.

The Weathering Effect: Impact on Health Outcomes

Geronimus's (1992) observations of racial variations in the relationship between maternal age and birth outcomes laid the foundation for the "weathering hypothesis." The weathering hypothesis offers an explanatory framework for health disparities and aids understanding of how stress experienced because of chronic exposure to socioeconomic disadvantage produces ill health. In sum, weathering posits that Black women may experience early health deterioration and acceleration of normal aging as a consequence of recurrent exposure to social and economic adversity, racism, discrimination, and political marginalization (Frazier et al. 2018; Geronimus 1992; Riggan, Gilbert, and Allyse 2021).

Although the weathering hypothesis was initially grounded in sociological observations, this framework has since been confirmed using biological theories such as the allostatic load model (Riggan, Gilbert, and Allyse 2021). **Allostatic load** refers to the cumulative impact of chronic stress and life events and the resulting "wear and tear" of the body following repeated exposure to stressors (McEwen and Stellar 1993). The allostatic load model calls attention to the health risks associated with cumulative biological dysfunction across systems (McEwen and Stellar 1993). **Allostatic overload** occurs when the physiological burden imposed by stress exceeds the individual's ability to cope or maintain allostasis, preserving homeostasis in response to stressors (Guidi et al. 2021; Riggan, Gilbert, and Allyse 2021).

Exposure to acute and chronic stressors results in physiological changes that are useful in characterizing an individual's allostatic load (Geronimus et al. 2006). The physiological stress response involves an intricate interaction between the hypothalamic–pituitary–adrenal axis, sympathetic–adreno–medullar axis, and the immune system (Chu et al. 2022). This results in elevated heart rate, blood pressure, and glucose production, and changes in the immune system to trigger a fight-or-flight response (Chu et al. 2022; Riggan, Gilbert, and Allyse 2021). Therefore, an individual's allostatic load can be assessed by observing deviations in biomarkers following prolonged exposure to stressors (Geronimus et al. 2006).

McEwen and Seeman (1999) categorized these biomarkers into three groups: primary, secondary, and tertiary **mediators of allostatic load** that proceed as a chain reaction. Primary mediators refer to the biomarkers that the body releases in response to stress such as cortisol, norepinephrine, epinephrine, and dehydroepiandrosterone sulfate (McEwen and Seeman 1999). Secondary mediators are byproducts of the actions of primary mediators including elevated levels of cholesterol, glycosylated hemoglobin, systolic and diastolic blood pressure, body mass index, and waist-hip ratio. Tertiary mediators of allostatic load refer to diseases that result from inability to attain homeostasis. It follows that repetitive high-effort coping with stress and adversity over the life course causes maladaptive reactions including inflammation, immunosuppression, and dysregulation of the cardiovascular and metabolic system, as well as the body aging prematurely (Frazier et al. 2018; Riggan, Gilbert, and Allyse 2021). The social and racial inequities that give rise to harmful biological mechanisms provide support for the weathering effect.

Black women experience chronic stress that flows from living in a racially hostile society that stigmatizes and discriminates against them. The resulting social adversity and marginalization accelerates physiological deterioration, increases allostatic load, predicts early onset of diseases, and facilitates racial disparities in health (Geronimus et al. 2006). In addition, research on inflammation, chronic stress, epigenetics, and telomere length provides support for weathering (Forde et al. 2019). Das (2013) uncovered a relationship between chronic inflammation, induced by cumulative stressors, and heightened risk for cardiovascular disease and diabetes. Another study found that Black women have a shorter telomere length and are biologically seven and a half years older than white women of the same chronological age—27% of this difference is due to poverty and perceived stress (Geronimus et al. 2010). Premature aging, another stress accumulation theory, refers to the body physically aging beyond a person's chronological age. At the level of the cell, premature aging refers to cell senescence. Sustained exposure to stressors promotes premature aging by increasing the number of old (or senescent) cells in tissues that build up over time (Campisi 2005; Frazier et al. 2018).

The impact of weathering on Black women's maternal and reproductive health outcomes is well documented. Researchers have repeatedly demonstrated a relationship between chronic stress due to racism and socioeconomic adversity and increased risk of preterm delivery or low birth weight in Black women (Barrett et al. 2018; Riggan, Gilbert, and Alyse 2021). Barrett et al. (2018) observed that a unit increase in allostatic load score, a measure of chronic physiological stress, four months before pregnancy yielded significant increases in the odds of preeclampsia (62%), preterm birth (44%), and low birth weight (39%).

Others have argued that mental and physical weathering helps explain disparities in the rates of unintended and early pregnancies among marginalized women. Specifically, experiencing discrimination is associated with increased risk of subsequent unintended pregnancy (Hall et al. 2015). Weathered bodies also may be programmed for pro-inflammatory dysregulation before pregnancy and/or carry a lower threshold for dysfunction signals to generate immune responses, placing them at risk of pregnancy failure (Frazier et al. 2018). This presents a plausible explanation for why Black women are at greater risk of experiencing spontaneous abortion than white women (Frazier et al. 2018). In addition, chronic stress is compounded by perceived lack of social support (e.g., family, friends, partners), social isolation, employment instability, unsafe living conditions, caring for family, and the mental and physical burden of socialized Black motherhood (Giurgescu et al. 2013; Jackson et al. 2001). These experiences and daily stressors accumulate, resulting in poor health outcomes (Giscombé and Lobel 2005; Giurgescu et al. 2013; Taylor 2020).

Determinants of Chronic Stress

Social Factors

To evaluate the effects of stress on Black women, one must consider one of the most impactful social determinants: chronic exposure to racism. A framework for understanding racism has been previously established by Camara P. Jones (2000) to aid in the understanding of race-associated differences in health outcomes and consists of three levels: institutionalized racism, personally mediated racism, and internalized racism. **Institutionalized racism** is the systemic, legal, and historical structures set in place to the detriment of marginalized communities (Jones 2000). This is seen in the lack of access to care because of sparse numbers of birthing centers in communities of color as well as poor-quality and underresourced health care when available (Carvalho et al. 2022). **Personally mediated racism** is the discrimination experienced by marginalized communities secondary to the perpetrator's conscious or subconscious thoughts, actions, and assumptions resulting in prejudice and implicit bias (Jones 2000). Personally mediated racism includes acts of commission as well as acts of omission. **Internalized racism** is the inherent belief and acceptance of society's imposed stereotypes leading to shame, self-doubt, and a perceived lack of autonomy (Jones 2000).

Experiences of racism have been linked to adverse birth outcomes including low birth weight and preterm birth (Dunkel Schetter 2011; Giscombé and Lobel 2005; Lima et al. 2018). This is due in part to a long history of mistreatment and experimentation on Black individuals perpetrated by the medical and research communities (Washington 2006). Still today, Black women often report experiences of mistreatment and discrimination when seeking medical care (Sakala et al. 2018; Taylor 2020). In the Listening to Mothers California study, authors found that 11% of Black women reported unfair treatment as an inpatient for peripartum care (Sakala et al. 2018). In addition, 7% of Black women reported the experience of both harsh language by health professionals and rough handling (Sakala et al. 2018). The aggregation of these varied thematic experiences causes women of color, particularly Black women, to feel misunderstood, disregarded, and, thus, invisible in the eyes of the health care system (Taylor 2020).

The collective physical and emotional trauma from these experiences results in mistrust and, thus, a hesitancy to self-advocate, leading to poor maternal health outcomes (Taylor 2020). Studies have found that racial concordance between physician and patient may have a positive effect on birth outcomes. When race of patient and physician differ, there is an increase in adverse outcomes (Greenwood et al. 2020). Correspondingly, racism triggers physiological responses, which can lead to poor chronic mental health outcomes and poor birth outcomes (Jackson, Rowley, and Curry Owens 2012).

Gendered racism has emerged from the construct of intersectionality as a particular kind of stressor that is more than the reports of perceived episodes of racism. For African American women, gendered racism occurs within the context of conditions where they feel the need to maintain a pervasive vigilance in anticipation of future racist events for themselves and their children (Nuru-Jeter et al. 2009). Countless investigations have concluded that chronic exposure to racial and gendered stress, which encompasses discrimination, is a key explanation for the racial health disparities and the poor birth outcomes seen among African American women (Jackson et al. 2001).

Partner-Related Factors

A leading cause of death for pregnant women in the United States is homicide. Pregnancy-related homicide disproportionately affects Black women and young women and girls aged 24 years and younger (Wallace et al. 2021). An inordinate number of pregnancy-related homicides are estimated to be at the hands of their partners (Kivisto, Mills, and Elwood 2021). A study by Kivisto et al. (2021) shows that while rates of non–pregnancy-associated intimate partner homicide did not differ across races, rates of pregnancy-associated intimate partner homicide was three times greater among Black women compared with white and Hispanic women. Black pregnant women were eight times more likely to be killed by intimate partners than Black nonpregnant women (Kivisto, Mills, and Elwood 2021).

While intimate partner homicide is the most severe form of intimate partner violence (IPV), the impact of a partner on the health and well-being of a pregnant person is evident beyond homicide victimization (Vignola-Lévesque and Léveillée 2021). IPV increases stress, affecting immune function during pregnancy (Chambliss 2008). In addition, a recent multistate Pregnancy Risk Assessment Monitoring System (PRAMS) phase 8 (2016-2018) analysis found that women who reported partner-related stressful events during pregnancy were more likely to experience hypertensive disorders of pregnancy, prenatal depression, and postpartum depression (Lawrence et al. 2022). Black women reported increased rates of all types of life stressors in this study. Furthermore, this study found that women who reported at least seven stressors were more likely to be Black, aged younger than 24 years, low-income women with no college education. Those who reported a history of partner-related abuse were more likely to experience stress during pregnancy (Lawrence et al. 2022).

Environmental Factors

Environmental factors such as neighborhood violence, redlining, maternity care deserts, and food insecurity are components of structural racism that negatively impact health outcomes in Black women. Redlining, a discriminatory practice of designating geographical areas with majority Black populations as hazardous and void of development, has historically oppressed the social and economic mobility of Black people (Collin et al. 2021; CDC 2017). Lack of resources in these neighborhoods limits employment opportunities and the quality of care at hospitals (Janevic et al. 2020; Riggan, Gilbert, and Allyse 2020). Pregnant Black women are four times more likely to live in disadvantaged neighborhoods with higher levels of violent crime; as such, they are more likely to report chronic stress compared with white women (Giurgescu and Misra 2018). As a consequence, individuals living in redlined neighborhoods have a higher risk of preterm birth, lower self-perceived health status, higher risk of injuries related to gun violence, and higher risk of experiencing chronic diseases such as stroke, diabetes, and hypertension (Lee et al. 2022). In fact, Black women in these neighborhoods have high ratings of perceived stress associated with increased allostatic load, premature aging, and disease risk (Lee et al. 2022).

Limited access to quality providers further impacts Black women's health, especially in rural areas. The ongoing closure of maternity care services in the rural United States has led to an estimated 54% of rural counties having zero hospital obstetrics-based services (Kozhimannil et al. 2019). Pregnant women who commute for more than an hour to access maternity care services are approximately 7.4 times more likely to experience higher stress levels than women who can access maternity care within proximity (Kornelsen, Stoll, and Grzybowski 2011). Thus, the persistent loss of rural maternal care has resulted in disproportionate adverse maternal health outcomes, especially for Black rural residents (Henning-Smith et al. 2019; Kozhimannil et al. 2019).

Nonetheless, a common occurrence in both urban and rural areas is food insecurity. Individuals who are affected by food insecurity often live in food deserts and/or food swamps. A **food desert** is a region with limited or low access to affordable, nutritious foods, while **food swamps** are areas with a high number of stores that sell high-caloric foods such as fast food (Hawkins and Panzera 2021). Living in food deserts or swamps contributes to poverty, chronic stress, and, ultimately, chronic diseases (CDC 2017; Kanfash 2018; Keith-Jennings, Llobrera, and Dean 2019; Sullivan et al. 2016).

Economic Factors

Financial instability negatively impacts essential medical care, access to transportation for prenatal appointments, safe and reliable childcare, and familial socioeconomic stability for pregnant and birthing people (Friedman, Heneghan, and Rosenthal 2009; Johnson et al. 2007). These economic concerns remain especially pertinent to Black individuals and families in the United States who continue to face income disparities. In a study of prenatal life stress, Black respondents had the highest report of economic stress, with about 31% reporting high financial stress (Liu et al. 2016). Respondents expressed the following financial stressors: moving to a new address, losing employment, and difficulty paying bills (Liu et al. 2016). Even when Black women have access to employment opportunities, they still face increased rates of workspace-based discrimination and stereotypes that lead to a hostile work environment and, ultimately, chronic diseases from repeated stress exposure (Pavalko, Mossakowski, and Hamilton 2003).

These financial stressors impact pregnant Black women's lived experiences and clinical outcomes (Novick et al. 2012; Zhao et al. 2015). Financial stress is linked to increased risks of both preterm birth and low birth weight (Almeida et al. 2018). Atkins et al. (2020) found that depressive symptomatology is linked to low access to financial resources and is highly prevalent among Black women, with about 36% reporting financial stress, 18% feeling stressed, and 12% struggling with parenting stress. These findings illuminate the systemic injustices that Black women continue to face in the United States as racial income gaps and financial-related concerns persist.

ADDRESSING THE DETERMINANTS OF CHRONIC STRESS IN BLACK WOMEN

Social Recommendations

Strategies for improving maternal health equity have been shown to be most successful when approached from a social justice perspective (Taylor et al. 2019). One aspect of the social justice perspective is the **theory of targeted universalism**, which is designed to directly address universal goals for all groups; it aims to correct the policies that nurture inequality as well as programs that inevitably exclude groups (Othering and Belonging Institute 2021; Bedayn 2022). From this standpoint, policy strategies that may promote Black women's health include expanding access to quality care, expanding access to maternal mental health services, investing in community programs and home visiting, and training health care professionals in cultural competency as well as diversifying the health care workforce.

Despite increased public awareness of the impact of racial discrimination on maternal health outcomes, there are still few proposed methods that exist to intervene (Siden et al. 2022). Personally mediated racism can occur either explicitly (consciously) or implicitly (subconsciously). Therefore, medical professionals should be provided with language or training that can alter explicit biases and messaging to patients (Siden et al. 2022). However, implicit bias is notably resistant to alteration, with many of the implicit bias trainings that are offered to clinicians only showing impacts immediately after training but not several days after the training (FitzGerald et al. 2019; Lai et al. 2016; Siden et al. 2022). Only one intervention that aims for "habit-breaking" of mental associations using strategies such as individuation and stereotype replacement has shown long-term effectiveness weeks after training completion (Devine 1989; Devine et al. 2012; Forscher et al. 2017). This model has been used with nonobstetric medical professionals and could be an effective implicit bias training for maternal health clinicians.

Partner-Related Recommendations

The impact of IPV and partner-related stress on pregnancy outcomes and experiences is clear. Interventions, including screening for and reduction of IPV, need to be developed and evaluated to provide necessary support to populations at greater risk. A systematic review from 2000 found that screening itself is an effective intervention to reduce IPV (McFarlane, Soeken, and Wiist 2000). Pregnancy can serve as an entry point to the medical system for many in their life course and, as such, a time when stressors including IPV can be found and help can be provided. Screening can be expanded from the clinical setting to mobile apps, as telehealth and telemedicine are on the rise (Krishnamurti et al. 2021). Empowerment counseling on IPV is the most frequently tested nonscreening intervention worldwide. This form of counseling provides information on types of abuse and the cycle of violence, includes a danger assessment, and creates a safety plan (World Health Organization 2011). While screening and psychological interventions are a step, there is a need for more research on prevention of IPV to reduce partner-related stress and homicide during the perinatal period.

There is growing evidence for the positive impact of paternal influence on birth outcomes Specifically, perceived strong partner support can decrease postpartum distress and improve mother and infant well-being (Battulga et al. 2021; Stapleton et al. 2012). Further research is needed to delineate the components of the positive social support received from spouses or partners that ameliorate the particular stressors for pregnant African American women (Jackson, Rowley, and Curry Owens 2012).

Environmental Recommendations

Solutions to environmental determinants of chronic stress in Black women must involve advocating for policies that undo the effects of redlining, including increased government funding to previously redlined neighborhoods, and that aim to develop communities while preventing gentrification. There is a need for policies that make it easier for Black families to obtain mortgages. To mitigate the racial wealth gap, an economics professor and public policy advisor, Dr. Darrick Hamilton, has proposed the idea of "baby bonds": a federal trust fund for every baby born in the United States to mitigate the racial wealth gap. Connecticut, New Jersey, Massachusetts, and the District of Columbia have been pushing forward baby bonds (Steverman 2017). In Atlanta, Georgia, the "In Her Hands" program addresses wealth disparities by providing a guaranteed income to Black women, in addition to basic income given to 300 people living under 200% of the federal poverty level (Alfonseca 2022).

Such recommendations focus on long-term solutions to decreasing chronic stress Black women experience, which contributes to adverse maternal health outcomes. For short-term strategies, more funding should be provided to hospitals and clinics in marginalized neighborhoods, such as federally qualified health centers, which provide accessible health care to underserved communities. Increased funding could help increase staff members and address financial barriers to care. In maternity care deserts, infrastructural changes are necessary to improve maternal health. This should include an emphasis on telehealth and maternity wards, as well as uplifting doula care and midwifery to create more points of support and contact in the health care system.

Economic Recommendations

At the core of improving Black maternal health outcomes is dismantling socioeconomic barriers that impede access to quality maternal care. Despite the passage of the Affordable Care Act, a significant proportion of Black women still cannot access quality and timely care largely because of cost (Long et al. 2021). Hence, it is pertinent to craft policies that provide financial subsidies or assistance like the COVID-19 federal childcare subsidies (Gurrentz 2021). Beyond federal policies, health system insurers should design mechanisms that address barriers in accessing care like transportation and childcare for doctor visits. Incorporating technologically based care could potentially mitigate these barriers (Wu, Lopez, and Nichols 2022). Furthermore, providing more comprehensive insurance coverage to enable uninterrupted care up to one year postpartum is ideal. Lastly, insurers should provide reimbursement and/or coverage for doula and midwifery services (which are often out-of-pocket expenditures). These forms of support are effective models of promoting positive maternal experiences (Gomez et al. 2021; Renfrew et al. 2014; Van Eijk et al. 2022).

Research Recommendations

Analysis of current evidence-based practices and maternal health interventions highlight the need for research directed for, by, and with Black women as well as the inclusion of assessment tools and frameworks developed and validated for, by, and with Black birthing populations (Black Mamas Matter Alliance 2019). Model instruments that offer guidance include the Jackson, Hogue, Phillips Contextualized Stress Measure, a race- and gender-validated tool grounded in the lived experiences of Black women designed to detect stress in populations of Black women (Jackson, Hogue, and Phillips 2005). The guiding principle for the research was that Black women are authorities on their lives, and, as such, their voices must be the source for uncovering stress and support in their lives (Jackson et al. 2001)

CONCLUSION

Chronic stress is a key driver of poor health outcomes, yet the detrimental effects of stress on maternal and reproductive health outcomes among Black women are less recognized. This chapter draws on qualitative and quantitative studies to depict the determinants of chronic stress for Black women and the resulting impact on their health. Despite the extensive literature that denotes that Black women shoulder the burden of adverse reproductive and maternal health outcomes, numerous attempts to explain the Black-white gap in health outcomes fail to adequately account for the overwhelming impact of chronic stress due to racism, economic disadvantage, neighborhood adversity, political marginalization, and partner-related stress, which predisposes Black women to early health deterioration. Eliminating disparities in maternal and reproductive health outcomes among Black women calls for multifaceted interventions. This can be achieved through increased screening for psychosocial stressors during pregnancy, timely referral to support and resources, training medical providers in cultural humility and trauma-informed care, and policy reforms to increase access to quality and inclusive reproductive health care.

REFERENCES

Alfonseca K. Guaranteed income experiment for Black women aims to tackle racial wealth gap. ABC News. January 12, 2022. Available at: https://abcnews.go.com/US/guaranteed-income-experiment-black-women-aims-tackle-racial/story?id=82073348

Almeida J, Bécares L, Erbetta K, Bettegowda VR, Ahluwalia IB. Racial/ethnic inequities in low birth weight and preterm birth: the role of multiple forms of stress. *Matern Child Health J.* 2018;22(8):1154–1163. https://doi.org/10.1007/s10995-018-2500-7

Atkins R, Luo R, Wunnenberg M, et al. Contributors to depressed mood in Black single mothers. *Issues Ment Health Nurs.* 2020;41(1):38–48. https://doi.org/10.1080/01612840.2019.1631414

Bailey ZD, Krieger N, Agenor M, Graves J, Linos N, Bassett MT. Structural racism and health inequities in the USA: evidence and interventions. *Lancet.* 2017;389(10077):1453–1463. https://doi.org/10.1016/S0140-6736(17)30569-X

Barrett ES, Vitek W, Mbowe O, et al. Allostatic load, a measure of chronic physiological stress, is associated with pregnancy outcomes, but not fertility, among women with unexplained infertility. *Hum Reprod.* 2018;33(9):1757–1766. https://doi.org/10.1093/humrep/dey261

Battulga B, Benjamin MR, Chen H, Bat-Enkh E. The impact of social support and pregnancy on subjective well-being: a systematic review. *Front Psychol.* 2021;12:3321. https://doi.org/10.3389/fpsyg.2021.710858

Bedayn J. Targeted universalism: A solution for inequality? *Cal Matters.* February 3, 2022. Available at: https://calmatters.org/california-divide/2022/02/targeted-universalism-racial-inequality

Black Mamas Matter Alliance Research Working Group; Aina A, Asiodu IV, Castillo P, et al. Black maternal health research reimagined: principles for conducting research in maternity care for Black mamas. 2019. Available at: https://blackmamasmatter.org/wp-content/uploads/2022/10/BMMA_RP_Report_1026.pdf

Bonilla-Silva E. Rethinking racism: toward a structural interpretation. *Am Sociol Rev.* 1997;62(3):465–480. https://doi.org/10.2307/2657316

Campisi J. Senescent cells, tumor suppression, and organismal aging: good citizens, bad neighbors. *Cell.* 2005;120(4):513–522. https://doi.org/10.1016/j.cell.2005.02.003

Carvalho K, Kheyfets A, Lawrence B, et al. Examining the role of psychosocial influences on Black maternal health during the COVID-19 pandemic. *Matern Child Health J.* 2022;26(4):764–769. https://doi.org/10.1007/s10995-021-03181-9

Centers for Disease Control and Prevention. African American health: creating equal opportunities for health. May 2017. Available at: https://www.cdc.gov/vitalsigns/pdf/2017-05-vitalsigns.pdf

Centers for Disease Control and Prevention. Racial and ethnic disparities continue in pregnancy-related deaths. June 9, 2019. Available at: https://www.cdc.gov/media/releases/2019/p0905-racial-ethnic-disparities-pregnancy-deaths.html

Chambliss LR. Intimate partner violence and its implication for pregnancy. *Clin Obstet Gynecol.* 2008;51(2):385–397. https://doi.org/10.1097/GRF.0b013e31816f29ce

Chappel A, Alley D, De Lew N, Fink D, Fulmer B, Hollis A. *Healthy Women, Healthy Pregnancies, Healthy Futures: Action Plan to Improve Maternal Health in America*. US Department of Health and Human Services. 2020. Available at: https://aspe.hhs.gov/sites/default/files/private/aspe-files/264076/healthy-women-healthy-pregnancies-healthy-future-action-plan_0.pdf

Chinn JJ, Eisenberg E, Dickerson SA, et al. Maternal mortality in the United States: research gaps, opportunities, and priorities. *Am J Obstet Gynecol*. 2020;223(4):486-492.e6. https://doi.org/10.1016/j.ajog.2020.07.021

Chu B, Marwaha K, Sanvictores T, Ayers D. Physiology, stress reaction. In: *StatPearls*. StatPearls Publishing. 2022. Available at: http://www.ncbi.nlm.nih.gov/books/NBK541120

Collin LJ, Gaglioti AH, Beyer KM, et al. Neighborhood-level redlining and lending bias are associated with breast cancer mortality in a large and diverse metropolitan area. *Cancer Epidemiol Biomarkers Prev*. 2021;30(1):53-60. https://doi.org/10.1158/1055-9965.EPI-20-1038

Das A. How does race get "under the skin"?: Inflammation, weathering, and metabolic problems in late life. *Soc Sci Med*. 2013;77:75–83. https://doi.org/10.1016/j.socscimed.2012.11.007

Davis D-A. Obstetric racism: the racial politics of pregnancy, labor, and birthing. *Med Anthropol*. 2019;38(7):560–573. https://doi.org/10.1080/01459740.2018.1549389

Devine P. Stereotypes and prejudice: their automatic and controlled components. *J Pers Soc Psychol*. 1989;56:5–18. https://doi.org/10.1037//0022-3514.56.1.5

Devine PG, Forscher PS, Austin AJ, Cox WTL. Long-term reduction in implicit race bias: a prejudice habit-breaking intervention. *J Experiment Soc Psychol*. 2012;48(6):1267–1278. https://doi.org/10.1016/j.jesp.2012.06.003

Dunkel Schetter C. Psychological science on pregnancy: stress processes, biopsychosocial models, and emerging research issues. *Ann Rev Psychol*. 2011;62(1):531–558. https://doi.org/10.1146/annurev.psych.031809.130727

Feagin JR, Ducey K. *Racist America*. New York, NY: Routledge; 2018.

FitzGerald C, Martin A, Berner D, Hurst S. Interventions designed to reduce implicit prejudices and implicit stereotypes in real world contexts: a systematic review. *BMC Psychol*. 2019;7(1):29. https://doi.org/10.1186/s40359-019-0299-7

Forde AT, Crookes DM, Suglia SF, Demmer RT. The weathering hypothesis as an explanation for racial disparities in health: a systematic review. *Ann Epidemiol*. 2019;33:1-18.e3. https://doi.org/10.1016/j.annepidem.2019.02.011

Forscher PS, Mitamura C, Dix EL, Cox WTL, Devine PG. Breaking the prejudice habit: mechanisms, timecourse, and longevity. *J Experiment Soc Psychol*. 2017;72:133–146. https://doi.org/10.1016/j.jesp.2017.04.009

Frazier T, Hogue CJR, Bonney EA, Yount KM, Pearce BD. Weathering the storm; a review of pre-pregnancy stress and risk of spontaneous abortion. *Psychoneuroendocrinology*, 2018;92:142–154. https://doi.org/10.1016/j.psyneuen.2018.03.001

Friedman SH, Heneghan A, Rosenthal M. Characteristics of women who do not seek prenatal care and implications for prevention. *J Obstet Gynecol Neonatal Nurs*. 2009;38(2):174–181. https://doi.org/10.1111/j.1552-6909.2009.01004.x

Geronimus AT. The weathering hypothesis and the health of African-American women and infants: evidence and speculations. *Ethn Dis*. 1992;2(3):207–221.

Geronimus AT, Hicken M, Keene D, Bound J. "Weathering" and age patterns of allostatic load scores among Blacks and whites in the United States. *Am J Public Health.* 2006;96(5):826–833. https://doi.org/10.2105/AJPH.2004.060749

Geronimus AT, Hicken MT, Pearson JA, Seashols SJ, Brown KL, Cruz TD. Do US Black women experience stress-related accelerated biological aging? *Hum Nat.* 2010;21(1):19–38. https://doi.org/10.1007/s12110-010-9078-0

Giscombé CL, Lobel M. Explaining disproportionately high rates of adverse birth outcomes among African Americans: the impact of stress, racism, and related factors in pregnancy. *Psychol Bull.* 2005;131(5):662–683. https://doi.org/10.1037/0033-2909.131.5.662

Giurgescu C, Kavanaugh K, Norr KF, et al. Stressors, resources, and stress responses in pregnant African American women: a mixed-methods pilot study. *J Perinat Neonat Nurs.* 2013;27(1):81–96. https://doi.org/10.1097/JPN.0b013e31828363c3

Giurgescu C, Misra DP. Psychosocial factors and preterm birth among Black mothers and fathers. *Am J Matern Child Nurs.* 2018;43(5):245–251. https://doi.org/10.1097/NMC.0000000000000458

Gomez AM, Arteaga S, Arcara J, et al. "My 9 to 5 job is birth work": a case study of two compensation approaches for community doula care. *Int J Environ Res Public Health.* 2021;18(20):10817. https://doi.org/10.3390/ijerph182010817

Greenwood BN, Hardeman RR, Huang L, Sojourner A. Physician-patient racial concordance and disparities in birthing mortality for newborns. *Proc Natl Acad Sci U S A.* 2020;117(35):21194–21200. https://doi.org/10.1073/pnas.1913405117

Guidi J, Lucente M, Sonino N, Fava GA. Allostatic load and its impact on health: a systematic review. *Psychother Psychosom.* 2021;90(1):11–27. https://doi.org/10.1159/000510696

Gurrentz B. Child care subsidies help married moms continue working, bring greater pay equity. US Census. October 2021. Available at: https://www.census.gov/library/stories/2021/10/measuring-impact-of-child-care-subsidies-on-working-moms.html

Hall KS, Kusunoki Y, Gatny H, Barber J. Social discrimination, stress, and risk of unintended pregnancy among young women. *J Adolesc Health.* 2015;56(3):330–337. https://doi.org/10.1016/j.jadohealth.2014.11.008

Hawkins M, Panzera A. Food insecurity: a key determinant of health. *Arch Psychiatr Nurs.* 2021;35(1):113–117. https://doi.org/10.1016/j.apnu.2020.10.011

Henning-Smith CE, Hernandez AM, Hardeman RR, Ramirez MR, Kozhimannil KB. Rural counties with majority Black or Indigenous populations suffer the highest rates of premature death in the US. *Health Aff (Millwood).* 2019;38(12), 2019–2026. https://doi.org/10.1377/hlthaff.2019.00847

Howell EA, Egorova NN, Janevic T, et al. Race and ethnicity, medical insurance, and within-hospital severe maternal morbidity disparities. *Obstet Gynecol.* 2020a;135(2):285–293. https://doi.org/10.1097/AOG.0000000000003667

Howell EA, Janevic T, Blum J, et al. Double disadvantage in delivery hospital for Black and Hispanic women and high-risk Infants. *Matern Child Health J.* 2020b;24(6):687–693. https://doi.org/10.1007/s10995-020-02911-9

Jackson FM, Hogue CR, Phillips MT. The development of a race and gender-specific stress measure for African-American women: Jackson, Hogue, Phillips contextualized stress measure. *Ethn Dis.* 2005;15(4):594–600.

Jackson FM, Phillips MT, Hogue CR, Curry Owens T. Examining the burdens of gendered racism: implications for the pregnancy outcomes of college-educated African American women. *Matern Child Health J.* 2001;5(2):95-107. https://doi.org/10.1023/a:1011349115711

Jackson FM, Rowley DL, Curry Owens T. Contextualized stress, global stress, and depression in well-educated, pregnant, African-American women. *Womens Health Issues.* 2012;22(3):e329-336. https://doi.org/10.1016/j.whi.2012.01.003

Janevic T, Zeitlin J, Egorova N, Hebert PL, Balbierz A, Howell EA. Neighborhood racial and economic polarization, hospital of delivery, and severe maternal morbidity. *Health Aff (Millwood).* 2020;39(5):768-776. https://doi.org/10.1377/hlthaff.2019.00735

Johnson AA, Hatcher BJ, El-Khorazaty MN, et al. Determinants of inadequate prenatal care utilization by African American women. *J Health Care Poor Underserved.* 2007;18(3):620-636. https://doi.org/10.1353/hpu.2007.0059

Jones CP. Levels of racism: a theoretic framework and a gardener's tale. *Am J Public Health.* 2000;90(8):1212-1215. https://doi.org/10.2105/ajph.90.8.1212

Kanfash N. *Examining the Role Dietary Habits Play With Food Access, Stress, and Chronic Conditions Among African-Americans.* Master's thesis. University of Maryland, College Park; 2018. https://doi.org/10.13016/M24M91D85

Keith-Jennings B, Llobrera J, Dean, S. Links of the Supplemental Nutrition Assistance Program with food insecurity, poverty, and health: evidence and potential. *Am J Public Health.* 2019;109(12):1636-1640. https://doi.org/10.2105/AJPH.2019.305325

Kivisto AJ, Mills S, Elwood LS. Racial disparities in pregnancy-associated intimate partner homicide. *J Interpers Violence.* 2021;37(13-17):NP10938-NP10961. https://doi.org/10.1177/0886260521990831

Kogler L, Müller VI, Chang A, et al. Psychosocial versus physiological stress—meta-analyses on deactivations and activations of the neural correlates of stress reactions. *Neuroimage.* 2015;119:235-251. https://doi.org/10.1016/j.neuroimage.2015.06.059

Kornelsen J, Stoll K, Grzybowski S. Stress and anxiety associated with lack of access to maternity services for rural parturient women: stress in rural pregnancy. *Aust J Rural Health.* 2011;19(1):9-14. https://doi.org/10.1111/j.1440-1584.2010.01170.x

Kozhimannil KB, Interrante JD, Henning-Smith C, Admon LK. Rural-urban differences in severe maternal morbidity and mortality in the US, 2007-15. *Health Aff (Millwood).* 2019;38(12):2077-2085. https://doi.org/10.1377/hlthaff.2019.00805

Krishnamurti T, Davis AL, Quinn B, Castillo AF, Martin KL, Simhan HN. Mobile remote monitoring of intimate partner violence among pregnant patients during the COVID-19 shelter-in-place order: quality improvement pilot study. *J Med Internet Res.* 2021;23(2):e22790. https://doi.org/10.2196/22790

Lai CK, Skinner AL, Cooley E, et al. Reducing implicit racial preferences: II. Intervention effectiveness across time. *J Exp Psychol Gen.* 2016;145(8):1001-1016. https://doi.org/10.1037/xge0000179

Lawrence B, Kheyfets A, Carvalho K, et al. The impact of psychosocial stress on maternal health outcomes: a multi-state PRAMS 8 (2016-2018) analysis. *J Health Disparities Res Prac.* 2022;15(2):article 7.

Lee EK, Donley G, Ciesielski TH, et al. Health outcomes in redlined versus non-redlined neighborhoods: a systematic review and meta-analysis. *Soc Sci Med.* 2022;294:114696. https://doi.org/10.1016/j.socscimed.2021.114696

Lima SAM, El Dib RP, Rodrigues MRK, et al. Is the risk of low birth weight or preterm labor greater when maternal stress is experienced during pregnancy? A systematic review and meta-analysis of cohort studies. *PLoS One.* 2018;13(7):e0200594. https://doi.org/10.1371/journal.pone.0200594

Liu CH, Giallo R, Doan SN, Seidman LJ, Tronick E. Racial and ethnic differences in prenatal life stress and postpartum depression symptoms. *Arch Psychiatr Nurs.* 2016;30(1):7–12. https://doi.org/10.1016/j.apnu.2015.11.002

Long M, Frederiksen B, Ranji U, Salganicoff A. Women's health care utilization and costs: findings from the 2020 KFF Women's Health Survey. KFF. April 21, 2021. Available at: https://www.kff.org/womens-health-policy/issue-brief/womens-health-care-utilization-and-costs-findings-from-the-2020-kff-womens-health-survey

McEwen BS, Seeman T. Protective and damaging effects of mediators of stress: elaborating and testing the concepts of allostasis and allostatic load. *Ann N Y Acad Sci.* 1999;896(1):30–47. https://doi.org/10.1111/j.1749-6632.1999.tb08103.x

McEwen BS, Stellar E. Stress and the individual: mechanisms leading to disease. *Arch Int Med.* 1993;153(18):2093–2101. https://doi.org/10.1001/archinte.1993.00410180039004

McFarlane J, Soeken K, Wiist W. An evaluation of interventions to decrease intimate partner violence to pregnant women. *Public Health Nurs.* 2000;17(6):443–451. https://doi.org/10.1046/j.1525-1446.2000.00443.x

Novick G, Sadler LS, Knafl KA, Ellen Groce N, Kennedy HP. The intersection of everyday life and group prenatal care for women in two urban clinics. *J Health Care Poor Underserved.* 2012;23(2):589–603. https://doi.org/10.1353/hpu.2012.0060

Nuru-Jeter A, Dominguez TP, Hammond WP, et al. "It's the skin you're in": African-American women talk about their experiences of racism: an exploratory study to develop measures of racism for birth outcome studies. *Matern Child Health J.* 2009;13(1):29–39. https://doi.org/0.1007/s10995-008-0357-x

Othering and Belonging Institute. *Targeted Universalism.* University of California, Berkeley. 2021. Available at: https://belonging.berkeley.edu/targeted-universalism

Pavalko EK, Mossakowski KN, Hamilton VJ. Does perceived discrimination affect health? Longitudinal relationships between work discrimination and women's physical and emotional health. *J Health Soc Behav.* 2003;44(1):18–33.

Renfrew MJ, McFadden A, Bastos MH, et al. Midwifery and quality care: findings from a new evidence-informed framework for maternal and newborn care. *Lancet.* 2014;384(9948):1129–1145. https://doi.org/10.1016/S0140-6736(14)60789-3

Riggan KA, Gilbert A, Allyse MA. Acknowledging and addressing allostatic load in pregnancy care. *J Racial Ethn Health Disparities.* 2021;8(1):69–79. https://doi.org/10.1007/s40615-020-00757-z

Sakala C, Declercq ER, Turon JM, Corry MP. *Listening to Mothers in California: A Population-Based Survey of Women's Childbearing Experiences, Full Survey Report.* National Partnership for Women and Families. September 2018. Available at: https://www.chcf.org/wp-content/uploads/2018/09/ListeningMothersCAFullSurveyReport2018.pdf

Schneiderman N, Ironson G, Siegel SD. Stress and health: psychological, behavioral, and biological determinants. *Ann Rev Clin Psychol.* 2005;1:607–628. https://doi.org/10.1146/annurev.clinpsy.1.102803.144141

Selye H. *The Stress of Life.* New York, NY: McGraw-Hill; 1956.

Siden JY, Carver AR, Mmeje OO, Townsel CD. Reducing implicit bias in maternity care: a framework for action. *Womens Health Issues.* 2022;32(1):3–8. https://doi.org/10.1016/j.whi.2021.10.008

Stapleton LRT, Schetter CD, Westling E, et al. Perceived partner support in pregnancy predicts lower maternal and infant distress. *J Fam Psychol.* 2012;26(3):453–463. https://doi.org/10.1037/a0028332

Steverman B. A once radical idea to close the wealth gap is actually happening. *Bloomberg.* March 2017. Available at: https://www.bloomberg.com/news/features/2022-03-17/baby-bonds-eyed-as-way-to-close-u-s-racial-wealth-gap

Sullivan SM, Peters ES, Trapido EJ, Oral E, Scribner RA, Rung AL. Assessing mediation of behavioral and stress pathways in the association between neighborhood environments and obesity outcomes. *Prev Med Rep.* 2016;4:248–255. https://doi.org/10.1016/j.pmedr.2016.06.012

Taylor JK. Structural racism and maternal health among Black women. *J Law Med Ethics.* 2020;48(3):506–517. https://doi.org/10.1177/1073110520958875

Taylor J, Novoa C, Hamm K, Phadke S. *Eliminating Racial Disparities in Maternal and Infant Mortality: A Comprehensive Policy Blueprint.* The Center for American Progress. May 2, 2019. Available at: https://www.americanprogress.org/article/eliminating-racial-disparities-maternal-infant-mortality

Tikkanen R, Gunja M, FitzGerald M, Zephyrin L. Maternal mortality and maternity care in the United States compared to 10 other developed countries. The Commonwealth Fund. November 18, 2020. https://doi.org/10.26099/411v-9255

Van Eijk MS, Guenther GA, Kett PM, Jopson AD, Frogner BK, Skillman SM. Addressing systemic racism in birth doula services to reduce health inequities in the United States. *Health Equity.* 2022;6(1):98–105. https://doi.org/10.1089/heq.2021.0033

Vignola-Lévesque C, Léveillée S. Intimate partner violence and intimate partner homicide: development of a typology based on psychosocial characteristics. *J Interpers Violence.* 2021;37(17–18):NP15874–NP15898. https://doi.org/10.1177/08862605211021989

Wallace M, Gillispie-Bell V, Cruz K, Davis K, Vilda D. Homicide during pregnancy and the postpartum period in the United States, 2018–2019. *Obstet Gynecol.* 2021;138(5):762–769. https://doi.org/10.1097/AOG.0000000000004567

Washington HA. *Medical Apartheid: The Dark History of Medical Experimentation on Black Americans From Colonial Times to the Present.* 1st paperback ed. New York, NY: Harlem Moon; 2006.

World Health Organization. Intimate partner violence during pregnancy. 2011. Available at: https://apps.who.int/iris/bitstream/handle/10665/70764/?sequence=1

Wu KK, Lopez C, Nichols M. Virtual visits in prenatal care: an integrative review. *J Midwifery Womens Health.* 2022;67(1):39–52. https://doi.org/10.1111/jmwh.13284

Zhao Y, Kershaw T, Ettinger AS, Higgins C, Lu MC, Chao SM. Association between life event stressors and low birth weight in African American and white populations: findings from the 2007 and 2010 Los Angeles Mommy and Baby (LAMB) surveys. *Matern Child Health J.* 2015;19(10):2195–2205. https://doi.org/10.1007/s10995-015-1734-x

5

Disrupting the System to Provide the Care Black Women Deserve: An Imperative for a Holistic Evidence-Based Systems Approach

Christy M. Gamble, JD, DrPH, MPH, and Osub Ahmed, MPH

For decades, Black women have experienced the brunt of health inequities in the United States, especially when it comes to their reproductive and sexual health. The reasons for this have been the focus of numerous academic papers and research studies. Indeed, a growing body of evidence is finding that the environments and conditions in which we are born, live, work, learn, play, age, and worship often have a profound impact on our health and our lives. What is more, these conditions have been shaped by racist, sexist systems and policies whose primary purpose has been to oppress and disenfranchise. The result is deeply entrenched health disparities, breaking down along racial and gender lines, with Black women facing some of the worst health outcomes.

Unfortunately, the approach to reducing or altogether eliminating reproductive and sexual health disparities has widely been limited to health care–based solutions. But given that the health disparities we seek to dismantle are not just the product of a broken health care system but also are shaped by all facets of our lives and society, the United States needs to move to a holistic evidence- and community-based systems approach if we want to see real change in Black women's health outcomes and well-being. This approach must be comprehensive, based on inclusive scientific research, and whole-person-centered—viewing a Black woman not as simply a patient but as a whole person whose life experiences, generational trauma, and physical, mental, spiritual, and social needs provide the basis for treatment or care provision. This also means incorporating complementary and alternative therapies that have been scientifically proven to work and have been a staple in the Black family. To deliver this type of care, cross-disciplinary collaborations—in which research, health care, public health, and social services work closely with the communities they are serving and are inclusive of community-based organizations—must be nurtured and serve as the central space where these solutions are developed and eventually scaled up.

SEXUAL AND REPRODUCTIVE HEALTH INEQUITIES AMONG BLACK WOMEN

Academic research and literature have clearly demonstrated that, when it comes to sexual and reproductive health, Black women in the United States routinely fare worse than other women in terms of incidence of diseases and conditions as well as health outcomes—and have for decades. There are numerous examples of health conditions for which this holds true, such as maternal morbidity and mortality, HIV/AIDS, fibroids, and reproductive cancers like cervical and breast cancer.

Recently, heightened attention to the maternal mortality crisis has shed light on a reality that many Black women have lived for years. In 2020, the National Center for Health Statistics reported that the US maternal mortality rate for Black women was almost three times the rate of white women, with more than 55 maternal deaths per 100,000 live births (Hoyert 2022). Black women are also more likely to suffer from severe maternal morbidity (SMM), or nonfatal "near misses" that can result in both immediate and long-term health consequences. While the topic of SMM remains less well-studied, particularly with regard to racial and ethnic disparities, Melillo (2020) did find that Black women experience SMM at about twice the rate of white women. The trend in racial disparities persists for HIV/AIDS: HIV remains among the top 10 causes of death for Black women between the ages of 20 and 54 years (Centers for Disease Control and Prevention 2020).

The same inequities hold true for another health condition that gets little attention and yet is prevalent in the general population—uterine fibroids. Uterine fibroids are noncancerous tumors that form in the wall of the uterus and are often detected through a routine pelvic exam (Office of the Assistant Secretary for Health 2021). While fibroids are common, Black women are three times more likely to develop them than white women (Al-Hendy, Myers, and Stewart 2017). Moreover, when Black women do seek treatment, they are more likely to be hospitalized or endure surgery to remove them and less likely to receive minimally invasive surgery compared to the general population (Marsh 2020).

SOCIAL DETERMINANTS OF HEALTH EQUITY

What is driving these disparate reproductive and sexual health outcomes for Black women? To begin answering this question, one must first analyze Black women's health outcomes through the lens of the social determinants of health equity. Over the past few decades, researchers have elucidated the profound effect that the social determinants of health—the environments and conditions in which people are born, live, work, learn, play, age, and worship—have on health outcomes and overall well-being. The social determinants of health are typically organized into five or six domains, which include economic stability (e.g., employment, job opportunities, income level), the built environment (e.g., housing quality, access to transportation and green spaces, neighborhood safety), social context (e.g., support systems, community engagement, exposure to stressors, policing/justice policy), education (e.g., early childhood as well as higher education), health care (e.g., health coverage, provider cultural competency, and quality of care; Drake and Rudowitz 2022).

Pathways through which social determinants affect sexual and reproductive health are numerous and depend on the outcome of interest. For instance, Lorch and Enlow (2016) developed a conceptual framework for perinatal health outcomes in which they posited that social determinants either directly affect perinatal outcomes or do so indirectly by leading to acute or chronic stress and that social determinants are themselves affected by race and ethnicity.

While traditional social determinants of health frameworks have afforded public health practitioners the opportunity to determine which factors could influence Black sexual and reproductive health outcomes, they have not been adequate in helping to explain why—that is, why Black women are consistently burdened by adverse social determinants when compared to their white counterparts and the general population. Inequities within social determinants of reproductive and sexual health are driven by pervasive structural systems, including racism, sexism, and xenophobia, meant to exploit and marginalize certain people. For Black women, whose multiple identities sit at the center of these overlapping systems of oppression, the compounding effects on social determinants lead to the significant health disparities previously noted.

To address this fundamental oversight, there has been a national movement to create a framework that emphasizes social justice and community power building to provide a more complete accounting of the forces at work that shape the health of members of marginalized populations such as Black women. The Praxis Project created the "social determinants of health equity" framework, which explicitly names the oppressive systems that "infect" the social determinants of health and places them in a framework that highlights the root causes of the social determinants from the perspective of social justice and community power building (The Praxis Project n.d.).

The visual framework, illustrated as a tree with soil, roots, a trunk, and fruit, depicts the systemic oppression that has led and continues to lead to inequitable health outcomes for marginalized populations (see image here: https://www.thepraxisproject.org/social-determinants-of-health). The "soil" represents the oppressive systems (heterosexism, capitalism, racism, sexism, ableism) that lead to inequities. The inequities at the "root" result in communities that have historically experienced and currently suffer oppression, represented by the "trunk." The poor state of the soil and roots of the tree result in fruit that is negatively impacted (or adverse health outcomes) even though the tree and its branches may appear strong and resilient. This illustration cleverly shows how systemic racism within the health care system has affected the sexual and reproductive health of Black women resulting in poor "fruit" or adverse health outcomes.

HOLISTIC SYSTEMS-THINKING APPROACH

Just as it is necessary to understand that multiple determinants are responsible for driving health outcomes—and inequities in said outcomes—one must also consider the systems within which these determinants operate and how they interact with one another to develop effective solutions. This is where systems thinking comes in: it permits the researcher to take a holistic view of a system while also investigating its components and their interconnectedness (Maloney 2020).

Specifically, systems thinking is "a set of synergistic analytic skills used to improve the capability of identifying and understanding systems, predicting their behaviors, and devising modifications to them in order to produce desired effects. These skills work together as a system" (Arnold and Wade 2016, p. 675).

Research has shown that using systems thinking in the design and delivery of health care can lead to improved patient and service outcomes—and that most of these improvements are driven by the design and integration of people into interventions, using strategies like stakeholder engagement, whole-person–centered and collaborative care, and a team-based approach (Komashie et al. 2021).

Systems thinking can also be viewed as a balance between the whole and its parts, which, in essence, represent two ends of a spectrum. Emergence—that is, studying a phenomenon as a product of a whole system—lies on one end of the spectrum, and reductionism—studying the individual components of a system in isolation—lies at the other (Maloney 2020). An overreliance on either an emergent or reductionist perspective can lead to ineffective or impractical solutions.

CROSS-DISCIPLINARY AND COMMUNITY COLLABORATION

Because of the complex nature of many health conditions as well as the degree to which oppressive systems are so deeply entrenched in the delivery of care, health issues faced by Black women cannot be solved by looking to one sector (e.g., health care) or discipline (e.g., public health). To properly and effectively address the inequities and the burden of disease carried by Black women, there needs to be cross-disciplinary collaboration, which is inclusive of varying sectors. This would involve, for example, key sectors such as research, public health, health care, and social services organizations working closely together with the individuals and communities they serve by integrating community-based organizations, particularly those centering and led by Black women, into the solution. Strategic partnerships with community-based organizations must occur in a way that individuals who are committed to the community and the specific health issue, preferably Black women in this case, are involved as experts to help achieve better outcomes, reduce redundancy, lower social costs, and foster innovation. For example, to address the Black maternal health crisis, Black doulas must be part of the solution and conversation on how best to deliver holistic care in a system that has racism engrained within it. The community must be nurtured and serve as the central space where solutions to these complex health issues are developed and eventually scaled up.

DISRUPTING THE NORMS OF TRADITIONAL HEALTH CARE DELIVERY

Standard Western medicine, as practiced in the United States, has tended to skew toward a reductionist approach, giving rise to a plethora of narrow medical specialties and subspecialties, a significant lack of care coordination within and between clinical and nonclinical practices, and an emphasis on the treatment of singular conditions. Holistic care, on the other hand, seeks to integrate conventional allopathic medicine with complementary practices, the latter of which utilizes an emergent approach to care for the whole person and honors the mind–body connection using a variety of clinically proven therapies to address physical, mental, spiritual, and social needs. Complementary, alternative, integrative, or holistic medicine (terms often used interchangeably) is rooted in the understanding that each of these needs can affect one's overall health and well-being and that deficiencies in one can translate to deficiencies throughout the whole system (Holland 2018). This is not to say that conventional medicine does not have a role in developing treatments or organizing health systems; rather, it is important that in continuing to improve conventional medical practices and systems, reductionist thinking cannot guide overall decision-making. Holistic medical practices and principles provide the necessary counterbalance to move away from these instincts.

Holistic medicine dates back centuries in other parts of the world and has recently made its way into the practice of Western medicine (Gore and Kaplan 2009), so much so that the National Institutes of Health created the National Center for Complementary and Integrative Health (NCCIH) in 1998 to determine the safety and usefulness of holistic approaches and the ways they can improve health and health care (NCCIH n.d.). Key to utilizing a holistic care approach is developing a strong patient–provider relationship based on mutual respect and trust. For providers to do this, they must be trained on the importance of methods for taking information about a patient's social, economic, psychological, and financial backgrounds into account—in essence, applying a social determinants of health equity lens.

Providers who adopt a holistic approach to health go beyond asking a patient about his or her symptoms or offering treatment options based on limited data—rather, these providers inquire about their patient's overall health and well-being to make effective and personalized treatment recommendations. Holistic practitioners also recognize the importance of educating and working with their patients in how to adopt healthy behaviors and treatment options to ensure that health improvements are effective and sustained. Holistic care is necessary to ensure that providers view a Black woman not simply as a patient but as a whole person whose life experiences, generational trauma, and physical, mental, spiritual, and social needs are the basis for any counseling, treatment, or care provision.

Holistic medical practices have been used within the Black community for centuries, and continue to this day (Johnson 2020). There are many reasons for this, including the preservation and transmission of medical knowledge through the generations as well as a deep-seated distrust of the medical institution in response to acts of medical exploitation and experimentation against Black people (Duke University 2021; Scharff et al. 2010; Miller and Miller 2021). In the first national study exploring the use of naturopathic medicine, a form of alternative medicine, among Black families between 1979 and 1980, Boyd et al. (2000) found that almost 70% of families reported using home remedies, herbal preparations, or nonprescription drugs. Barner et al. (2010) also concluded that, among Black individuals who responded to the 2002 National Health Interview Survey, nearly 70% had used complementary or alternative medicine for treatment or prevention purposes in the past year. The most popular therapies among survey respondents included alternative medical systems approaches (e.g., naturopathy), manipulative and body-based therapies (e.g., acupuncture), biologically based therapies (e.g., folk medicine), and mind–body therapies (e.g., yoga/tai chi/qigong, biofeedback; Barner et al. 2010).

Holistic care can help to address the inequities in reproductive and sexual health outcomes experienced by Black women. For example, despite myths that Black women are hyperfertile, some studies suggest Black women are twice as likely to experience infertility (Wellons et al. 2008). According to the Society for Assisted Reproductive Technology (SART), the average cost for in vitro fertilization (IVF), one of the most successful forms of assisted reproductive technology, in the United States is between $10,000 and $15,000 per cycle (SART n.d.). But there are some evidence-based holistic approaches to addressing infertility such as dietary and lifestyle changes, homeopathy, reversing vitamin deficiencies, acupuncture, and Chinese herbal medicine (Murray and Pizzorno 1998; Frawley and Lad 1986). Moreover, many of the approaches to naturally treat infertility have been shown to be effective in treating uterine fibroids (Njaka 2019).

However, there are numerous barriers to accessing holistic care, with inadequate or nonexistent health coverage and high out-of-pocket costs topping the list. While the popularity of certain holistic therapies within the United States has risen over the past couple decades, coverage for services is variable and usually limited to certain modalities. For example, one visit to a naturopathic doctor can cost up to $400 for an initial 90-minute visit and up to $200 for follow-ups (Gengler and Levine 2014), and insurance plans typically do not cover naturopathic services. It is no wonder then that, according to the 2012 National Health Interview Survey, out-of-pocket spending for holistic therapies topped $30.2 billion each year—more than 9% of all out-of-pocket health care spending (NCCIH 2016). Interestingly, increases in alternative medical utilization rates seem to be concentrated among people whose insurance plans do not cover these services, even though more insurers are choosing to cover some complementary therapies (Nahin et al. 2016). This may be because coverage of these therapies is more likely to be partial (Nahin et al. 2016), potentially leaving patients with unexpected medical expenses that make it less likely for them to use them again.

BROADENING EVIDENCE AND REPRESENTATION IN RESEARCH

It is also of the utmost importance to address the need for continuing evidence to support the call for a holistic, systems-thinking approach to delivering care to Black women. It is critical that Black women are better represented in clinical research studies to ensure that any interventions and treatments that are proposed or developed are effective among Black women patients. An example of a failure to do so was in the drug trials for the human papillomavirus (HPV) vaccine (Brooks n.d.). Moreover, there is a need to conduct more research on systems-thinking approaches to discover other ways to address the complex and longstanding issues produced by the normative ways that oppressive systems have continued to withstand numerous attempts at change.

Looking to The Praxis Project's social determinants of health equity framework would provide the necessary information on which disciplines or sectors ("roots") to involve in the delivery of care to improve health outcomes and which gaps in the research must be filled to provide evidence-based solutions to improve the "fruit" that is produced by the "tree" of the resilient Black woman.

CONCLUSION

While Black women have faced inequities and injustices related to their reproductive and sexual health and outcomes, it is imperative that we begin to address the needs in these areas. To do so, we need a different approach—one that disrupts the current delivery of health care. A holistic, systems-thinking approach that is built on the foundation of Black women–led and –centered community-based organizations and inclusive research is the answer. We should look to the most accurate model of the factors that impact the health of Black women—The Praxis Project's social determinants of health equity framework— if we are to truly break down the power structures and oppressive systems that have adversely affected Black women's reproductive and sexual health care.

REFERENCES

Al-Hendy A, Myers ER, Stewart E. Uterine fibroids: burden and unmet medical need. *Semin Reprod Med.* 2017;35(6):473–480. https://doi.org/10.1055/s-0037-1607264

Arnold RD, Wade JP. A definition of systems thinking: a systems approach. In: *Procedia Computer Science: 2015 Conference on Systems Engineering Research.* 2015;44(2015):669–678. https://doi.org/10.1016/j.procs.2015.03.050

Barner JC, Bohman TM, Brown CM, Richards KM. Use of complementary and alternative medicine for treatment among African-Americans: a multivariate analysis. *Res Soc Adm Pharm.* 2010;6(3):196–208. https://doi.org/10.1016/j.sapharm.2009.08.001

Boyd EL, Taylor SD, Shimp LA, Semler CR. An assessment of home remedy use by African Americans. *J Natl Med Assoc.* 2000;92(7):341–353. Available at: https://www.ncbi.nlm.nih.gov/pmc/articles/PMC2608585

Brooks M. Black women may benefit less from current HPV vaccines: study. Consultant360. Available at: https://www.consultant360.com/story/black-women-may-benefit-less-current-hpv-vaccines-study

Centers for Disease Control and Prevention. HIV Surveillance Report, 2018 (updated); vol. 31. May 2020. Available at: http://www.cdc.gov/hiv/library/reports/hiv-surveillance.html

Drake P, Rudowitz R. Tracking social determinants of health during the COVID-19 pandemic. Kaiser Family Foundation. April 21, 2022. Available at: https://www.kff.org/coronavirus-covid-19/issue-brief/tracking-social-determinants-of-health-during-the-covid-19-pandemic

Duke University Medical Center Library and Archives. Black history month: a medical perspective: folk medicine. February 14, 2021. Available at: https://guides.mclibrary.duke.edu/blackhistorymonth/folkmed

Frawley D, Lad V. *The Yoga of Herbs: An Ayurvedic Guide to Herbal Medicine.* Silver Lake, WI: Lotus Press; 1986.

Gengler A, Levine H. Take the sting out of alternative medicine costs. *Money.* November 14, 2014. Available at: https://money.com/alternative-medicine-costs-insurance

Gore J, Kaplan E. Infertility: A holistic approach. Center for Holistic Medicine. June 2, 2009. Available at: https://holistic-medicine.com/infertility-a-holistic-approach

Holland TM. What is holistic health care, anyway? Dignity Health. January 24, 2018. Available at: https://www.dignityhealth.org/articles/what-is-holistic-health-care-anyway

Hoyert DL. Maternal mortality rates in the United States, 2020. National Center for Health Statistics. 2022. Available at: https://www.cdc.gov/nchs/data/hestat/maternal-mortality/2020/maternal-mortality-rates-2020.htm

Johnson C. Black distrust for modern medicine drives movement to holistic health. *The Spokesman.* December 2, 2020. Available at: https://themsuspokesman.com/11746/showcase/black-distrust-for-modern-medicine-drives-movement-to-holistic-health

Komashie A, Ward J, Bashford T, et al. Systems approach to health service design, delivery and improvement: a systematic review and meta-analysis. *BMJ Open.* 2021;11(1):e037667. https://doi.org/10.1136/bmjopen-2020-037667

Lorch SA, Enlow E. The role of social determinants in explaining racial/ethnic disparities in perinatal outcomes. *Pediatr Res.* 2016;79(1–2):141–147. https://doi.org/10.1038/pr.2015.199

Maloney M. Systems thinking: a balance between reductionism and emergence. *Intelligent Speculation.* May 19, 2020. Available at: https://www.intelligentspeculation.com/blog/systems-thinking

Marsh E. Understanding racial disparities for women with uterine fibroids. University of Michigan Institute for Healthcare Policy and Innovation. August 12, 2020. Available at: https://ihpi.umich.edu/news/understanding-racial-disparities-women-uterine-fibroids

Melillo G. Racial disparities persist in maternal morbidity, mortality and infant health. *Am J Manag Care*. June 13, 2020. Available at: https://www.ajmc.com/view/racial-disparities-persist-in-maternal-morbidity-mortality-and-infant-health

Miller F, Miller P. Transgenerational trauma and trust restoration. *AMA J Ethics*. 2021;23(6):E480–E486. https://doi.org/10.1001/amajethics.2021.480

Murray MT, Pizzorno J. *The Encyclopedia of Natural Medicine*. Rocklin, CA: Prima Communications Inc; 1998.

Nahin RL, Barnes PM, Stussman BJ. Insurance coverage for complementary health approaches among adult users: United States, 2002 and 2012. National Center for Health Statistics Data Brief, No. 235. January 2016. Available at: https://www.cdc.gov/nchs/data/databriefs/db235.pdf

National Center for Complementary and Integrative Health. The NIH Almanac. Available at: https://www.nih.gov/about-nih/what-we-do/nih-almanac/national-center-complementary-integrative-health-nccih

National Center for Complementary and Integrative Health. Paying for complementary and integrative health approaches. June 2016. Available at: https://www.nccih.nih.gov/health/paying-for-complementary-and-integrative-health-approaches

Njaka N. Black women and fibroids part 2: holistic treatments and preventative health. *Blood & Milk*. June 13, 2019. Available at: https://www.bloodandmilk.com/black-women-and-fibroids-part-2-holistic-treatments-and-preventative-health

Office of the Assistant Secretary for Health, Office on Women's Health. Uterine fibroids. February 2021. Available at: https://www.womenshealth.gov/a-z-topics/uterine-fibroids

The Praxis Project. Social determinants of health. Available at: https://www.thepraxisproject.org/social-determinants-of-health

Scharff DP, Mathews KJ, Jackson P, Hoffsuemmer J, Martin E, Edwards D. More than Tuskegee: understanding mistrust about research participation. *J Health Care Poor Underserved*. 2010;21(3):879–897. https://doi.org/10.1353/hpu.0.0323

Society for Assisted Reproductive Technology. Frequently asked questions: what is the cost of IVF? Available at: https://www.sart.org/patients/frequently-asked-questions

Wellons MF, Lewis CE, Schwartz SM, Richman J, Sites CK, Siscovick DS. Racial differences in self-reported infertility and risk factors for infertility in a cohort of Black and white women: The CARDIA Women's Study. *Fertil Steril*. 2008;90(5):1640–1648. https://doi.org/10.1016/j.fertnstert.2007.09.056

Appendix I: From the Archives

- Geronimous AT. The weathering hypothesis and the health of African American women and infants: evidence and speculations. *Ethn Dis.* 1991;2(3):207–221.

As a possible explanation for racial variation in maternal age patterns of births and birth outcomes, Geronimous proposed the "weathering hypothesis," which posits that the health of Black women may begin to deteriorate in early adulthood as a physical consequence of cumulative exposure to experiences of social, economic, and political adversity.

- Jackson FM, Phillips MT, Hogue CJ, Curry-Owens TY. Examining the burdens of gendered racism: implications for pregnancy outcomes among college-educated African American women. *Matern Child Health J.* 2001;5(2):95–107.

This study, including focus groups, interviews, and the administration of a pilot stress instrument, examined how African American college-educated women experience racism linked to their identities and their roles as African American women (gendered racism). The findings revealed that the stressors of gendered racism preceding and accompanying pregnancy may be risk factors for adverse birth outcomes. Additionally, a felt sense of obligation for protecting children from racism and other women from workplace racism was a significant stressor.

- Black Women Scholars and the Research Working Group of the Black Mamas Matter Alliance. Black maternal health research re-envisioned: best practices for the conduct of research with, for, and by Black Mamas. *Harvard Law Policy Rev.* 2020;14:393–415. https://harvardlpr.com/wp-content/uploads/sites/20/2020/11/BMMA-Research-Working-Group.pdf

This article provides an overview of the principles that should underpin the ethical design of clinical and epidemiological public health research and health services, specifically those, with, for, and by Black Mamas. The full report referenced by this article presents recommendations for improving research on maternal health outcomes for Black Mamas.

II. REEMBODIMENT OF THE SELF: DISPELLING MYTHS IN MEDIA AND SOCIETY

6

Reframing Historical Narratives, Images, and Beliefs About the Sexuality of Black Women

Regina Davis Moss, PhD, MPH

Throughout history, Black women have been unfairly subjected to myths and stereotypes. Black women have been ascribed negative and inferior images as the result of a long-lived legacy of racism, sexism, and oppression. The distorted representation of the Black woman was extremely important for the creation and maintenance of the political, economic, and social structure of America, particularly during slavery. To justify their dehumanization, the conceptualization of narratives that continuously discredited and "othered" Black women became the foundation for framing Black women's identities. Prevailing stereotypes of Black womanhood include the Jezebel, mammy, tragic mulatto, Sapphire, matriarch, welfare mother, and strong Black woman.

JEZEBEL

The Jezebel is depicted as an attractive seductress who is governed by her libido and matters of the flesh (Gray White 1999). She is a hypersexual woman with voracious, animalistic passions and, therefore, is able to appease the insatiable desires of white men. The historical portrayal of the Jezebel was diametrically opposed to the idealized passionlessness of the "true woman" who was chaste, delicate, pure, and white. The stereotype of sexual promiscuity also defined Black women as bad mothers who procreate with abandon and who can never be trusted to be constant or loyal (Roberts 2017).

It is important to note that the construct of the licentious temptress served to justify the sexual abuse of slave women by their owners and, thus, the jealousy and resentment of white women (Hill Collins 2000; Villarosa 1994). American society widely believed Black women drew on their sexual relationships with their white masters not only to satisfy their own desires but also to gain freedom and other privileges (Stephens and Phillips 2003). This reinforced the myth that Black women are responsible for their own rape and sexual coercion. Indeed, from the moment they set foot in America, Black women have been vulnerable to rationalized sexual exploitation.

The image of the devious and lascivious Black woman has been systematically perpetuated long after the ending of slavery (Roberts 2017). Black women are often portrayed in modern society as more sexually aggressive (Leath et al. 2022), and the outdated stereotype is reinforced in mass media. Images of promiscuous Black women have been featured in movies, television, music, the internet, and magazines—most notably, Black exploitation films during the post–Civil Rights Era, video vixens of the 1980s to 2000s, and voluptuous models across digital media platforms.

Some Black actresses and entertainers are using their eroticism to self-define their sexuality and exercise agency. Whether performative, an authentic depiction of their sexual liberty, savvy marketing, or all of the above, many are monetizing their sexuality—perhaps, believing Black women should profit from what they were forced to give away for too long. Their deployment of double-edged eroticism is a classic Josephine Baker-esque release of exploitation tension with the special twist of Black dance, music, and fashion that soon becomes copied and distorted by global culture. While this approach may make some respectability ideologists uncomfortable, their message of reclamation has sparked a unique space for Black women to resist oppression, subvert objectification, and assert sex positivity. Messages of sexual empowerment and Black womanhood also fuel its popularity.

Research indicates that Black women's awareness of the Jezebel stereotype can inform their sexual agency. The stereotype may lead Black women to subscribe to sexual scripts that objectify them, champion sexual passivity, and decrease regard for their own sexual desires (Leath et al. 2022; Crooks et al. 2019; French 2013; Stephens and Phillips 2003). Black women with a stronger awareness of the Jezebel stereotype were more likely to demonstrate more emotional avoidance behaviors, have a tendency to participate in sexual distancing, display significant feelings of sexual objectification, and have poorer sexual outcomes (Leath et al. 2022). Conversely, when Black women rejected the Jezebel stereotype and embraced positive feelings about their identity as a Black woman, they experienced more sexual satisfaction (Leath et al. 2022; Crooks et al. 2019).

MAMMY

In direct contradiction to the Jezebel, the obsequious and matronly mammy represented the embodiment of the ideal Black woman. Generally pictured as dark-skinned, thick-lipped, rotund, and handkerchiefed, the mammy portrayed the obedient servant, skilled cook, devoted housekeeper, and capable caretaker of the master's children (Roberts 2017). She was also depicted as asexual and nonthreatening to her mistress's femininity due to her old age, physical strength, and obesity.

The mammy archetype highlighted the social prestige of Southern white families, the South's romanticization of the Black–white relationship, and a historical legitimation for slavery and segregation (Morton 1991). The image preserved the convenient script of the happy, docile, Black female servant during a period when Black women were transitioning from unpaid house slaves to paid domestic workers (Stephens and Phillips 2003).

The mammy was an image of the ideal Black woman and mother, but only in relation to her care for her white family, not for her Black children, Black family, or Black community. Despite evidence affirming that the mammy was a largely mythical figure with little basis in the lived experiences of Black women (Walker-Barnes 2014), the caricature became a cult figure during the Jim Crow Era. The mammy was embodied in Aunt Jemima for the Chicago Columbia Exposition in 1893 and appeared on pancake boxes for decades (Roberts 2017). There have been many calls to retire the name and character, asserting its origins are based on a racial stereotype. The mammy image, however, continues to proliferate, whether partly disguised or totally unchanged, today. Black male comedians and actors donning wigs and fat suits to portray modern-day mammies further demean and dehumanize Black women just as its earlier representations did.

TRAGIC MULATTO

As slaves or as free domestic servants, Black females' proximity to their white masters made them more likely to be sexually harassed or raped. One result of interracial rape was the emergence of mulattos (Mgadmi 2009). The mulatto is the offspring of a white slaveholder and his Black female slave. Despite her mixed Black and white ancestry, the mulatto was considered Black in the light of the pervasive "one-drop rule," which held that "a single drop of 'Black blood'" made a person Black (Davis 1991).

Being "whitish" and regarded, thus, as more beautiful than full-blooded Black women, during slavery, many mulattas were also sold for the exclusive purpose of prostitution and concubinage. The mulatta's imagery was conspicuously dichotomized between "good" and "bad," between the elevated "whitish" and degraded "Blackness," and capable of progress (Mgadmi 2009).

Most strikingly, the mulatto was perceived as the product of an unnatural relationship committed by either Blacks or whites, and miscegenation was considered the greatest sin of all (Frederickson 1987). She was loathed by white society for being living proof that the color line had been crossed and stigmatized in the Black community for being born of a mother who had not exhibited standards of sexual purity. All these factors were contributory to the emergence of the image of "the tragic mulatto," who is figured as an unstable, dangerous person who despised her descent, her family, and herself (Morton 1991).

SAPPHIRE

The Sapphire image is a loud, bitter, and domineering female who controls men and usurps their role. She is characterized as an angry, disagreeable, hypersensitive, and emasculating woman whose berating is directed at her partners and children

(Stephens and Phillips 2003). The Sapphire caricature is a harsh label used to punish Black women who violate the societal norms that encourage them to be passive, servile, nonthreatening, and unseen. This image became the prelude to the matriarch and the angry Black woman, which is so ingrained in society that the tag gets slapped on many professional Black women or any Black woman in a position of power.

MATRIARCH

The matriarch is the unwed mother whose overbearing attitude is insinuated to be the cause of family instability. The stereotype holds that Black women's independence damages their families in two ways: they demoralize Black men, and they transmit a pathological lifestyle to their children, perpetuating generational poverty and antisocial behavior (Roberts 2017). Assistant Secretary of Labor Daniel Patrick Moynihan popularized this myth when he commissioned a 1965 report, *The Negro Family: The Case for National Action,* which stated that the African American experience was problematized by a family structure that was under the sexual controls of its women (Moynihan 1967). Through his use of the term "matriarch," Moynihan presented African American women as emasculating and contemptuous females who did not need a man beyond using his seed for childbearing (Stephens and Phillips 2003). The physical appearance of the matriarch has been portrayed as "undefined and unnecessary" (Roberts 2017). Mainstream imagery of Black women has reinforced these body images.

WELFARE MOTHER

The welfare mother archetype is one that is lazy, uneducated, and purposefully breeding children to take advantage of public assistance programs (Hill Collins 2000; Stephens and Phillips 2003). Black mothers are portrayed as calculating, unable to adequately care for their children, a burden on taxpayers, and deserving of harsh discipline (Roberts 2017). They are deemed "not useful" to the needs of white culture, and their physical appearance is similarly "undefined and unnecessary."

Despite white and working people always having comprised the majority of those receiving government assistance, this stigmatizing stereotype has been attributed to the Black female. This shift in narrative has enabled those in power to continue to monitor and regulate the reproductive lives of Black women under the guise of assistance (Roberts 2017).

STRONG BLACK WOMAN

In an attempt to project an image of strength and, in part, push back against negative stereotypes such as Jezebel, mammy, or welfare mother, Black women created the narrative of the strong Black woman (SBW). The SBW role, also often referred to as the superwoman, obligates Black women to present an image of strength, suppress emotions, resist dependence on others, succeed despite limited resources, and prioritize caregiving over self-care (Woods-Giscombé 2010).

In her book *Too Heavy a Yoke: Black Women and the Burden of Strength*, Walker-Barnes (2014) contends, "The myth of Black women's strength is dangerously seductive in that it imbues Black women with a certain moral and emotional superiority, providing a psychic balm against the daily insults incurred from social injustice" (p. 21). Accordingly, Black women consider emotional strength a birthright, and moments of deviation cultural flaws or failure.

The stereotype of the SBW may be an emblem of a Black woman's value to her community, but it can also compromise her well-being. The need for Black women to constantly project themselves as strong is so pervasive that it may limit Black women's ability to cope healthily and exacerbate negative mental health outcomes of stress. In addition, reinforcing the idea that a "Black woman must perform as though she is superhuman conceals her vulnerabilities, isolation, and dissociation from any suffering" (Bryant 2018, p. 356).

Taken together, these prevailing stereotypes represent limited sexual scripts that have been written for Black women for centuries. Regardless of their circumstance or appearance, Black women are presumed to be without sexual control, without sexuality, or available at some price. Black women are simultaneously fetishized and desexualized. On one hand, they experience others as being attracted to them because of their physical appearance while, on the other hand, they are confined to negative sexual scripts reflective of a patriarchal society and culture. Sexual scripts are schema used to categorize ideas about appropriate sexual beliefs, behaviors, and experiences. The everyday reinforcement of limited scripts has a direct impact on Black women's sexual self-concept, behaviors, and decision-making processes (Morton 1991).

THE POLITICS OF RESPECTABILITY

Although the demeaning stereotypical perception of Black women was conditioned by patriarchal white middle-class American ideals, Black women's efforts to counter these negative images were paradoxically based on the very values that condemned and degraded them. The "politics of respectability," a term coined by Dr. Evelyn Higginbotham (1992), was at the heart of a strategy within the Black community to survive the racial terrorism of the United States and "uplift" the race (Mgadmi 2009). Black women felt respectable behavior earned esteem from white America, and placed an exaggerated importance on industriousness, thrift, cleanliness, refined manners, and Victorian mores (Wolcott 2001). Conservative morality was the blueprint for Black integration. Many participated in domestic training courses and were instructed to be good Christians and wear modest, subdued clothing.

Black intellectuals, activists, and institutions for racial reform such as the Urban League, the National Association for the Advancement of Colored People, and the National Association of Colored Women actively promoted respectability (Mgadmi 2009). However, elites of the period such as Booker T. Washington, W.E.B. Du Bois, and members of "The Talented Tenth," often perpetuated negative stereotypes about Black women by emphasizing domesticity, monogamy, sexual restraint, and other white patriarchal values known as the Cult of True Womanhood (Hammonds 1997; Welter 2012). In their view, it reframed the "bad" image of Black women into a "good" feminine picture and capable of rise in status. Yet, it also reflected a legitimization and internalization of such representations, a yielding to cultural inferiority, and a narrow identity for Black female sexuality. More current representations of Black women who have achieved middle-class status include the Black lady (Collins 2005) a role developed to speak to respectability politics and disrupt narratives of Black women's promiscuity.

THE POLITICS OF SILENCE

Despite the "sexually respectable" identity projected upon them, Black women of all classes were distinctly left to contend with its day-to-day actualization. Working-class Black women may have been able to use this approach as a shield against the continuing sexual harassment, exploitation, and rape in private homes, while aspiring or middle-class Black women may have had to endure these incidences to appeal to whites and gain status. In both cases, Black women were ushered into a cult of secrecy and silence even when sexually abused and harassed (Hine 1994). In addition to dissemblance defining much of their public life, Black women's silence was a denial and sacrifice of their own sexuality and emotions. Hammonds argues the "politics of silence" surrounding Black sexuality did little to deconstruct the notion of hypersexuality associated with Black Americans, and the ideologies have negative implications for sexual development, health-seeking behaviors, sexual communication, and mental well-being. (Hammonds 1997; Crooks 2019).

SPIRITUALITY AND FAITH

Religious concepts related to spirituality and faith have long been important sources of hope and resilience for many Black women. Their strong faith in God gave enslaved women the strength to endure—and has also been from which many draw the fortitude needed to continue the struggle against racism, sexism, classism, and white supremacy (In Our Own Voice: National Black Women's Reproductive Justice Agenda 2021). At the same time, religion has long been weaponized to stigmatize, blame, and control Black women's reproductive and sexual health. The Black church has used religion to classify "good" versus "bad" Black women and promote oppressive theological teachings that deny bodily autonomy (Toni M. Bond, PhD, written communication, May 2023).

The consequences of violating covenants about sex are grim—going to hell, being labeled a whore, and being ostracized from the church and even from one's family (Wyatt 1997). Body awareness is also limited by cultural and religious prohibitions against body touching, condom and contraceptive use, and certain sexual practices.

Religious institutions provide informal scripts for sexual taboos and when sex is and is not appropriate. Because religion holds such an important role in the lives of Black women and girls, its influence may extend to sexual attitudes, behaviors, pleasure, and satisfaction.

INFLUENCE OF MEDIA

Although there are more representations of Black women available in the mass media than ever before, the substance of these images has changed little over the past century (Wyatt 1997; Stephens and Phillips 2003). The exoticizing of African American women as wild, sexually promiscuous, and amoral continues to be normalized by descriptors that are widely circulated, accepted, and used to frame ideas about Black women (hooks 1992; Stephens and Phillips 2003).

Media impacts our environments by influencing our beliefs, value systems, public ideology, and relation to one another. Information the media presents to the general public regarding a particular group of people becomes how the public learns to understand the behaviors, expectations, and image of others. When audiences do not possess direct knowledge or experiences with such a group, they become particularly reliant upon the media to inform them.

Throughout history, mass media in various forms has tended to support the power of the dominant group by presenting highly negative, emotion-evoking images of minority groups (Luther, Ringer Lepre, and Clark 2011). This includes news, network television series, reality TV, advertisements, music videos, and social media that portray Black women in ways that reify stereotypical gendered schemas. With these considerations in mind, it is important to understand the social consequences of narratives as a result of media-biased content. For example, during the 1980s' "War on Drugs," babies who had been exposed to drugs in utero were always depicted as crack babies who were Black and on welfare, sparking widespread paranoia of a rising generation of criminals and violent predators. Yet, over the past two decades, there has been a substantial increase in the national rate of maternal opioid use disorder and a starkly different approach from the media. Prescription drug abuse is viewed as an activity concentrated in white, suburban neighborhoods, as opposed to crack cocaine, which is presumed to be abused primarily in Black, urban communities.

Although the choice to take drugs while pregnant conflicts with social mores, the difference in race, class, and choice of drug is precisely what influences the tolerance and tone of the conversation surrounding infants and their mothers. According to Roberts (2017), infants impacted by prescription drug abuse are treated with much more sympathy and without the same moral panic, and there is concern about the humanity of the mother and the mother's needs. The mainstream media's narrative of Black mothers with substance abuse problems has consistently been punitive and vilifying. The story is different, because the profile of the woman is different, and the kinds of social questions that the concern is responding to are, therefore, very different (Cadet 2012).

The media sets up an assumption that all Black American girls grow up in the projects or city streets, and all Black women, often regardless of their socioeconomic status, get placed in the same societal categorization. This stereotype is not a real person but a uni-dimensional stick figure who lives in the public imagination (Lamb 2001).

Certainly, not all media portrayals of Black women are negative or disempowering. However, it is particularly troubling that the images available for emulation exceedingly portray Black women in such limited and frequently offensive ways. Current findings, along with past evidence of the damaging effects of societal stereotypes, underscore the importance of diversifying images of Black women in media and including more positive, complex, and dynamic portrayals (Mastro 2015). The extent to which audiences perceive negative, and often uncontested, portrayals as realistic are associated with endorsement of social scripts and decreased agency.

Research has shown that television, particularly entertainment programming, is the most important source of information and socialization for African American adolescents. Educators must be intentional about designing media literacy curricula that help Black adolescent girls and young women think critically about the ways they internalize and embody stereotypes, interact with one another, and navigate imbalances of power in gender, race, and socioeconomics (Flowers 2018). Young women who have not yet developed a sense of self strong enough to withstand the influences of negative stereotypes frequently attempt to emulate them (Wyatt 1997).

It has also been found that when comparing by race and gender, Blacks and women spend the greatest amount of time watching television (Stephens and Phillips 2003). How television media content is formed, selected, and presented is heavily subjected to the opinions of those involved in the industry. Content not only activates and reinforces stereotypical beliefs of consumers who have little contact with Black women, but persistent exposure may also shape how Black women come to feel about themselves. As consumers of media, it is important that Black women challenge the dominant discourse and hold creators of content that promote stereotypical images accountable.

IMPACT ON REPRODUCTIVE HEALTH AND SEXUALITY

It is important to explore the effects of myths and stereotypes on health behaviors and reproductive outcomes. There is evidence that stereotypes can be harmful to the well-being of Black women through at least two mechanisms: (1) stereotype threat and

(2) stereotyping leading to discrimination (Rosenthal and Lobel 2016). Stereotype threat is when an individual is worried or anxious about the possibility of confirming or being judged according to stereotypes about their group (Steele and Aronson 1995). Patients who feel judged by health care workers are more likely to mistrust their health providers and delay treatment of health problems. They are also less likely to access available preventive care and follow medical instructions (Jones et al. 2013). Stereotype threat related to unique stereotypes about African American women have led Black women to experience greater distress throughout their lifetimes and specifically during pregnancy (Rosenthal and Lobel 2016). A large body of research supports the idea that chronic stress predicts greater risk of adverse birth outcomes for Black women, including maternal mortality, preterm birth, and low birth weight (Geronimus 1992; Giscombé and Lobel 2005; Parker Dominguez et al. 2008).

Stereotypes of Black women held by health care providers leading to conscious or unconscious discrimination and biases has been found to affect provision of care (Rosenthal and Lobel 2016). In ample quantitative and qualitative studies, Black women report receiving lower quality of care including poor or disrespectful communication, rushed care, dismissed concerns, denial of treatment, and invasive procedures without consent, regardless of socioeconomic status.

Some health care stereotyping may be an unintended consequence of health awareness campaigns that often communicate and reinforce negative stereotypes about Black women. Examples include education campaigns about contraception, sexual risk taking, and prevention of sexually transmitted infections. This does not assert certain health concerns should not be addressed among Black women. However, messaging and interventions tend to focus on adverse sexual and reproductive outcomes and seldom include sex-positive data, rendering Black women's sexuality invisible. Black women are inundated with messages of how to have sex, with whom to have sex, and where to have sex. Few have heard sex and emotional pleasure discussed in the same breath (Stephens and Phillips 2003).

Many Black researchers and feminists (Wyatt 1997; Hill Collins 2000; hooks 1992) have long noted that Black female sexuality is stereotypically represented as inherently "abnormal," "excessive," and "disproportionate." Black women and girls are unable to escape the ways in which culture has used their gender and race to shape a monolithic image of deviant sexuality.

Reframing negative images of US Black women will only be accomplished by critically exploring the fallacies on which they are constructed and confronting the social and institutional structures connected to their maintenance. In the face of repressive stereotypes, Black women's resilience prevails, and we continue to define ourselves through our own eyes instead of through the eyes of others. We continue to write our own narrative filled with self-love, empowerment, admiration, and liberation.

REFERENCES

Bryant C. Remembering ourselves: confession as a pathway to conscientization. *Meridians.* 2018;16(2):351–362. https://doi.org/10.2979/meridians.16.2.16

Cadet D. Crack babies' comparison to neonatal drug withdrawal ignores racist rhetoric of 1980s, experts argue. *HuffPost.* September 4, 2012. Available at: https://www.huffpost.com/entry/crack-babies-neonatal-drug-withdrawal_n_1847712

Collins P. *Black Sexual Politics: African Americans, Gender, and the New Racism.* New York, NY: Routledge; 2005.

Crooks N, King B, Tluczek A, Sales JM. The process of becoming a sexual Black woman: a grounded theory study. *Perspect Sex Reprod Health.* 2019;51(1):17–25. https://doi.org/10.1363/psrh.12085

Davis F. *Who Is Black? One Nation's Definition.* University Park, PA: Pennsylvania State University Press; 1991.

Flowers SC. Enacting our multidimensional power: Black women sex educators demonstrate the value of an intersectional sexuality education framework. *Meridians.* 2018;16(2):308–325. https://doi.org/10.2979/meridians.16.2.11

Frederickson G. *The Black Image in the White Mind: The Debate on Afro-American Character and Destiny 1817–1914.* Hanover, NH: Wesleyan University Press; 1987.

French B. More than Jezebels and freaks: exploring how Black girls navigate sexual coercion and sexual scripts. *J Afr Am Stud.* 2013;17(1):35–50. https://doi.org/10.1007/s12111-012-9218-1

Geronimus AT. The weathering hypothesis and the health of African-American women and infants: evidence and speculations. *Ethn Dis.* 1992;2(3):207–221.

Giscombé CW, Lobel M. Explaining disproportionately high rates of adverse birth outcomes among African Americans: the impact of stress, racism, and related factors in pregnancy. *Psychol Bull.* 2005;131:662–683. https://doi.org/10.1037/0033-2909.131.5.662

Gray White, D. *Ar'n't I a Woman: Female Slaves in the Plantation South,* New York, NY: Norton; 1999.

Hammonds E. Toward a genealogy of Black female sexuality: the problematic of silence. In: Price J, Shildrick M, eds. *Feminist Theory and the Body: A Reader.* New York, NY: Routledge; 1997: 93–104.

Higginbotham EB. African-American women's history and the metalanguage of race. *Signs.* 1992;17(2):251–274. http://www.jstor.org/stable/3174464

Hill Collins P. *Black Feminist Thought: Knowledge, Consciousness, and the Politics of Empowerment.* 2nd ed. New York, NY: Routledge; 2000.

Hine, D. Rape and the inner lives of Black women in the middle west: preliminary thoughts on the culture of dissemblance. In: Ruiz VL, Du Bois EC, eds. *Unequal Sisters: A Multicultural Reader in US Women's History.* New York, NY: Routledge; 1994.

hooks B. *Black Looks: Race and Representations.* Toronto, ON: Between the Lines Press; 1992.

In Our Own Voice: National Black Women's Reproductive Justice Agenda. Black Reproductive Justice Policy Agenda. June 2021. Available at: https://blackrj.org/blackrjpolicy

Jones PR, Taylor DM, Dampeer-Moore J, et al. Health-related stereotype threat predicts health services delays among Blacks. *Race Soc Probl.* 2013;5(2):121–136. https://doi.org/10.1007/s12552-013-9088-8

Lamb S. *The Secret Lives of Girls: What Good Girls Really Do—Sex Play, Aggression, and Their Guilt.* New York, NY: Free Press; 2001.

Leath S, Jones M, Jerald MC, Perkins TR. An investigation of Jezebel stereotype awareness, gendered racial identity and sexual beliefs and behaviours among Black adult women. *Cult Health Sex.* 2022;24(4):517–532. https://doi.org/10.1080/13691058.2020.1863471

Luther C, Ringer Lepre C, Clark N. *Diversity in US Mass Media.* Hoboken, NJ: John Wiley and Sons; 2011.

Mastro D. Why the media's role in issues of race and ethnicity should be in the spotlight. *J Soc Issues.* 2015;71(1):1–16. https://doi.org/10.1111/josi.12093

Mgadmi M. Black women's identity: stereotypes, respectability and passionlessness (1890-1930). *Revue LISA.* 2009;7(1). https://doi.org/10.4000/lisa.806

Morton P. *Disfigured Images: The Historical Assault on Afro-American Women.* New York, NY: Praeger; 1991.

Moynihan DP. The Negro family: a case for national action. In: Rainwater L, Yancey WL, eds. *The Moynihan Report and the Politics of Controversy.* Cambridge, MA: MIT Press; 1967: 41–124.

Parker Dominguez T, Dunkel-Schetter C, Glynn L, Hobel C, Sandman C. Racial differences in birth outcomes: the role of general, pregnancy, and racism stress. *Health Psychol.* 2008;27:194–203. https://doi.org/10.1037/0278-6133.27.2.194

Roberts D. *Killing the Black Body.* New York, NY: Vintage Books; 2017.

Rosenthal L, Lobel M. Stereotypes of Black American women related to sexuality and motherhood. *Psychol Women Q.* 2016;40(3):414–427. https://doi.org/10.1177/0361684315627459

Steele CM, Aronson J. Stereotype threat and the intellectual test performance of African Americans. *J Pers Soc Psychol.* 1995;69(5):797–811. https://doi.org/10.1037//0022-3514.69.5.797

Stephens DP, Phillips LD. Freaks, gold diggers, divas, and dykes: the sociohistorical development of adolescent African American women's sexual scripts. *Sex Cult.* 2003;7(1):3–49. https://doi.org/10.1007/BF03159848

Villarosa L. *Body & Soul: The Black Women's Guide to Physical Health and Emotional Well-Being.* New York, NY: HarperCollins; 1994.

Walker-Barnes C. *Too Heavy a Yoke: Black Women and the Burden of Strength.* Eugene, OR: Cascade Books; 2014.

Welter B. The cult of true womanhood: 1820–1860. In: Nancy FC, ed. *Domestic Ideology and Domestic Work.* Vol. 4/1. Munich, Germany: K.G. Saur; 2012:48–71.

Wolcott V. *Remaking Respectability: African American Women in Interwar Detroit,* Chapel Hill, NC: University of North Carolina Press; 2001.

Woods-Giscombé CL. Superwoman schema: African American women's views on stress, strength, and health. *Qual Health Res.* 2010;20(5):668–683. https://doi.org/10.1177/1049732310361892

Wyatt G. *Stolen Women: Reclaiming Our Sexuality, Taking Back Our Lives.* New York, NY: Wiley; 1997.

7

Black Feminist Digital Erotic Resistance as a Harm-Reduction Strategy to Positively Impact the Sexual Health Behaviors of Black Women

Shawna G. Shipley-Gates, MA, MPH

Black women[1] have poor sexual health outcomes, such as HIV/AIDS, unplanned pregnancy, and sexual abuse, due to historical interlocking oppressions, such as gendered racism, misogynoir, and homophobia, that relegate their bodies as targets of sexual injury instead of sources of pleasure. Previous sexual health efforts have focused more on deficiency and sex risks (i.e., violence, disease, and pregnancy prevention) and less on the erotic aspects of sexual health that promote safety, liberation, and pleasure. According to Townes et al. (2021),

> Most often, research related to Black women's sexualities is focused on the prevention of sexually transmitted infections (STIs) and pregnancy [which] prevents a holistic approach to Black women's sexualities…Black sexualities have a narrow focus in the literature and lack a broad and expansive investigation of various sexual experiences that would enhance sexual health promotion efforts among and for Black women. (p. 2)

The World Health Organization (WHO) provides a definition of sexual health that includes "the possibility of having pleasurable and safe sexual experiences, free of coercion, discrimination and violence" (para. 1). In addition, the American Sexual Health Association describes a sexual health that promotes "being able to experience sexual pleasure, satisfaction, and intimacy when desired" (para. 4). However, traditional gender roles and heterosexism prevent Black women from embracing their eroticism by promoting the prioritization of their partners' pleasure (Thorpe et al. 2021, p. 2). Without negating the importance of preventing pregnancy and disease, Black women who are not prioritizing their eroticism are not holistically engaging in positive sexual health behaviors.

---

[1] According to Moya Bailey, "misogynoir is deployed because of social beliefs about Black women, and those of us who are read as Black women—despite our self-identification—get caught in the crosshairs" (Bailey 2021, p. 20). Throughout this chapter, when I refer to Black women or girls, this includes queer, cisgender, transgender, nonbinary femmes, and other minoritized genders who experience misogynoir.

While Black women have prioritized their eroticism in many ways including intimacy during slavery, Black lesbian feminist organizing, pornography, and blues music (Johnson 2020; Combahee River Collective 1979; Miller-Young 2014; Davis 1998), there has been an increase in Black feminist resistance focusing on eroticism in digital landscapes such as social media, blogs, and podcasts. Using self-naming, digital alchemy, and harm reduction, digital erotic resistance is an essential strategy to fight against sexual oppressions including homophobia, misogynoir, and controlling images to impact sexual health behaviors among Black women.

SEXUAL HEALTH ROOTED IN EROTICISM

Eroticism is broadly defined as one's desire for pleasure, but Black feminists have theorized that eroticism can be powerful in transforming Black women from hypersexualized objects to erotic subjects. Audre Lorde's (1984) foundational essay "Uses of the Erotic" describes the erotic as

> a measure between the beginnings of our sense of self and the chaos of our strongest feelings. It is an internal sense of satisfaction to which, once we have experienced it, we know we can aspire. For having experienced the fullness of this depth of feeling and recognizing its power, in honor and self-respect we can require no less of ourselves. (p. 54)

While Lorde's influential essay views the erotic as a source of power, Jennifer Nash (2018) emphasizes the sexual tone of the term as a

> tender space of sanctuary, self-imagination, intimacy and creative play, a vibrant space of collective world-making that takes the violence of the ordinary and turns it on its head, mobilizing it to unleash sexual pleasures, erotic longings and disrespectable desires. (p. 3)

In comparison to Nash who calls attention to eroticism's ability to shift from violence to pleasure, bell hooks (2015) explains that

> when black women relate to our bodies, our sexuality, in ways to place erotic recognition, desire, pleasure and fulfillment at the center of our efforts to create radical black female subjectivity, we can make new and different representations of ourselves as sexual subjects. (p. 76)

Lastly, Patricia Hill Collins argues that this shift from violence to reclamation and self-definition of Black women's eroticism is a form of resistance. Collins (2002) describes that

> when self-defined by Black women ourselves, Black women's sexualities can become an important place for resistance. Just as harnessing the power of the erotic is important for domination; reclaiming and self-defining that same eroticism may constitute one path toward Black women's empowerment. (p. 138)

As a powerful form of resistance against sexual oppression, sexual health rooted in eroticism encourages subjectivity, self-definition, and sexual empowerment.

SEXUAL OPPRESSION AMONG BLACK WOMEN

Historically, Black female sexuality has been silenced, ignored, and deemed invisible by sexual oppressions that have manifested in many forms, including sexual violence, politics of respectability, negative sexual tropes, and toxic masculinity. In *Sisters of the Yam: Black Women and Self-Recovery,* bell hooks (2014b) bluntly states that Black women have been used as "breeding machines, as receptacles for pornographic desires, [and] as 'hot pussies' to be bought and sold" (p. 90). Hooks explains how the use of Black women as sexual chattel and other sexual oppressions can cause erotic estrangement, which deters them from embracing their erotic power. According to hooks,

> their estrangement is just as intense as that of Black females who have learned from childhood on that they can protect themselves from objectification, from commodification by repressing erotic energy, and by denying any sensual or sexual dimension in themselves. (p. 87)

hooks understands the detrimental impact that sexual oppression has on the erotic power of Black women. Lorde (1984) articulates how oppression suppresses the erotic:

> The erotic is a resource within each of us that lies in a deeply female and spiritual plane, firmly rooted in the power of our unexpressed or unrecognized feeling. In order to perpetuate itself, every oppression must corrupt or distort those various sources of power within the culture of the oppressed that can provide energy for change. For women, this has meant a suppression of the erotic as a considered source of power and information within our lives. (p. 53)

Sexual oppressions including heterosexism, homophobia, hypersexual controlling images, and misogynoir have the potential to suppress Black women's erotic power.

In *Feminist Theory: From Margin to Center*, hooks argues that Black female sexuality is oppressed by heterosexism and homophobia. Specifically, she discusses how lesbian women have worked the hardest to end heterosexist oppression:

> They have shown many heterosexual women that their prejudices against lesbians support and perpetuate compulsory heterosexuality. They have also shown women that we can find emotional and mutual sexual fulfillment in relationships with one another. Some lesbians have suggested that homosexuality may be the most direct expression of pro-sex politics, since it is unconnected to procreation. Feminist movement to end sexual oppression is linked to lesbian liberation. The struggle to end prejudice, exploitation, and oppression of lesbians…is a crucial feminist agenda. It is a necessary component of the movement to end female sexual oppression. Affirming lesbianism, women of varied sexual preferences resist the perpetuation of compulsory heterosexuality. (hooks 2014a, pp. 152-153)

Black feminist critic Barbara Smith (1983/2000) reiterates hooks's urgent call for a Black feminist movement that aims to eliminate sexual oppression among Black women of all sexual preferences, especially lesbian women who suffer from heterosexism.

Black women's sexual oppression also manifests in hypersexual controlling images. In *Black Feminist Thought: Knowledge, Consciousness, and the Politics of Empowerment*, Patricia Hill Collins (2002) describes controlling images as when "racist and sexist ideologies permeate the social structure to such a degree that they become hegemonic, namely, seen as natural, normal, and inevitable…[and] certain assumed qualities that are attached to Black women are used to justify oppression" (p. 7). Collins discusses how controlling images of the Jezebel and "hoochie" portray Black women as sexually deviant:

> Her insatiable sexual desire helps define the boundaries of normal sexuality…On this border, the hoochie participates in a cluster of 'deviant female sexualities,' some associated with the materialistic ambitions where she sells sex for money, others associated with so-called deviant sexual practices such as sleeping with other women, and still others attached to 'freaky' sexual practices such as engaging in oral and anal sex. (p. 92)

Due to these promiscuous labels, hooks (2015) argues in *Black Looks: Race and Representation* that

> the vast majority of Black women in the United States, more concerned with projecting images of respectability than with the idea of female sexual agency and transgression, do not often feel we have the 'freedom' to act in rebellious ways in regards to sexuality without being punished. (p. 160)

According to Collins and hooks, Black women are reluctant to represent their erotic power in fear of being called Jezebels, hoochies, and other sexually controlling images.

Black female eroticism is also oppressed by hypersexual, controlling images in digital spaces. Safiya Umoja Noble (2018), author of *Algorithms of Oppression: How Search Engines Reinforce Racism*, explores sexual oppressions as "algorithmically data failures that are specific to people of color and women and to underscore the structural ways that racism and sexism are fundamental" (p. 25). Noble shares her story about searching for fun activities for "Black girls" on the Google search engine and being met with an overwhelming amount of pornography. She decided to research how "'hot,' 'sugary,' or any other kind of 'black pussy' can surface as the primary representation of Black girls and women on the first page of a Google search" (p. 25). Such representations are "dehumanizing them as commodities, as products and as objects of sexual gratification" (p. 18). Noble's work focuses on how these pornographic representations perpetuate the adultification, commodification, and objectification of Black girls and women online.

Another example of digital sexual oppression targeting Black women is "Hotep Twitter." Feminista Jones (2019), author of *Reclaiming Our Space: How Black Feminists Are Changing the World From the Tweets to the Streets*, defines Hotep Twitter as a group of people within the Black Twitter community who focus on sharing their so-called Pan-Africanism that maintains that "Africans across the diaspora are supreme, regal, originators of everything, and are all descendants of kings and queens with Egyptian hieroglyphs encoded into their DNA" (p. 106). Despite its affirmed Blackness, Hotep Twitter is antifeminist, "violently anti-LGBTQ, and their queerphobia and transmisogyny is antithetical to Black liberation" (p. 107).

For example, Jones points out that the three founders of the Black Lives Matter movement identify with the lesbian, gay, bisexual, transgender, and queer or questioning (LGBTQ) community and "once a person is known to identify as queer, their whole life is picked apart and whatever good they do or whatever important ideas they share are subjected to microscopic criticism simply because they exist openly as a nonheterosexual or transgender person" (p. 107). Hotep Twitter's blatant misogyny and homophobia sexually oppresses Black women's sexuality and erotic liberation.

Misogyny against Black women in digital landscapes is an oppression that exists beyond Hotep Twitter. In her book, *Misogynoir Transformed: Black Women's Digital Resistance*, Moya Bailey (2021) discusses her coined term misogynoir—or anti-Black misogyny—particularly in relation to the digital presence of queer and transgender Black women. Bailey explains that misogynoir is "a portmanteau of 'misogyny,' the hatred of women, and 'noir,' the French word for 'black,' which also carries a specific meaning in film and other media" (p. 1). She delves deeper into the definition of misogynoir:

> Misogynoir is not simply the racism that Black women encounter, nor is it the misogyny Black women negotiate. Misogynoir describes the uniquely co-constitutive racialized and sexist violence that befalls Black women as a result of their simultaneous and interlocking oppression at the intersection of racial and gender marginalization. (p. 1)

Even though misogynoir existed before digital media, its current manifestation in digital platforms, including Facebook, among others, has "transcended borders to describe an unfortunately global phenomenon…and has found a home in each of the communication advancements of the last two centuries" (p. 1). Misogynoiristic digital media perpetuates the "hegemony of 'white supremacist capitalist patriarchy' by controlling the way society views marginalized groups and how we view ourselves," especially pertaining to the eroticism of Black women (p. 11). Sexual oppressions including misogynoir, biased algorithms, controlling images, and homophobia all contribute to the suppression of Black women's eroticism.

DIGITAL EROTIC RESISTANCE AGAINST SEXUAL OPPRESSION

According to L.H. Stallings (2007), author of *Mutha' Is Half a Word: Intersections of Folklore, Vernacular, Myth, and Queerness in Black Female Culture*, it is not enough for Black cultural producers to identify and analyze sexual tropes and other oppressions forced upon Black women: "[i]nstead of disregarding work that might be considered vulgar or profane," she argues, "we should observe them for their strategies of creating radical black female sexual subjectivity and a discourse for that subjectivity" (p. 294). Bailey (2021) argues that

> [w]hile memes circulate through social media platforms such as YouTube, Facebook, Instagram, Tumblr, and others that depict Black women as more ugly, dirty, deficient, hypersexual, and unhealthy than their white or non-black women of color counterparts, Black women employ these same platforms in ways that subvert negative stereotypes through processes that can be their own health-affirming practice. (p. 11)

As a sexual health-affirming practice, digital erotic resistance is defined as the utilization of erotic cultural production in digital spaces as a form of resistance against sexual oppression.

Black women need to embrace eroticism in digital landscapes—regardless of how it is perceived—as a form of resistance against oppression to prioritize their own erotic desires and rewrite their own sexual narratives. Stallings (2007) further explains that discourses that focus on desire "lead to languages of sexual rights that Black females need to know and embrace for their own sake" (p. 293). Digital erotic resistance against sexual oppression has the potential to encourage Black women to self-define, embrace, and subjectify their sexual desires, thus improving their sexual health behaviors.

Catherine Knight Steele (2021), author of *Digital Black Feminism*, offers a significant concept relevant for digital erotic resistance called "self-naming" where Black women—who are often called out of their names—"use their rhetorical skills to name themselves, rename, and rebrand others" (p. 131). Steele (2021) explains that digital spheres "provide an opportunity to resist external naming structures and controlling images of Black women" (p. 131). Similarly, Bailey (2021) introduces an important praxis called "digital alchemy" where Black women "transform everyday digital media into valuable social justice media that recode the failed scripts that negatively impact their lives" (p. 24). Digital erotic resistance as a strategy to fight against sexual oppressions—especially misogynoir and controlling sexual scripts—to rewrite sexual narratives can be seen and used in many ways including social media, hashtags, blogs, and YouTube.

Using Evelynn Hammonds's (1994) concept of politics of articulation, Dominique Adams-Santos (2020) conducted a narrative analysis on the coming-out YouTube videos of 50 queer Black women "to understand how their social positionalities as racialized sexual minority women affect their narrative strategies on a hypervisible digital platform" (p. 1435). Adams-Santos noticed two distinct strategies for the coming-out stories: one that used normative and respectable scripts and one that countered politics of respectability using "intimate candor" (p. 1435). Adams-Santos argues that

> using intimate candor—the performative and discursive strategy of publicly revealing interior, often sexually explicit, aspects of the self—enables queer Black women to (1) center desire and queerness, (2) articulate a vision of queer Black womanhood not tethered to respectability, and (3) complicate the coming-out formula. (p. 1435)

Adams-Santos contends that politics of articulation explains the intimate candor and digital erotic presence of some queer Black women.

Feminista Jones (2019) exemplifies digital erotic resistance through her digital presence and call for a paradigm shift, "in which we stop assigning women value based on their sexual activity and we stop suggesting that there are universally accepted appropriate and consensual behaviors for anyone" (p. 79). Using #TalkLikeSex as a hashtag and as the title for her Ebony.com column, Jones reclaims the graphic and degrading song "Talk Like Sex" by hip-hop artist Kool G Rap as a way of "subverting his 'talk' about sex—and other degrading depictions of sex and sexual abuse and disregard of women in hip hop music—changing the way we, Black women, particularly those raised on hip hop culture, talk about sex" (p. 57). Jones also used Twitter hashtag #KSFem to complement her blog website "Knob-Slobbing Feminism" and encourage Black women to "feel comfortable in their enjoyment of sex and pleasing their men, and that doing so does not make one any less a feminist" (p. 71). As the Love & Sex section editor at BlogHer.com, Jones was a proud "Black face on the sex-positive movement" (p. 72) that is usually controlled by white women. Jones, Adams-Santos, and Bailey represent the importance of digital erotic resistance to subvert the erasure of Black women in both erotic and digital spaces that privilege their white counterparts.

THE IMPACT OF DIGITAL EROTIC RESISTANCE ON THE SEXUAL HEALTH OF BLACK WOMEN

With the rise of social media and other digital environments, Black women have the ability to "challenge the stereotypes that negatively impact their health and well-being" using harm-reduction efforts (Bailey 2021, p. 10). Harm-reduction is a public health strategy that assumes that harm is inevitable, "but one can reduce harm by engaging in small transformative interventions" (p. 28). As a form of harm reduction, Black women's digital erotic resistance cannot eradicate sexual oppression on its own but, rather, it "mitigates its harm through the promotion of images and narratives Black women want to see" (p. 28). Through web shows, blogs, and digital storytelling projects, digital erotic resistance is utilized to reduce the harm of sexual oppressions and provide uplifting sexual representations, thus positively impacting sexual health behaviors among Black women.

According to Bailey, Black queer women and femmes create web shows that highlight sexual pleasure, consensual nonmonogamy, and the destigmatization of STIs. For example, the web show "Skye's the Limit," created by Black queer writer and producer Blue Telusma, follows the lives of Black queer women in the District of Columbia. She defends the use of this platform for digital erotic resistance:

> Web shows both reinforce and challenge dominant ideas about sexuality. They can become a space where sexual pleasure, gender expression, and desire can be pushed beyond the limits of mainstream television. When a range of gender expressions and sexual possibilities is presented, sexual health expands to include discussions of kink, consent, and fluidity. (Bailey 2021, p. 111)

Bailey articulates that the purpose of Black women's digital resistance is not to create positive and respectable counternarratives but, rather, for Black women to be their authentic erotic selves while engaging in pleasure-based sexual health practices.

Carter et al. (2021) created the feminist digital storytelling project "Live and Love With HIV," which collects 43 stories written by 12 women living with HIV in Kenya, South Africa, Nigeria, and the United States, among other countries, to address sexual health disparities in a way that promotes pleasure rather than foregrounds disease, risk, and pathology:

> We envisioned a collection regarding sexuality and relationships that drew together stories and blog posts from around the world as well as research and guidance for women and couples living with HIV, and that was a tool that could empower and educate. Whether people were having sex or not, single or in relationship(s), wanting to learn more about sexuality, or just curious, we wanted to create a space that was safe, inclusive, and accessible to all and supported by the latest scientific evidence. (p. 86)

In the first 1.5 years of the study, researchers used feedback from a pop-up survey on the website, readers' comments on actual blog posts, and Google analytics to capture the following results:

> Our social media community grew to 1600, and our website received approximately 300 visits per month, most by women (70%) and people aged 25–44 years (65%), from more than 50 cities globally, with shifts in use and demographics over time. Qualitative data indicated the power of feminist digital storytelling for opportunity, access, validation, and healing. (p. 83)

By "regaining control of HIV narratives and asserting their right to have pleasurable, fulfilling, and safer sexual lives," this digital storytelling project demonstrates the importance of digital erotic resistance to improve sexual health disparities (p. 83).

Demetria Lucas, founder of the blog "A Belle in Brooklyn," channels digital erotic resistance that impacts sexual health among Black women by dedicating space for pleasure-based sexual health messaging. For example, Lucas wrote a blog post that simultaneously celebrated Beyoncé as a "sexual but not sexualized" icon and advertised Oraquick, an at-home HIV testing kit. Lucas took advantage of the opportunity to not only profit from the advertisement but also discuss Black women's eroticism, "promote ideals of sexual health and reverse the stigma around HIV in the Black community" (Steele 2021, p. 70). Like many Black women digital cultural producers, Lucas is "repurposing the capitalist tools of social media into tools that allow them to grow community, share resources, and even advocate for each other's safety and health" (Bailey 2021, p. 71). Lucas, Bailey, Carter and colleagues provide a gateway for further exploration regarding the impact of digital erotic resistance on the sexual health behaviors of Black women.

THE FUTURE OF DIGITAL EROTIC RESISTANCE

The future of digital erotic resistance and its impact on sexual health relies upon Black feminist theorizing, community, training, and policy change for Black women sexuality professionals. First, Black women sexuality professionals should intentionally cite Black feminist scholars who support the idea that the unique embodied experiences of Black women heavily influence their sexual health behaviors.

Second, there is a need for more well-trained Black women sexuality professionals who create digital safe spaces for different aspects of sexuality including sexual health, religion/spirituality, disability, body positivity, politics, and pleasure. Such spaces for Black women allow accessibility, anonymity, and community to facilitate pleasure-based sexual health conversations on social media platforms, online private forums, virtual workshops, and resource websites.

Third, Black women sexuality professionals would benefit from training about current and upcoming digital platforms, tools, and strategies to create timely and relevant sexual health content for Black female followers.

Lastly, digital erotic resistance requires sex-positive and antimisogynoiristic content guidelines and policies that permit provocative yet informative sexual health content by, for, and about Black women without the threat of being flagged, shadowbanned, and/or permanently deleted from digital platforms. All in all, digital erotic resistance has the potential to fight against sexual oppression, empower sexual subjectivity, and impact the sexual health behaviors of Black women.

REFERENCES

Adams-Santos, D. "Something a bit more personal": digital storytelling and intimacy among queer Black women. *Sexualities*. 2020;23(8):1434–1456. https://doi.org/10.1177/1363460720902720

American Sexual Health Association. What is sexual health? Available at: https://www.ashasexualhealth.org/sexual-health

Bailey M. *Misogynoir Transformed: Black Women's Digital Resistance*. New York, NY: New York University Press; 2021.

Carter A, Anam F, Sanchez M, et al. Radical pleasure: feminist digital storytelling by, with, and for women living with HIV. *Arch Sex Behav.* 2021;50:83–103. https://doi.org/10.1007/s10508-020-01822-8

Collins PH. *Black Feminist Thought: Knowledge, Consciousness, and the Politics of Empowerment.* New York, NY: Routledge; 2002.

Combahee River Collective. A Black feminist statement. *Off Our Backs.* 1979;9(6):6–8.

Davis AY. *Blues Legacies and Black Feminism.* New York, NY: Vintage Books; 1998.

Hammonds E. Black (w)holes and the geometry of Black female sexuality. *Differences.* 1994;6(2–3):126–145. https://doi.org/10.1215/10407391-6-2-3-126

hooks b. *Black Looks: Race and Representation.* New York, NY: Routledge; 2015.

hooks b. *Feminist Theory: From Margin to Center.* New York, NY: Routledge; 2014a.

hooks b. *Sisters of the Yam: Black Women and Self-Recovery.* New York, NY: Routledge; 2014b.

Johnson JM. *Wicked Flesh: Black Women, Intimacy, and Freedom in the Atlantic World.* Philadelphia, PA: University of Pennsylvania Press; 2020.

Jones F. *Reclaiming Our Space: How Black Feminists Are Changing the World From the Tweets to the Streets.* Boston, MA: Beacon Press; 2019.

Lorde A. Uses of the erotic: the erotic as power. In: *Sister Outsider: Essays and Speeches.* Trumansburg, NY: Crossing Press; 1984:53–59.

Miller-Young M. *A Taste for Brown Sugar: Black Women in Pornography.* Durham, NC: Duke University Press; 2014.

Nash J. Black sexualities. *Feminist Theory.* 2018;19(1):3–5. https://doi.org/10.1177/14647001177428

Noble SU. *Algorithms of Oppression: How Search Engines Reinforce Racism.* New York, NY: New York University Press; 2018.

Smith B, ed. *Home Girls: A Black Feminist Anthology.* New Brunswick, NJ: Rutgers University Press; 2000.

Stallings LH. *Mutha' Is Half a Word: Intersections of Folklore, Vernacular, Myth, and Queerness in Black Female Culture.* Columbus, OH: The Ohio State University Press; 2007.

Steele CK. *Digital Black Feminism.* New York, NY: New York University Press; 2021.

Thorpe S, Dogan JN, Townes A, Malone N, Jester JK, Hargons CN. Black women's pleasure mapping. *J Black Sex Relationships.* 2021;7(4):1–23. https://doi:10.1353/bsr.2021.0008

Townes A, Thorpe S, Parmer T, Wright B, Herbenick D. Partnered sexual behaviors, pleasure, and orgasms at last sexual encounter: findings from a US probability sample of Black women ages 18 to 92 years. *J Sex Marital Ther.* 2021;47(4):353–367. https://doi:10.1080/0092623X.2021.1878315

World Health Organization. Sexual health. Available at: https://www.who.int/health-topics/sexual_health#tab=tab_1

8

Black Women's Experiences With Infertility: Messages About Reproductive Health on the *Being Mary Jane* Television Show

DaKysha Moore, PhD, MHS, MS, and Elijah O. Onsomu, PhD, MPH, MS

There is a long history of negative stereotypes in the media of Black women and pregnancy. Some of the most common images of Black women include young single parents such as what the audience witnessed in the 2009 film *Precious*. Media representations of Black women's fertility must go beyond the female who can conceive at a young age.

One realistic image is Mary Jane Paul, the main character on *Being Mary Jane*, which aired on Black Entertainment Television (BET) from 2013 to 2019 (IMDB n.d.) and currently runs on streaming services. Mary Jane is a successful professional in the television industry who confronts her fertility issues when she turns to assisted reproductive technology, which is a much-needed discussion in the media given that statistics show Black women have high rates of infertility. The series also features the character Niecy Patterson, Mary Jane's niece, who is young and single with two young kids. In the context of Black females' reproductive health, these are two distinct portrayals. This chapter will explore images of Black women's fertility on network television and discuss the reproductive experiences of two main Black female characters in the series *Being Mary Jane*.

BLACK FEMALE FERTILITY

The United States experiences some of the highest rates of negative health outcomes associated with childbirth. Annually, approximately 700 women die due to a complication associated with pregnancy, and, compared to white women, Black women are more likely to die from a pregnancy-related cause (Centers for Disease Control and Prevention [CDC] 2022, para. 2). Black women experience other challenges related to giving birth, including infertility, defined as not being able to conceive after a year of unprotected sex. While Black women are two times as likely as white women to be infertile (Eichelberger et al. 2016; Wellons et al. 2008), this fact is not a common part of their image in the media.

BLACK FEMALE SEXUAL AND REPRODUCTIVE IMAGES IN THE MEDIA

There are multiple sexual images of Black women in the media and popular culture. Among the most discussed female stereotypes is the young, poor, hypersexual, and very fertile Black woman. The 2009 film *Precious* presents it through a Black adolescent mother struggling with two kids (Menzies and Ryalls 2020). Starring representations of Black women in popular serialized television dramas are rare. Jefferies and Jefferies (2015) assert images of Black feminist characters on *Scandal* (ABC) and *Being Mary Jane* (BET) are portrayed as sexual even when they are successful in their careers. Siebler (2019) discusses the characters' sexual and reproductive images through their relationships and experiences of an unplanned pregnancy. Both television shows address abortions, depicting Black professional women making their own choices about having a baby.

Mara Brock Akil is credited with creating *Being Mary Jane*, and Salim Akil is the executive producer. The show features a television journalist and anchor, Mary Jane Paul, played by Gabrielle Union, who is single and in her late 30s. She has a close relationship with her family, including both parents, her brothers, and nieces. During her quest for romance and love, Mary Jane discusses her desire to have a child.

We conducted a thematic analysis of series episodes to gain a perspective of the characters' interactions in the context of their reproductive health. The scenes, pertaining to reproductive health, in episode five, season two, were transcribed, which is an important phase for becoming more aware of data (Braun and Clarke 2006). Of note, "No Eggspectations," which first aired during March 2015, highlighted such reproductive issues as in vitro fertilization (IVF) and adolescent pregnancy. Conversations among Mary Jane; her mother, Helen Patterson; and her niece, Niecy, addressed egg freezing, fertility, and mothering. After identifying reproductive health dialogue and images, we grouped the content into themes. We used the thematic analysis method to develop patterns within the data and to define representations of Black women's reproductive health to the public (Braun and Clarke 2006).

The research was guided by the critical framework of Black feminist thought (Collins 1990). In discussing the oppression of Black women, Collins (2000) finds that some oppression continues from images of slavery that persist in a certain form throughout society:

> From the mammies, jezebels, and breeder women of slavery to the smiling Aunt Jemimas on pancake mix boxes, ubiquitous Black prostitutes, and ever-present welfare mothers of contemporary popular culture, negative stereotypes applied to African-American women have been fundamental to Black women's oppression. (p. 5)

Other studies also use Black feminist thought as a lens for understanding how the media frames images of Black women (Griffin 2014; Meyers 2004).

THE REALITY

The "reality" theme is based on images and conversations about Mary Jane's struggles during the IVF process. Throughout the first season, Mary Jane's reproductive health is a topic of discussion. Mary Jane has conversations with her family members and boyfriends about the possibility of having children. However, during season two's "No Eggspectations," Mary Jane is doing a segment of a live show, called "Modern Day Motherhood" and decides to show viewers the journey toward freezing her eggs for a future pregnancy. During the live follicle count, her ultrasound shows unexpected results. Her physician states, "Mary Jane, it is not what we were hoping for. They are measuring, I would say on average about six millimeters. That's far short of what I expect to see at this stage." Mary Jane becomes concerned, asking, "What are you telling me?" The physician replies, "This is abnormal, but you can always try again" (Akil et al. 2015).

The scene should not be a surprise to Black women. According to the American Pregnancy Association (2021), women in their mid-30s and 40s are still able to conceive, but their age may create problems, including a reduction in the "quantity and quality" (para. 3) of their eggs, fibroids, and other health conditions, such as diabetes, that create barriers. As portrayed in the episode, even with medical assistance, Mary Jane might not be able to produce the number of follicles anticipated for egg retrieval.

The scene represents an undiscussed reality for some Black women, and studies show Black women are having fewer children (Bogue 2010). Similar to other women from different cultures, some are waiting to become mothers because of social factors such as more education and working more (Livingston 2018). At age 38, Mary Jane may be experiencing a decline in fertility. Seifer et al. (2008) studied differences in outcomes among women who used assisted reproductive therapy and demonstrated that Black women had less success with the treatment but tended to start the process later than white women. Black women like Mary Jane, who wait until almost 40 to try to freeze their eggs, have lower rates of success than younger women.

Later in the episode and still in the physician's office, Mary Jane questions what went wrong with the procedure. The doctor suggests she might need to modify her hormone medication and/or her lifestyle (Akil et al. 2015). The message creates a health education opportunity to inform all women, especially Black women, to seek counseling about fertility preservation, IVF, and other reproductive therapies. Heyward et al. (2021) show that, compared to white women, Black women have less success in achieving pregnancy and live births after frozen embryo transfers. Even in Massachusetts, where barriers, such as insurance coverage, are fewer, Black and other minority women used infertility services less than white women (Jain and Hornstein 2005).

EMBARRASSMENT, SHAME, AND STIGMA

The second theme related to the topic of reproductive health is embarrassment. Mary Jane is uncomfortable with the public display of her reproductive health and seems ashamed about not producing quality eggs for freezing. During a conversation with her coworker Mark, she asks why he allowed her to do a segment that puts her in such a position. He assures her that the embarrassment will pass. She says, "it does not compare to being told live on air that you are broken" (Akil et al. 2015). After conducting interviews with Black women about infertility, Ceballo, Graham, and Hart (2015) found that a diagnosis could play a role in the woman's self-worth. This type of reaction is not atypical when women face the possibility of infertility. A woman might feel responsible for the couple's infertility (Fledderjohann 2012). Already feeling pressured to conceive and become a mother, Black women could feel additional stress. Missmer, Seifer, and Jain (2011) found Black women were concerned about disappointing their spouses when faced with infertility.

Mary Jane is not the only character demonstrating a sense of embarrassment. During the episode, her mother, Helen Patterson, is on the telephone discussing Mary Jane's television segment and is clearly upset about her daughter's reproductive health. She says, "She can't have babies, and now the whole damn world knows…I heard the man just now tell my baby that she is abnormal, and I have never raised my children to be abnormal" (Akil et al. 2015). Helen's reactions may surprise the television audience, yet research shows that Black women are concerned about negative reactions to their infertility struggles. Chin et al. (2015) found that Blacks were less likely to pursue help from a physician for assistance with pregnancy because of concerns about family and those in their social circles learning about their medical affairs. Missmer, Seifer, and Jain's (2011) results show Black and Asian American women, especially Chinese, were more concerned about stigma from infertility.

STEREOTYPICAL IMAGES

Although Mary Jane is not a mother, she can be viewed as acting like a matriarchal presence in her family, caring for many of her relatives both emotionally and financially. During the first episode of the series, the audience is introduced to Niecy Patterson, Mary Jane's niece. She is still an adolescent, has a son, and is pregnant with her second child. The character can be viewed as the stereotypical hyperfertile Black woman. In the season two episode "No Eggspectations," she is shown disagreeing with Cameron, the father of her first child, about their son (Akil et al. 2015). One could argue that the character also embodies the stereotypical Sapphire and Jezebel. According to West (1995), in a historical context, these stereotypes are associated with speaking, sometimes combatively, with authority (Sapphire) and sexualization (Jezebel).

In another scene in the episode, Niecy and her grandmother talk about Niecy's life trajectory—the struggles she encounters as a young Black single mother with two kids. The grandmother says she can do better for herself and tells her, "Keep your legs closed" (Akil et al. 2015). Other episodes, especially during season one, show Niecy speaking with her doctor about contraception. According to the National Partnership for Women and Families (2018), Black women are less likely to receive counseling on different options for contraception, which contributes to unintended pregnancies.

Being Mary Jane portrays two sides of Black women's reproductive health: Mary Jane, who struggles with issues of getting pregnant, and Niecy, the adolescent mother. Statistics about the latter may be more familiar to the public, but most are unaware of Black female infertility statistics, even Black women (Wiltshire et al. 2019).

Portraying Black women in this situation is important; as Taylor (2018) asserts, their stories are not prevalent in the media, and research on the experiences of Black couples who face infertility must continue. Moore and Onsomu (2021) interviewed a small group of Black female college students about infertility and social egg freezing and found the participants knew little about either. Moreover, their attitudes about Black women's fertility were mainly based on stereotypes that Black women usually get pregnant easily. Therefore, when Black women find themselves facing infertility, they may be inclined to cope in silence. Ceballo, Graham, and Hart (2015) stressed the importance of making sure the public understands that Black women can experience a diverse set of circumstances pertaining to their reproductive health, including infertility. These discussions could help to reduce their feelings of "isolation," that they are not living up to the image of Black women of being fertile or strong, and hesitancy to discuss problems trying to conceive.

Black women use assisted reproductive technology less than white women, but when given more knowledge and access to treatment, their use increases (Feinberg et al. 2006). It is imperative that Black women see images of women who look like them and struggle with infertility. Lee (2019) conducted interviews in the United States among 54 women who were described as mainly white, Black, and Asian. The findings showed participants, especially Black women, lacked awareness about infertility issues. Moreover, the women in the study felt regret about their lack of awareness and counseling on the subject. In the television episode, Mary Jane is not aware that the procedure may not happen as planned. She tries to retrieve her eggs and, while sad and embarrassed, is still more fortunate than many. A study by Missmer, Seifer, and Jain (2011) shows that social problems, such as the cost of treatment, can deter women of all backgrounds from seeking treatment.

It is important to represent the diverse set of sexual and reproductive circumstances Black women face in media and popular culture. The image of Mary Jane, a professional Black woman who tries to take control of her fertility, differs radically from a representation of a very young Black mother who needs public assistance. Studies refer to this persona as the "welfare mother" and imply she may not have wanted to get pregnant (James and Rashid 2013). According to Collins (2000), "both the matriarch and the welfare mother are sexual beings. But their sexuality is based on their fertility, and this link forms one fundamental reason they are negative images" (p. 84).

Television shows not only entertain but also inform the audience about societal and medical issues—in this case, fertility concerns. As Black women have a higher rate of infertility diagnosis compared to white women (Eichelberger et al. 2016; Wellons et al. 2008), the media might help increase awareness levels of these medical issues among Black women by showing the complexities of their reproductive health. Storylines about assisted reproductive technology and social egg freezing could act as a catalyst to get Black women who are waiting to have children for various reasons to consider their options for future children and their overall reproductive health. Infertility messages through different media outlets could help Black women become more aware of the health disparities and options to start a family. At the end of series, Mary Jane does get pregnant from the embryos she had transferred and gives birth.

In the future, researchers should continue to monitor messages about Black women's reproductive health on television shows, films, online, and through news outlets. In addition, media executives, directors, and producers could collaborate with physicians and agencies who specialize in assisted reproductive technology to help create interesting and factual storylines about Black women's health issues surrounding infertility. The messages created through the collaboration would not only educate the public about the health disparity but also reduce any stigma associated with infertility in the Black community.

REFERENCES

Akil MB, Brown N, Rivera M [writers], Akil S [director]. No Eggspectations. Transcript. *Being Mary Jane*. Akil Productions. March 3, 2015.

American Pregnancy Association. Trying to conceive after age 35. 2021. Available at: https://americanpregnancy.org/getting-pregnant/trying-to-conceive-after-age-35

Bogue DJ. Contraception, attitude-practice, and fertility differentials among US Hispanic, African American and white women. *J Popul Res*. 2010;27(4):275–292. https://doi.org/10.1007/s12546-011-9052-7

Braun V, Clarke V. Using thematic analysis in psychology. *Qual Res Psychol*. 2006;3(2):77–101. https://doi.org/10.1191/1478088706qp063oa

Ceballo R, Graham ET, Hart J. Silent and infertile: an intersectional analysis of the experiences of socioeconomically diverse African American women with infertility. *Psychol Women Q*. 2015;39(4):497–511. https://doi.org/10.1177/0361684315581169

Centers for Disease Control and Prevention. Working together to reduce Black maternal mortality. April 6, 2022. Available at: https://www.cdc.gov/healthequity/features/maternal-mortality/index.html

Chin HB, Howards PP, Kramer MR, Mertens AC, Spencer JB. Racial disparities in seeking care for help getting pregnant. *Pediatr Perinat Epidemiol.* 2015;29(5):416–425. https://doi.org/10.1111/ppe.12210

Collins PH. *Black Feminist Thought: Knowledge, Consciousness, and the Politics of Empowerment.* Boston, MA: Unwin Hyman; 1990.

Collins PH. *Black Feminist Thought: Knowledge, Consciousness, and the Politics of Empowerment.* 2nd ed. New York, NY: Routledge; 2000.

Eichelberger KY, Doll K, Ekpo GE, Zerden ML. Black Lives Matter: claiming a space for evidence-based outrage in obstetrics and gynecology. *Am J Public Health.* 2016;106(10): 1771–1772. https://doi.org/10.2105/AJPH.2016.303313

Feinberg EC, Larsen FW, Catherino WH, Zhang J, Armstrong AY. Comparison of assisted reproductive technology utilization and outcomes between Caucasian and African American patients in an equal-access-to-care setting. *Fertil Steril.* 2006;85(4):888–894. https://doi.org/10.1016/j.fertnstert.2005.10.028

Fledderjohann JJ. "Zero is not good for me": implications of infertility in Ghana. *Hum Reprod.* 2012;27(5):1383–1390. https://doi.org/10.1093/humrep/des035

Griffin RA. Pushing into Precious: Black women, media representation, and the glare of the white supremacist capitalist patriarchal gaze. *Crit Stud Media Commun.* 2014;31(3):182–197. https://doi.org/10.1080/15295036.2013.849354

Heyward Q, Walter JR, Alur-Gupta S, et al. Racial disparities in frozen embryo transfer success. *J Assist Reprod Genet.* 2021;38(12):3069–3075. https://doi.org/10.1007/s10815-021-02348-1

IMDB. *Being Mary Jane*: episode list. Available at: https://www.imdb.com/title/tt2345481/episodes?-season=1&ref_=ttep_ep_sn_pv

Jain T, Hornstein MD. Disparities in access to infertility services in a state with mandated insurance coverage. *Fertil Steril.* 2005;84(1):221–223. https://doi.org/10.1016/j.fertnstert.2005.01.118

James EA, Rashid M. "Welfare queens" and "teen moms": how the social construction of fertile women impacts unintended pregnancy prevention policy in the United States. *Policy Polit Nurs Pract.* 2013;14(3–4):125–132. https://doi.org/10.1177/1527154413510408

Jefferies D, Jefferies R. Mentoring and mothering Black femininity in the Academy: an exploration of body, voice and image through Black female characters. *West J Black Stud.* 2015;39(2): 125–133.

Lee M. I wish I had known sooner: stratified reproduction as a consequence of disparities in infertility awareness, diagnosis, and management. *Women Health.* 2019;59(10):1185–1198. https://doi.org/10.1080/03630242.2019.1593283

Livingston G. They're waiting longer, but US women today more likely to have children than a decade ago. Pew Research Center. April 20, 2018. Available at: https://www.pewresearch.org/social-trends/2018/01/18/theyre-waiting-longer-but-u-s-women-today-more-likely-to-have-children-than-a-decade-ago

Menzies AL, Ryalls ED. Depicting Black women, the politics of respectability, and HIV in *Precious. Howard J Commun.* 2020;31(5):481–492. https://doi.org/10.1080/10646175.2019.1707134

Meyers M. African American women and violence: gender, race, and class in the news. *Crit Stud Media Commun.* 2004;21(2):95–118. https://doi.org/10.1080/07393180410001688029

Missmer SA, Seifer DB, Jain T. Cultural factors contributing to health care disparities among patients with infertility in Midwestern United States. *Fertil Steril.* 2011;95(6):1943–1949. https://doi.org/10.1016/j.fertnstert.2011.02.039

Moore D, Onsomu EO. Waiting to conceive: young Black women discuss media messages about infertility and egg freezing. *J Mother Stud.* 2021;6. Available at: https://jourms.wordpress.com/dakysha-moore-elijah-o-onsomu

National Partnership for Women and Families. Black women's maternal health: a multifaceted approach to addressing persistent and dire health disparities. April 2018. Available at: https://www.nationalpartnership.org/our-work/resources/health-care/maternity/black-womens-maternal-health-issue-brief.pdf

Seifer DB, Frazier LM, Grainger DA. Disparity in assisted reproductive technologies outcomes in Black women compared with white women. *Fertil Steril.* 2008;90(5):1701–1710. https://doi.org/10.1016/j.fertnstert.2007.08.024

Siebler K. Black feminists in serialized dramas: the gender/sex/sexuality/race politics of *Being Mary Jane* and *Scandal. J Popular Film Television* 2019;47(3):152–162. https://doi.org/10.1080/01956051.2018.1540395

Taylor LC. The experience of infertility among African American couples. *J Afr Am Stud.* 2018;22:357–372. https://doi.org/10.1007/s12111-018-9416-6

Wellons MF, Lewis CE, Schwartz SM, et al. Racial differences in self-reported infertility and risk factors for infertility in a cohort of Black and white women: The CARDIA Women's Study. *Fertil Steril.* 2008;90(5):1640–1648. https://doi.org/10.1016/j.fertnstert.2007.09.056

West CM. Mammy, Sapphire, and Jezebel: historical images of Black women and their implications for psychotherapy. *Psychother Theory Res Pract Training.* 1995;32(3):458–466. https://doi.org/10.1037/0033-3204.32.3.458

Wiltshire A, Brayboy LM, Phillips K, Matthews R, Yan F, McCarthy-Keith D. Infertility knowledge and treatment beliefs among African American women in an urban community. *Contracept Reprod Med.* 2019;4:16. https://doi.org/10.1186/s40834-019-0097-x

Appendix II: From the Archives

- Collins PH. The social construction of Black feminist thought. *Signs.* 1989;14(4): 745–773.

Patricia Hill Collins's classic text provides a lens into the experiences of Black women and the ways in which they interact with society. In this article, the author challenges matrices of oppression pertaining to race, class, and gender and confronts the structures causing oppression.

- Walker A. *In Search of Our Mothers' Gardens: Womanist Prose.* Boston, MA: Houghton Mifflin Harcourt; 2004:401–409.

Alice Walker coined the term "womanism" in her collection of essays first published in 1983. At the beginning of her book, she gives a definition of this "feminist, Afrocentric, healing, embodied, and spiritual" concept:

> **Womanist.** A black feminist or feminist of color…A woman who loves other women, sexually and/or nonsexually. Appreciates and prefers women's culture, women's emotional flexibility (values tears as natural counterbalance of laughter), and women's strength. Sometimes loves individual men, sexually and/or nonsexually. Committed to survival and wholeness of entire people, male and female. Not a separatist, except periodically, for health. Loves music. Loves dance. Loves the moon. Loves the Spirit. Loves love and food and roundness. Loves struggle. *Loves* the Folk. Loves herself. *Regardless.* Womanist is to feminist as purple to lavender.

- Douglas KB. *Sexuality and the Black Church: A Womanist Perspective.* Maryknoll, NY: Orbis Books; 1999.

This book tackles the taboo subject of sexuality in the Black church, a topic it has long avoided. Kelly Brown Douglas argues that this view of Black sexuality has frustrated healthy female/male relationships, interfered with constructive responses to the AIDS crisis and teenage pregnancies, fostered intolerance of sexual diversity, and rendered Black and womanist theologians silent on sexual issues.

- **Wyatt GE.** *Stolen Women: Reclaiming Our Sexuality, Taking Back Our Lives.* **New York, NY: Wiley; 1997.**

Gail Wyatt's groundbreaking research illuminates the intersections of race, gender, ethnicity, and religion as it relates to Black women's expression of sexuality. The book provides an in-depth analysis of the sexual experiences of African American women through a discussion of sociohistorical influences, dating back to Africa, the middle passage through slavery, Jim Crow segregation, institutionalized racism, and the resulting internalized racism and sexism.

III. REVOLUTIONIZING JUSTICE, ACTIVISM, AND POLICY: CREATING MOVEMENTS OF TRUE LIBERATION

9

Using Justice-Oriented Frameworks to Understand Black Women's Reproductive Health

Dawn Godbolt, PhD, MS, and Hena Wadhwa, PhD, MS, MA

In the United States, three critical concepts are embedded in the timeline of the nation's history and are responsible for the reproductive health inequities experienced by Black women, femmes, girls, and gender-expansive birthing people[1]: first, racism, bias, and discrimination are engrained in public policy and the health care system; second, the states have a vested economic interest in the reproductive health of Black birthing people; and, third, the persistent violation of reproductive freedom is a key policy tactic for oppression.

The United States is experiencing an ongoing maternal health crisis that disproportionately impacts Black birthing people. In comparison to white women, Black women are more likely to die from pregnancy-related complications, more likely to die from preventable causes, and more likely to experience severe maternal morbidity (Centers for Disease Control and Prevention 2019; Creanga et al. 2017). Black women are also more likely to experience preeclampsia, postpartum hemorrhage, placental eruption, and many other maternal health complications. The onset of these conditions tends to present earlier and with more severity for Black women in comparison to white women (Howell 2018).

There are a number of underlying and interlocking nonclinical factors that influence maternal health outcomes, including social and structural determinants of health and barriers to the full range of reproductive health care including contraception and abortion that are created by policy (Hayes, Sufrin, and Perritt 2020; Thompson and Seymour, 2017). Hundreds of years of harmful policy decisions have resulted in social conditions that obstruct reproductive freedom and ultimately result in poor reproductive health outcomes (Taylor 2020).

Efforts to equitably and holistically address these adverse outcomes requires the utilization of justice-oriented frameworks that can contribute to large-scale social

---

[1] We use gender-neutral language such as "birthing people" and "pregnant people" to be inclusive and affirming across all gender identities. We also use the term "women" throughout this chapter but recognize that people of many gender identities—transgender, nonbinary, and cisgender alike—need and receive maternity care.

change that contributes toward longer-term systemic change and, ultimately, self-determination. This chapter begins with a brief overview of justice-oriented reproductive frameworks, followed by an examination of how systemic racism impacts reproductive health for Black people and how policymaking impacts maternal health outcomes. We make the case that justice-oriented frameworks are the appropriate tools for addressing America's Black maternal health crisis and can be used to build comprehensive policy solutions as demonstrated by the Black Maternal Health Momnibus Act of 2021.

HISTORY OF JUSTICE-ORIENTED REPRODUCTIVE HEALTH FRAMEWORKS

In 1989, the Supreme Court upheld *Webster v. Reproductive Health Services*, weakening access to reproductive rights protected by *Roe v. Wade* (Webster 1989; Roe 1973). This ruling, coupled with a lack of policies aimed at improving health and well-being, added to the historical legacy of reproductive oppression of Black women. In response, Black women policymakers and advocacy leaders developed a call to action for the reproductive freedom of Black women. The collective statement, "We Remember," articulates a protest against the history of racism, slavery, and control that Black women have been subjected to in the United States (National Council of Negro Women 1989). The document consists of 11 key points that define the core principles of reproductive freedom, including the rights to access high-quality, safe, comprehensive reproductive health services and the freedom to make reproductive health choices.

Building on the foundation of reproductive freedom, in 1994, a group of Black women met and determined that the Women's Rights Movement did not represent the needs of Black, Indigenous, and transgender people, nor did it allow space for Black women's leadership in the development of agenda priorities. The Reproductive Justice Movement was developed to steer policy conversations toward the comprehensive reproductive health needs of Black women. Reproductive justice is defined as "the human right to maintain personal bodily autonomy, have children, not have children, and parent children in safe and sustainable communities" (Julian et al. 2020; Ross and Solinger 2017; SisterSong 2022). The cross-disciplinary framework identifies how socio-political systems play a role in restricting Black women's reproductive autonomy.

In a parallel framework, *birth justice* focuses on expanding Black women's reproductive rights throughout the course of a pregnancy into the postpartum period (Southern Birth Justice Network 2020). Birth justice focuses on empowerment of birthing people in response to the medicalization of the birthing process, which decenters autonomy and choice in favor of institutional practice and policy. Obstetric violence coupled with medical racism, the eradication of granny midwives, and the use of coercion in medical decision-making has had a detrimental impact on the experiences and outcomes of Black birthing people and includes experiences of harm, discrimination, disrespect, and a lack of gained consent before procedures (Mena-Tudela et al. 2020; Scott, Britton, and McLemore 2019). Birth justice draws on the long history of holistic and culturally appropriate, person-centered care models led by midwives and doulas. Birth justice promotes self-advocacy and is predicated on the belief that Black communities are stronger when Black women are given the freedom to make their own decisions across the entire spectrum of birth outcomes.

RACISM IN THE HEALTH CARE SYSTEM

The health care system is built on a web of oppression with intersecting axes of structural and interpersonal racism, classism, and genderism. These dimensions influence access to care, quality of care, and patient-physician interactions. For example, 75% of Black women give birth at hospitals that serve predominantly Black populations, which are underresourced, underfunded, and understaffed in comparison to hospitals that serve predominantly white populations. These hospitals have higher rates of maternal health complications and perform worse on 12 of 15 outcome measures including nonelective cesarean births and mortality (Howell et al. 2016). However, there is no standardized data-collection process, and quality improvement initiatives need to be expanded.

In maternity care settings, Black birthing people are harmed by obstetric racism, defined as the phenomenon by which Black birthing people are mistreated, neglected, and harmed by both clinical and nonclinical factors, and it is a direct threat to birth outcomes (Davis 2019). Explicit and implicit bias operate at both the conscious and subconscious levels and influence medical decision-making, treatment course, and the physician-patient relationship (Agrawal and Enekwechi 2020; Hardeman, Karbeah, and Kozhimannil 2020). This history of racism within health care has led to a legacy of mistrust between Black birthing communities and the medical system and, ultimately, impeded reproductive health and well-being.

There is also a severe lack of Black perinatal birth workers. During a time when health care was highly segregated, granny midwives served Black women as their main source of care. However, the erasure of the granny midwives in the early part of the 20th century due to the medicalization of childbirth nearly destroyed the long traditions of midwifery care in Black communities (Luke 2018). Culturally concordant care is associated with better maternal and infant health outcomes for Black people, and the lack of Black birth workers results in a lack of culturally concordant care (Hardeman, Karbeah, and Kozhimannil 2020). Black birthing people are also more likely than their white counterparts to live in maternity care deserts, defined as counties where access to maternity care services is limited or absent, which impedes access to adequate care (Noursi, Saluja, and Richey 2021; March of Dimes 2020). Community-based organizations attempt to fill gaps in the health care system, but they are underresourced due to inequities in funding (Dorsey et al. 2020).

A HISTORICAL ANALYSIS OF REPRODUCTIVE OPPRESSION THROUGH POLICYMAKING

From its inception, policy in the United States has been used to control the reproductive health and well-being of Black women. In 1662, legal doctrine established "*partus sequitur ventrem*," which deemed that children born to enslaved women assumed the legal status of their mothers (Brown et al. 2021). This law was established to expand the population of slaves during the colonial period. During the period of American slavery, the reproductive health outcomes of Black women were critical to sustaining the capitalist economic system. Once laws prohibited the importation of slaves to the United States, enslaved Black children were forced to mate upon the onset of menarche as they were valued for their procreant potential (Brown et al. 2021; Nelson 2007; Deyle 2005).

In the early part of the 20th century, governmental eugenics programs were developed with the goal to control the reproduction of women of color and low-income women as they were frequently deemed socially undesirable or unfit. Approximately 60,000 forced sterilizations were performed in government-based organizations across seven decades with race, ethnicity, and socioeconomic status as key factors for determination of sterilization (Brown et al. 2021). In particular, Indigenous women were targeted for sterilization as a government-sponsored effort to reduce populations within this community, and Black women were given unnecessary hysterectomies (Fofana 2021). State-sanctioned eugenics programs continued until 2003, when the California prison system came under investigation for its forced sterilization program (Schaffner 2019; Cohn 2020).

Throughout the period of Jim Crow and the post–Civil Rights Era, Black women continued to experience reproductive oppression due to racism in policymaking. In the 1930s, the Home Owners' Loan Corporation, a government-sanctioned program, was developed to fuel the segregation of neighborhoods and the systematic divestment of Black communities in favor of white neighborhoods (Mendez, Hogan, and Culhane 2011). This process held great implications for access to education, employment opportunities, and the accumulation of intergenerational wealth through home ownership. Redlining is understood to be a key influencer of health inequities as the policy maintains barriers to accessing high-quality health care and is associated with poor infant and maternal health outcomes including preterm birth and low birth weight (Mehra, Boyd, and Ickovics 2017).

The economic disenfranchisement of Black people has implications for health care access: Black people are more likely to be uninsured or underinsured than white people and disproportionately rely on Medicaid (Garfield, Damico, and Orgera 2020; Snowden and Graaf 2019). In 1973, the Supreme Court ruled in the landmark case, *Roe v. Wade*, 410 US 113, that access to abortion care was a constitutional right; however, the Hyde Amendment, passed in 1976, restricted the use of Medicaid funds for abortion care, leaving low-income people without access to a critical component of health care. Furthermore, the failure to expand Medicaid across the entire country led to Black women disproportionately falling into insurance coverage gaps and the defunding of Title X programs, which undermines sustainable family planning (Taylor 2020). Many states have also failed to extend Medicaid postpartum coverage from the typical 60 days to at least one year postpartum, per clinical guidelines (American College of Obstetricians and Gynecologists 2018).

In 2021, states across the country enacted more than 100 abortion restrictions in a concerted effort to restrict reproductive autonomy (Nash 2021). Abortion restrictions are associated with poor reproductive health outcomes, undermine reproductive autonomy, and disproportionately harm Black women (National Partnership for Women and Families 2019; Thompson and Seymour 2017). In *Dobbs v. Jackson Women's Health Organization*, the Supreme Court deliberated the constitutionality of *Roe v. Wade*. This decision effectively, once again, simultaneously stripped Americans of their reproductive autonomy and codified discrimination into the law of the land (Dobbs 2022; Roe 1973).

APPLYING JUSTICE-ORIENTED FRAMEWORKS TO HEALTH CARE POLICY

In response to the ongoing Black maternal health crisis, the Black Maternal Health Caucus, led by Rep. Lauren Underwood (D-IL) and Rep. Alma S. Adams (D-NC), re-introduced the Black Maternal Health Momnibus Act of 2021. This set of 12 bills incorporates a justice-oriented framework in efforts to provide a broad range of policy solutions to address reproductive health, and, more specifically, maternal and infant health inequities faced by Black birthing people. The application of a justice-oriented framework to the Momnibus Act provides a mechanism to connect the various clinical and nonclinical factors that impact health with policy solutions. This comprehensive approach links many factors, including racism, social determinants of health, and gaps in research and funding to meet the key tenets of justice-oriented frameworks. This section pulls out six key concepts that embody justice-oriented frameworks from the Momnibus that demonstrate the importance of an expansive approach to addressing a complex public health crisis.

Concept 1: Public Policy Must Address Systemic Racism at the Structural and Interpersonal Levels to Improve Black Maternal Health Outcomes

A growing body of research demonstrates that structural and interpersonal racism have a particularly harmful impact on maternal health outcomes (Julian et al. 2020; Thompson et al. 2022). The Momnibus recognizes that racism is a contributing factor to the Black maternal health crisis and seeks to address it directly by providing a number of antiracism solutions:

- S. 1042/H.R. 1212 (117th Cong. [2021–2022]), the **Kira Johnson Act**, sponsored by Sen. Raphael G. Warnock (D-GA) and Rep. Alma S. Adams (D-NC), supports bias and racism training and the establishment of Respectful Maternity Care Compliance programs. These programs are designed to address racism and bias and to promote accountability mechanisms within the maternal health space.

Concept 2: Systems and Structures of Disadvantage Must Be Alleviated to Reduce Inequities in Maternal Health

A growing body of research demonstrates that exposure to adverse social risk factors, including hazardous living environments, a lack of nutritious and affordable food, and unreliable transportation, all have harmful impacts on reproductive health outcomes (Prather et al. 2018; Jones 2002). The Momnibus considers the structured disadvantage of underserved Black communities and proposes a range of efforts aimed at improving the conditions in which pregnant and postpartum people exist:

- S. 851/H.R. 943 (117th Cong. [2021–2022]), the **Social Determinants for Moms Act**, sponsored by Sen. Richard Blumenthal (D-CT) and Rep. Lucy McBath (D-GA), establishes a federal taskforce dedicated to addressing social determinants of health for pregnant and postpartum people. It also addresses inequitable access to healthy and nutritious foods by funding and expanding programs that deliver essentials like nutritious food, infant formula, clean water, and diapers to pregnant and postpartum people who live in underserved areas. The bill reaches across cabinets, including Health and Human Services (HHS), Housing and Urban Development, and the Department of Transportation, as well as programs like the Supplemental Nutrition Assistance Program and the Special Supplemental Nutrition Program for Women, Infants, and Children.
- S. 484/H.R. 909 (117th Cong. [2021–2022]), the **Moms Matter Act**, sponsored by Sen. Kirsten E. Gillibrand (D-NY) and Rep. Lisa Blunt Rochester (D-DE) is designed to support moms with mental health conditions and substance use disorder by awarding grants from HHS and the Substance Abuse and Mental Health Services Agency.

The bill invests in community-based programs that provide mental and behavioral health support through collaborative and group care models, suicide prevention programs, and destigmatization campaigns.

- S. 334 (117th Cong. [2021–2022]), the **IMPACT to Save Moms Act,** sponsored by Sen. Robert P. Casey Jr. (D-PA), establishes a new Centers for Medicare and Medicaid Services demonstration project, which includes diverse stakeholders, designed to promote equity and improve maternal health outcomes among birthing people covered by Medicaid. The bill ensures continuity of coverage by developing strategies that increase and maintain health insurance coverage through Medicaid and the Children's Health Insurance Program while also removing barriers to insurance access.

Concept 3: The Maternal Health Field Needs More Perinatal Birth Workers and More Black Birth Workers

There are a number of barriers to maternity care training pathways. The credentialing process is often expensive and time-consuming and has application processes and curriculums steeped in bias. As a result, Black people are underrepresented in maternity care settings. The Momnibus addresses this shortage by providing a range of investments in the perinatal workforce:

- S. 287/H.R. 6164, the **Perinatal Workforce Act**, sponsored by Sen. Tammy Baldwin (D-WI) and Rep. Gwen Moore (D-WI), requires HHS to provide guidance on the growth and diversification of maternity care teams. It facilitates the study of entryway barriers to maternity care professions and provides funding to establish and support programs that will grow and diversify the perinatal workforce. It also supports the incorporation of midwifery practice, doula care, lactation consultants, and other community health workers into maternity care teams.

Concept 4: Community-Based Organizations Must Have the Proper Support to Fill Gaps in the Health Care System and the Social Safety Net

Community-based organizations provide holistic, person-centered care that addresses systemic racism and structural disadvantage. They offer enhanced care models, wraparound services, and increased access to midwives, doulas, and other perinatal birth workers. However, these organizations are historically underfunded and underresourced. The Momnibus provides supports to community-based organizations through

- S. 1042/H.R. 1212 (117th Cong. [2021–2022]), the **Kira Johnson Act**, sponsored by Sen. Raphael G. Warnock (D-GA) and Rep. Alma S. Adams (D-NC), mandates HHS to provide funding to community-based organizations to support addressing social determinants of health and mental health and substance use disorder, and supports expansion of midwifery practices and other perinatal health workers into maternity care teams.

Concept 5: Equitable Maternal Health Requires Innovation in Quality Improvement and Standardized Data-Collection Processes Disaggregated by Race and Ethnicity

The health care delivery system provides a lower quality of care to Black birthing people and there is no standardized data collection process that disaggregates mortality, morbidity, or patient satisfaction by race and ethnicity. Quality-improvement initiatives, robust data collection processes, and the leveraging of technology are key drivers of health equity and an accountability mechanism for reproductive justice. The Momnibus addresses the lack of standardized data collection and the need for innovative quality improvement measures by proposing several initiatives that leverage the use of data and technology:

- S. 347/H.R. 925 (117th Cong. [2021–2022]), the **Data to Save Moms Act**, sponsored by Sen. Tina Smith (D-MN) and Rep. Sharice Davids (D-KS), conducts a comprehensive review of maternal health data-collection processes and quality measures. It incorporates community members and the lived experiences of birthing people into Maternal Mortality Review Committees and evaluates the incorporation of culturally appropriate maternity care into maternity care models.
- S. 893/H.R. 937 (117th Cong. [2021–2022]), the **Tech to Save Moms Act**, sponsored by Sen. Robert Menendez (D-NJ) and Rep. Eddie Bernice Johnson (D-TX) requires the Centers for Medicare and Medicaid Services to consider the integration of telehealth services in maternal health. The bill also provides funding from HHS for technology that enables collaborative learning models that build capacity around a number of issues, including safety and quality improvement and the use of remote monitoring tools to monitor common complications during the perinatal period. It also establishes a grant to promote tools that address racial and ethnic disparities and studies bias in the use of new technologies in maternity innovations.

Concept 6: Solutions to the Black Maternal Health Crisis Must De-silo Overlapping Social Issues

Solutions to the Black maternal health crisis must address overlapping social issues to be impactful. The Momnibus addresses these overlapping social issues in a variety of ways, such as recognizing that incarcerated mothers deserve dignity and respect during the birthing process and that veteran moms deserve special consideration from Veterans Affairs. It also considers the impact of climate change and environmental risks and promotes strategies to mitigate risks from COVID-19 and to raise vaccination rates for birthing people:

- S. 341/H.R. 948 (117th Cong. [2021–2022]), the **Justice for Incarcerated Moms Act**, sponsored by Sen. Cory A. Booker (D-NJ) and Rep. Ayanna Pressley (D-MA), commissions a study to better understand how the maternal health crisis impacts incarcerated pregnant and postpartum people, provide funding to expand maternity care teams for birthing people, and use financial incentives to end the practice of shackling pregnant people.
- S. 796/H.R. 958 (117th Cong. [2021–2022]), the **Protecting Moms Who Served Act**, sponsored by Sen. Tammy Duckworth (D-IL) and Rep. Lauren Underwood (D-IL) coordinates maternity care programs at Veterans Affairs in efforts to promote improved maternal health among veterans. The bill facilitates access to community-based resources and childbirth and parenting supports, and commissions a study on the extent of maternal mortality and morbidity among veterans.
- S. 423/H.R. 957 (117th Cong. [2021–2022]), the **Protecting Moms and Babies Against Climate Change Act**, sponsored by Sen. Edward J. Markey (D-MA) and Rep. Lauren Underwood (D-IL), centers climate change as a reproductive health issue by allocating funding from HHS for initiatives that raise awareness of climate-related risks, providing pregnant people with air conditioning units, air filtration systems, and other weather supports, as well as promoting research and the development of climate-change professionals. It also commissions the National Institutes of Health (NIH) and CDC to develop climate change research and solutions.
- S. 4769/H.R. 8027 (116th Cong. [2019–2020]), the **Maternal Health Pandemic Response Act**, sponsored by Sen. Elizabeth Warren (D-MA) and Rep. Lauren Underwood (D-IL), advances research on maternal health during the COVID-19 pandemic, ensures a standardized data collection process disaggregated by race on the pandemic's impact, and commissions a study on public health emergency preparedness. The bill commissions HHS to standardize data collection processes and provides funding to CDC for pregnancy surveillance programs and NIH research initiatives.
- S. 345/H.R. 951 (117th Cong. [2021–2022]), the **Maternal Vaccination Act**, sponsored by Sen. Tim Kaine (D-VA) and Rep. Terri A. Sewell (D-AL), provides funding to increase vaccine awareness and vaccine rates for pregnant people. The bill requires CDC to partner with community-based stakeholders in efforts to increase vaccination rates.

CONCLUSION

For far too long, Black birthing people in the United States have experienced reproductive oppression and shouldered an undue reproductive health burden created by bad policy decisions. Over the past 300 years, the government has maintained inhumane control over the reproductive health of Black birthing people. Through the application of justice-oriented frameworks and comprehensive legislation, we can address the vestiges of racism in policymaking and health care and meaningfully improve reproductive health for Black birthing people.

REFERENCES

Agrawal S, Enekwechi A. It's time to address the role of implicit bias within health care delivery. *Health Affairs Blog.* January 15, 2020:10. https://doi.org/10.1377/forefront.20200108.34515

American College of Obstetricians and Gynecologists. ACOG redesigns postpartum care. 2018. Available at: https://www.acog.org/news/news-releases/2018/04/acog-redesigns-postpartum-care#:~:text=ACOG%20now%20recommends%20that%20postpartum,women%20with%20chronic%20medical%20conditions

Brown HL, Small MJ, Clare CA, Hill WC. Black women health inequity: the origin of perinatal health disparity. *J Natl Med Assoc.* 2021;113(1):105–113. https://doi.org/10.1016/j.jnma.2020.11.008

Centers for Disease Control and Prevention, National Center for Health Statistics. Maternal mortality. November 20, 2019. Available at: https://www.cdc.gov/nchs/maternal-mortality/index.htm

Cohn E. Belly of the beast. Presented at: the American Public Health Association's 2020 Virtual Annual Meeting and Expo; October 24–28, 2020.

Creanga AA, Syverson C, Seed K, Callaghan WM. Pregnancy-related mortality in the United States, 2011–2013. *Obstet Gynecol.* 2017;130(2):366–373. https://doi.org/10.1097/AOG.0000000000002114

Davis DA. Obstetric racism: the racial politics of pregnancy, labor, and birthing. *Med Anthropol.* 2019;38(7):560–573. https://doi.org/10.1080/01459740.2018.1549389

Deyle S. *Carry Me Back: The Domestic Slave Trade in American Life.* New York, NY: Oxford University Press; 2005.

Dobbs v Jackson, No. 19-1392, 597 US ___ (2022).

Dorsey C, Kim P, Daniels C, Sakaue L, Savage B. Overcoming the racial bias in philanthropic funding. *Stanford Social Innovation Review.* May 4, 2020. Available at: https://ssir.org/articles/entry/overcoming_the_racial_bias_in_philanthropic_funding

Fofana MO. Time and time again: the reincarnations of coerced sterilisation. *J Med Ethics.* 2022;48(11):805–809. https://doi.org/10.1136/medethics-2020-106924

Garfield R, Damico A, Orgera K. The coverage gap: uninsured poor adults in states that do not expand Medicaid. Peterson KFF-Health System Tracker. San Francisco, CA: Kaiser Family Foundation; January 2020.

Hardeman RR, Karbeah JM, Kozhimannil KB. Applying a critical race lens to relationship-centered care in pregnancy and childbirth: an antidote to structural racism. *Birth.* 2020;47(1):3–7. https://doi.org/10.1111/birt.12462

Hayes CM, Sufrin C, Perritt JB. Reproductive justice disrupted: mass incarceration as a driver of reproductive oppression. *Am J Public Health.* 2020;110(suppl 1):S21–S24. https://doi.org/10.2105/AJPH.2019.305407

Howell EA. Reducing disparities in severe maternal morbidity and mortality. *Clin Obst Gynecol.* 2018;61(2):387. https://doi.org/10.1097/GRF.0000000000000349

Howell EA, Egorova N, Balbierz A, Zeitlin J, Hebert PL. Black-white differences in severe maternal morbidity and site of care. *Am J Obstet Gynecol.* 2016;214(1):122e1–122e7. https://doi.org/10.1016/j.ajog.2015.08.019

Jones CP. Confronting institutionalized racism. *Phylon.* 2002;50(1–2):7–22.

Julian Z, Robles D, Whetstone S, et al. Community-informed models of perinatal and reproductive health services provision: a justice-centered paradigm toward equity among Black birthing communities. *Semin Perinatol.* 2020;44(5):151267. https://doi.org/10.1016/j.semperi.2020.151267

Luke JM. *Delivered by Midwives: African American Midwifery in the Twentieth-Century South.* Jackson, MS: University Press of Mississippi; 2018.

March of Dimes. Nowhere to go: maternity care deserts across the US 2020 report. 2020. Available at: https://www.marchofdimes.org/peristats/assets/s3/reports/archives/2020-Maternity-Care-Report.pdf

Mehra R, Boyd LM, Ickovics JR. Racial residential segregation and adverse birth outcomes: a systematic review and meta-analysis. *Soc Sci Med.* 2017;191:237–250. https://doi.org/10.1016/j.socscimed.2017.09.018

Mena-Tudela D, González-Chordá VM, Soriano-Vidal FJ, et al. Changes in health sciences students' perception of obstetric violence after an educational intervention. *Nurse Educ Today.* 2020;88:104364. https://doi.org/10.1016/j.nedt.2020.104364

Mendez DD, Hogan VK, Culhane J. Institutional racism and pregnancy health: using Home Mortgage Disclosure Act data to develop an index for mortgage discrimination at the community level. *Public Health Rep.* 2011;126(suppl 3):102–114. https://doi.org/10.1177/00333549111260S315

Nash E. For the first time ever, US states enacted more than 100 abortion restrictions in a single year. Guttmacher Institute. October 2021. Available at: https://www.guttmacher.org/article/2021/10/first-time-ever-us-states-enacted-more-100-abortion-restrictions-single-year

National Council of Negro Women. We remember: African American women are for reproductive freedom. Washington, DC: National Council of Negro Women; 1989.

National Partnership for Women and Families. Maternal health and abortion restrictions: how lack of access to quality care is harming Black women. October 2019. Available at: https://www.nationalpartnership.org/our-work/resources/health-care/repro/maternal-health-and-abortion.pdf

Nelson CA. American husbandry: legal norms impacting the production of (re) productivity. *Yale J L Feminism.* 2007;19:1.

Noursi S, Saluja B, Richey L. Using the ecological systems theory to understand Black/white disparities in maternal morbidity and mortality in the United States. *J Racial Ethn Health Disparities.* 2021;8(3):661–669. https://doi.org/ 10.1007/s40615-020-00825-4

Prather C, Fuller TR, Jeffries IV WL, et al. Racism, African American women, and their sexual and reproductive health: a review of historical and contemporary evidence and implications for health equity. *Health Equity.* 2018;2(1):249–259. https://doi.org/10.1089/heq.2017.0045

Roe v Wade, 410 US 113 (1973).

Ross L, Solinger R. *Reproductive Justice: An Introduction.* Oakland, CA: University of California Press; 2017.

Schaffner KJ. Reckoning with the past—eugenic sterilization in the United States. Seinan Gakuin University Academic Research Institute. Departmental bulletin paper. 2019;33(3):1–26.

Scott KA, Britton L, McLemore MR. The ethics of perinatal care for Black women: dismantling the structural racism in "mother blame" narratives. *J Perinat Neonatal Nurs.* 2019;33(2):108–115. https://doi.org/10.1097/JPN.0000000000000394

Sister Song. What is reproductive justice? 2022. Available at: https://www.sistersong.net/reproductive-justice

Southern Birth Justice Network. Birth justice bill of rights. 2020. Available at: https://southern-birthjustice.org/birth-justice

Snowden L, Graaf G. The "undeserving poor," racial bias, and Medicaid coverage of African Americans. *J Black Psychol.* 2019;45(3):130–142. https://doi.org/10.1177/0095798419844129

Taylor JK. Structural racism and maternal health among Black women. *J Law Med Ethics.* 2020;48(3):506–517. https://doi.org/ 0.1177/1073110520958875

Thompson TA, Seymour J. Evaluating priorities: measuring women's and children's health and wellbeing against abortion restrictions in the states. Cambridge, MA: Ibis Reproductive Health; 2017:1–66.

Thompson TAM, Young YY, Bass TM, et al. Racism runs through it: examining the sexual and reproductive health experience of Black women in the South: study examines the sexual and reproductive health experiences of Black women in the South. *Health Aff (Millwood).* 2022;41(2):195–202. https://doi.org/10.1377/hlthaff.2021.01422

Webster v Reproductive Health Services, 492 US 490 (1989).

10

#MeToo: Changing the Narrative for Black Women Experiencing Sexual Violence, Intimate Partner Violence, and Sexual Aggression

Camille A. Clare, MD, MPH, and Torie Comeaux Plowden, MD, MPH

Black activist Tarana Burke originated the #MeToo movement in 2006 as a platform to empower survivors of sexual violence, especially young and vulnerable women of color. The continuum of sexual violence includes attempted or completed rape, sexual coercion, unwanted contact, and noncontact unwanted experiences, such as harassment, which often intersects sex and race (Clare 2020). Intimate partner violence (IPV) is defined as violence or aggression that occurs in a close relationship between current and/or former intimate partners, and includes physical and sexual violence, stalking, and verbal and psychological aggression (Centers for Disease Control and Prevention [CDC] 2022). Reproductive coercion is a behavior that interferes with the autonomous decision-making in reproductive health, including forced abortions, pregnancy coercion, and contraception sabotage (Grace and Anderson 2018).

This chapter discusses the history of sexual violence experienced by Black women, the socio-political factors that shape how Black girls and women cope with sexual trauma, the influence of the #MeToo movement in the cultural context of the lives of Black women and girls, and the public health impact of intimate partner and gender-based violence in Black women, relative to sexual and reproductive health.

SEXUAL VIOLENCE

The context of sexual freedom and expression, autonomy, and ownership of one's body as a Black woman has been debated since they were brought to the first and second stops along the triangle trade in the 1600s as enslaved people. Several distinct historical time periods over more than 400 years characterize the experiences of sexual violence and trauma of Black women in the United States and have impacted their current reproductive and sexual health status (Prather et al. 2018).

Enslavement of Black Women (1619–1865): 246 Years

Dating back to the enslavement of Black women, sexual freedom and the presence of the Black body laid a background for repeated experiences of genital trauma by the enslaved's masters (Brown et al. 2021). Black women were sexual property and not protected from sexual assault, rape, and sexual exploitation. Since the economic worth of Black women and girls was based on their ability to procreate, they often were forcibly subjected to public displays of nudity with physical auction examinations, without consent, to determine reproductive ability. This view was a justification for the enslavement and lack of human rights of Black women.

Saartjie (Sara or Sarah) Baartman (1789-1815) was one of the first Black women known to be subjugated to human sexual trafficking. Derisively known as "Hottentot Venus," her life demonstrates the earliest reports of the existing and negative sexual fascination of white Europeans with African bodies. Born in 1789 at the Gamtoos River, now known as the Eastern Cape in South Africa, Baartman and her family were members of the Gonaquasub group of the Khoikhoi. Her parents died when she was a child, and she married as an adolescent. Her husband, with whom she had a baby that died, was murdered by Dutch colonizers. Brought to Europe seemingly on false pretenses, she was ultimately enslaved, and her body was put on display with exhibits of animals in England, Ireland, and France. She was also allowed to be sexually abused by the patrons of the exhibits at the hands of her enslaver. Baartman died at the young age of 26 (Howard 2018). However, a plaster cast was made of her body before it was dissected, and her exploitation continued.

Black Codes/Jim Crow Era (1865–1965): 100 Years

Rape, lynching, genital and reproductive mutilation of Black women and men, uncertain and unequal civil rights, continuation of stereotypes, negative media portrayals, and generational poverty were commonplace in this era (Prather et al. 2018). Nonconsensual medical experiments continued. There was poor or no health care for impoverished Black individuals. Furthermore, Jim Crow laws enforced the lack of access to quality health care services and opportunities, such as segregated hospitals and health care settings, and discriminatory practices against Black physicians, who were denied hospital privileges.

The effects of the "US Public Health Service (PHS) Study of Untreated Syphilis in the Male Negro," better known as the Tuskegee Study, on women, in addition to men, outline the repeated sexual trauma and disparate health care experiences of Black women during the Jim Crow Era. Black men were recruited to this study beginning in 1932 through 1972 by the US Public Health Service. These men, who were intentionally left untreated even after the discovery of penicillin as an effective treatment, passed syphilis to their partners, some of whom subsequently delivered children with congenital syphilis (Prather et al. 2018).

Civil Rights Era (1955–1975): 20 Years

The Civil Rights Movement arose out of the efforts of Black women to demand control over their bodies and lives, in protest of Black men being killed for protecting Black women, and in the fight for Black women's agency over their bodies and against the white supremacist acts of rape and assault (Barlow 2020). In 1944, Recy Taylor was walking home from a church meeting in Abbeville, Alabama, with two other churchgoers when she was terrorized by a group of white men in a green Chevrolet truck, taken to a secluded area, and assaulted and raped, being told to "act like you do, with your husband or I'll cut your damn throat" (as recounted by Recy Taylor in McGuire 2010).

The National Association for the Advancement of Colored People (NAACP) sent Rosa Parks to what was her father's hometown of Abbeville to investigate what happened. Her efforts resulted in the formation of the Committee for Equal Justice, which later became known as the Montgomery Improvement Association. The 1955 Montgomery bus boycott, often heralded as the opening scene of the Civil Rights Movement, was in many ways the last act of a decades-long struggle to protect Black women like Taylor from sexualized violence and rape (McGuire 2010). Parks asserted her authority and autonomy over her body as a Black woman by refusing to sit in the back of the bus. This was more than sitting in the "wrong place on the bus." Parks, as the best investigator and organizer of the NAACP, launched a movement that exposed a ritualized history of sexual assault against Black women and ignited the growing call for change (McGuire 2010).

The eugenics movement intersected at this time with more Black women being subjected to forced hysterectomies and offered more intrauterine devices compared to their white counterparts for long-term contraception. After the Jim Crow Era, there were limited educational opportunities afforded to Black women, stemming from slavery when laws prohibited them from formal education. Studies demonstrate poverty and other community-level factors such as lack of employment or low-income jobs with limited opportunities for advancement influence sexual decision-making, including survival sex for the acquisition of basic needs such as shelter and food. Black women living in poverty are more likely to have experienced childhood sexual abuse. A personal history of sexual violence can influence overall health. Reproductive coercion lowers self-esteem, leading to high stress, feelings of inferiority, and vulnerability to risky sexual behaviors (Prather et al. 2018).

Post–Civil Rights (1975–Present Day): 50+ Years

Sexualization is the practice of excessively sexualizing individuals (Moses 2020). Dr. Dionne Stephens (n.d.) explains that the experiences, narratives, formulated beliefs, and interactions of the sexuality of Black women have been based on a sociocultural context of these experiences and imagery, which are rooted in American history and culture. The social script and context of sexuality is learned and acted out in social spheres, which may change based on circumstances.

Sexuality and Black womanhood include being at greater risk for sexual violence, rape, victimization, sexual assault, and murder by intimate partners than their white counterparts. In addition, Black girls and young women are more likely to be threatened or injured with a weapon on school property and subjected to forced sexual intercourse and dating violence than their white peers (Lindsay-Dennis, Williams, and Pomeroy 2019). This includes being subjected to daily intersectional barriers of racism, sexism, misogyny, economic and educational inequalities, and threats to physical and mental well-being.

One in four Black girls are sexually abused before the age of 18 years (CDC 2022). However, Black women and girls are often less likely to report sexual violence due to historic and current unfairness in the justice system and are less likely to participate in the criminal prosecution of their perpetrators (Lindsay-Dennis, Williams, and Pomeroy 2019). The engagement of Black girls and women with the US criminal justice system (CJS) is fraught with inequalities. Many have a sense of mistrust toward law enforcement, a heightened sense of legal cynicism, and an overall negative outlook on the CJS. As such, often Black girls and women are not seen as victims of sexual offenses, but as noncompliant offenders. Within families, they are socialized to survive (Jones-DeWeever 2009). Many survivors suffer in silence for years—some for decades.

In the "three-staged model" of victim notification of the police, three elements are needed: the victim must first label the event as a crime; second, evaluate its seriousness; and finally, decide what to do (Greenberg and Ruback 1985). These steps may take on a whole other layer as a Black woman or girl when previous negative or unfair experiences with the CJS may lead to hesitation toward an already stressful process. The race and ethnicity of women and girls who are raped or sexually assaulted heavily impacts the outcome of arrest or prosecution by the police (Morabito, Williams, and Pattavina 2019). Stacey, Martin, and Brick (2017) found that white women who reported sexual assault had slightly lower rates of attrition—that is, dropping out at each stage of the CJS process—than Black women. When the victim is a Black woman, the arrest of the perpetrator is more likely when a weapon has been used or due to the race of the alleged perpetrator as opposed to a commitment to safety and justice for Black girls and women (Morabito, Williams, and Pattavina 2019).

Zero-tolerance school policies and the use of law enforcement officers to address school safety issues greatly impact these interactions (Morris 2012; Crenshaw, Ocen, and Nanda 2015). The racialized experiences of Black girls and young women in the school system demonstrates stark differences when compared to those of other groups. Black girls and young women are often victimized and criminalized in educational settings. Widely disseminated images on social media footage show Black girls as young as 5 years of age having tantrums in the classroom and subsequently being handcuffed, arrested, and detained for displaying "inappropriate behavior" or "questioning authority."

Over the past 20 years, school suspension and juvenile confinement rates have increased for Black girls, who are 5.3 times more likely than girls from any other racial group to be suspended from school (Morris 2012). In addition, Black girls are disproportionately tracked to the school-to-prison pathway according to a 2012 African American policy report (Moses 2020). This report further describes the lived experiences of Black boys and girls in this "school-to-prison pipeline" framework, which refers to the "collection of policies, practices, conditions, and prevailing consciousness that facilitate both the criminalization within educational environments and the processes by which this criminalization results in the incarceration of youth and young adults" (Morris 2012, p. 1).

These unique experiences of Black girls cannot be overlooked. When we hear about Black girls being subjected to extreme exclusionary, disciplinary actions, the assumption is that they are just "being bad" versus "good" and are from bad neighborhoods (Morris 2012). There is often no inquiry into victimization histories (Lindsay-Dennis, Williams, and Pomeroy 2019). The African American policy report notes that Black girls were the fastest growing segment of the juvenile population in secure confinement between 1985 and 1997, and, by 2010, Black girls comprised 36% of juvenile females in residential placement (Morris 2012). Actions such as these highly impact the educational completion and future economic opportunities for Black girls and young women in society.

The reproductive justice framework has arisen in the context of colonialism, slavery, and the government, which have regulated the reproductive capacity of Black women (Ross and Solinger 2017). The traditional understanding of the identity of a woman may limit the access of Black women and girls to bodily autonomy, health care services, and legal protections. Intersectionality reconceptualizes individual identity (Collins and Bilge 2020); for Black women, it is impossible to separate out these identities, making them vulnerable to sexual violence.

#MeToo MOVEMENT: ITS ORIGINS AND CONTEXT

Black activist and sexual assault survivor Tarana Burke coined the phrase #MeToo in 2006 to increase awareness of the pervasiveness of sexual violence that women and girls face in society (Wellesley Centers for Women 2019). The movement was created as a pathway toward the healing of Black girls and women and was one of the programs of Just Be, Inc., a "youth organization focused on the health, well-being and wholeness of young women of color" (Maule 2020). In October 2017, #MeToo went viral after millions of survivors of sexual assault and harassment around the world made a courageous decision to share their stories on Twitter.

Social media hashtags have been increasingly utilized for advocacy and awareness. However, it is uncertain to what extent a complete understanding of the nuanced experiences of Black women survivors of sexual assault may be captured in a hashtag (Wellesley Centers for Women 2019). According to Burke (2022), the movement was about reimagining safety, understanding bodily autonomy, and shifting culture.

While the US Congress passed a complete overhaul of the workplace sexual misconduct law in 2022, initially introduced during the rise of #MeToo, Black women and girls have seen the least amount of change. Eight decades later, Black women still need protection from sexual violence, despite the Civil Rights and #MeToo movements. The complex and intersecting roles of victimization and criminalization in the lives of Black girls and women have been mapped out in several examples in digital and social media. Black girls and young women are exposed to social injustice, racial trauma, and sexual violence through these platforms, and witnessing the violation and death of Black young people in public spaces and spheres over the past 10 years has led to the creation of other movements such as Black Lives Matter (BLM). While BLM has exposed such acts of violence as the victimization of Black girls and women in police custody, it has not addressed other forms of victimization, such as commercial sexual exploitation and sex trafficking (Lindsay-Dennis, Williams, and Pomeroy 2019).

BLACK WOMEN'S CULTURALLY SITUATED RESPONSES TO SEXUAL TRAUMA

The current framework of #MeToo has been analyzed by scholars within the historical and socio-political context in which Black women's and girls' victimization has occurred, which has not been in a vacuum. Black girls are socialized as "kin-keepers" as a self-protection strategy and in an effort to armor them against race and gender discrimination. They are taught to be strong, develop racial pride, and cope with their double-minoritized status of being Black and women.

These different socialized experiences are utilized to cope with victimization and prepare for racial and gender devaluation. For example, learning to be strong has allowed Black girls and women to withstand the vestiges of enslavement, segregation, and persistent racial and gender discrimination; however, qualities of self-reliance, independence, and caretaking also mean withholding or suppressing emotions. The psychological, educational, and social costs of suppressing emotions for some Black girls are great (Lindsay-Dennis, Williams, and Pomeroy 2019). Having a façade of strength and toughness is often perceived as being aggressive and uncooperative by law enforcement.

This is in accord with the findings of Williams, Pattavina, and Morabito (2017), who note that Black women and adolescents reporting sexual assault are more likely to be perceived as noncooperative with the police and prosecutors (Lindsay-Dennis, Williams, and Pomeroy 2019). The delay or lack of reporting of sexual violence is often with the knowledge of the harsher CJS responses to Black male suspects and perpetrators. Black male perpetrators often receive more punitive sentences than white male perpetrators for similar crimes. In the case of violence perpetrated by Black men against Black women and girls, there can be pressure not to speak up for fear of damaging the reputations of Black men by playing into oppressive stereotypes. In addition, Black women must be seen as the "ideal victim of sexual assault"—someone who fits the stereotype of hegemonic femininity—for criminal prosecution to be pursued by the US justice system (Lindsay-Dennis, Williams, and Pomeroy 2019).

Understanding the decision-making process that Black girls and women negotiate to come forward with a report of sexual assault, despite being in the #MeToo Era, requires a more comprehensive understanding of the socio-cultural experiences by Black women, who are often racialized, gendered, or othered. For every Black woman who reports rape, at least 15 Black women do not. We must respect Black girls' and women's decisions to report or not report sexual assault and create safe spaces in which they can explain their experiences in their own voices. One in five Black women are survivors of rape (Barlow 2020). Allowing for Black girls and women from diverse economic and social backgrounds to deal with their trauma in what is perceived to be socially and culturally unacceptable ways as a consequence of their structural conditions and historical experiences should be welcomed (Lindsay-Dennis, Williams, and Pomeroy 2019).

Furthermore, Lindsay-Dennis, Williams, and Pomeroy (2019) noted that supporters of the #MeToo movement should bring more attention to the challenges of Black girls and young women by including them in the dialogue about sexual violence. This movement was thought to be "silent" during #Clemency4CyntoiaBrown in which Cyntoia Brown, a Black female adolescent, was forced into human sex trafficking and sentenced to life in prison for killing a man who paid her for sex. At that time, celebrities and BLM protested the fact that Ms. Brown's rape and molestation was not discussed during her trial. She subsequently received clemency.

INTIMATE PARTNER VIOLENCE AND BLACK WOMEN

Intimate partner violence (IPV) is defined as violence or aggression that occurs in a close relationship between current and/or former intimate partners and includes physical and sexual violence, stalking, and verbal and psychological aggression (CDC 2022). Common risk factors for perpetration of IPV include (1) substance abuse; (2) growing up in a violent home/witnessing violence at an early age; (3) gendered motivations to aggressive behavior, socioeconomic norms, and conditioning; and (4) access to firearms. Demographics that place partners at risk for IPV include age, gender, socioeconomic status, race/ethnicity, acculturation, stress, and neighborhood, community, and school factors. IPV is common in both straight and same-sex relationships (Clare et al. 2021).

According to the 2010-2012 National Intimate Partner and Sexual Violence Survey, 45% of Black women experienced contact sexual violence, physical violence, and/or stalking by an intimate partner in their lifetime. Based on this same survey, approximately 41% of Black women have experienced physical violence by an intimate partner during their lifetime compared to 31% of white women, 30% of Hispanic women, and 15% of Asian or Pacific Islander women. Risk factors for recent experiences of IPV included having children, being younger, or being born in the United States (Hargrove 2018). The National Center for Victims of Crime found that 53.8% of Black women had experienced psychological abuse, and 41.2% of Black women experienced physical abuse. Black women are 2.5 times more likely to be murdered than white women, and 56% of these murders were committed by a current or former partner (The Blackburn Center 2020), usually with the use of a firearm (West 2004). Thirty-seven percent of Black women experienced reproductive coercion compared to 18% of white women.

Racial inequities are illustrated in how Black women cope with IPV. For example, Black women are more likely to have posttraumatic stress disorder, depression, anxiety, suicidality, stress, and somatic complaints (Futures Without Violence 2019; West 2004). They are also less likely to seek behavioral or physical support for injuries sustained because of IPV due to racism and discrimination and the lack of culturally responsive support systems. Black women are more likely to be convicted of killing their abusive partners than are white women. They are also more likely to be subject to mandatory arrest policies leading to "dual arrest" (Futures Without Violence 2019).

Closely aligned with IPV, reproductive coercion is associated with elevated risks for HIV and sexually transmitted infections, as well as unintended pregnancies. Low-income Black women report reproductive coercion experiences at disproportionate rates compared to women of other races, ethnicities, or socioeconomic backgrounds (Grace and Anderson 2018).

RACIAL AND GENDER-BASED SEXUAL VIOLENCE AGAINST SEX WORKERS

The trajectory of Black female bodies in sex work has been a historical site of abuse and a reclamation of autonomy. Black women's sex work from the late 19th century to the Depression Era and World War II provided an arena for Black women to exhibit economic self-reliance and individual self-respect. In applying the principles of Black feminist theory, capitalism has been used to sideline Black women's societal contributions and realities. Rejecting this notion of capitalism has elevated Black women and other marginalized groups in a similar social stratum (i.e., poor, noncisgender, nonwhite, disabled women), especially as it applied to Black sex work, which is even more apparent for Black transgender women. According to Zee Xaymaca (2022), "sex workers, Black women, and Black sex workers of all/no genders are seen as less deserving of respect because they transgress societal boundaries by choice of employment and/or by existing outside of whiteness."

There is a stigmatized narrative that because adult sex workers exchange money for consensual erotic performances or sexual services, they are not allowed to refuse or reject the sexual advances of others. Sex work has a long history of being criminalized, and, because of limited legality, workers are rarely protected from harassment and assault. By denying sex workers protections, they are less likely to report to law enforcement because of potential arrest or further assault. As a result, Black women, femmes, and gender-expansive persons are particularly vulnerable to sexual violence and assault from both clients and police (Flores et al. 2021).

Globally, immigrant and migrant (im/migrant) communities face heightened criminalization and profiling on the basis of race, gender, class, and national origin, and greater barriers to contacting authorities for protection or recourse after experiencing any form of crime, especially sex workers or victims of human trafficking. Racialized and im/migrant women, despite facing higher rates of gender-based violence, are less likely to seek redress through criminal justice systems. In Canada, for example, current literature on racialized policing suggests that the outcomes of racialized women's justice system interactions are often unsatisfactory or lead to experiences of re-victimization (McBride et al. 2022).

Black transgender women are often profiled whether or not they are actually sex workers. When we take a further look at the criminalization of sex work, we discover that Black transgender women are disproportionately criminalized and thrust into a prison system that denies them gender-affirming care. This increases the risk for further harm such as misgendering, targeted sexual assault, and prison systems denying health care and medications. Police policies, such as presence of condoms as evidence of intent to engage in sex work, perpetuates discrimination and deters many sex workers from carrying condoms, placing them at risk of contracting HIV and other sexually transmitted infections (Wurth et al. 2013). Sex workers sometimes forgo medical care out of fear of arrest or poor treatment by medical staff if it is discovered that they are a sex worker (Sawicki et al. 2019).

The National LGBTQ Task Force indicates that Black transgender people have a 26% unemployment rate, which is twice as high as the unemployment rate for transgender people of all racial and ethnic backgrounds, and four times as high as the unemployment rate in the general population (Forestiere 2020). In addition, 41% of Black transgender people have been homeless (>5 times the general population), 34% of Black transgender people have household incomes less than $10,000 (>8 times the general population), and nearly half of the Black transgender population has attempted suicide. Although these statistics apply to the Black transgender population in general and not to Black transgender women specifically, it may reasonably be assumed that Black transgender women experience these more than other transgender populations (Forestiere 2020). Because of these limited economic opportunities and high rates of poverty and homelessness, Black transgender women often resort to sex work as a means of income.

Congress has consistently failed to pass The Equality Act, a bill that would provide more sweeping protections for the entire lesbian, gay, bisexual, queer, and questioning plus (LGBTQ+) community, including requiring prisons to "house transgender individuals in facilities that match their gender identity," a protection that is currently lacking and that leaves incarcerated transgender people 13 times more likely to experience sexual assault in prison (Forestiere 2020). Black transgender women are particularly vulnerable to violence at the hands of law enforcement. Twenty-eight states have dangerous hate crime laws that do not include protections for transgender people, and several states recognize the "trans panic defense," a claim that a defendant was driven to violence due to their volatile emotional state after discovering that someone is transgender, as a valid legal defense for violence against transgender women. As a result, online lists exist, such as "Where to Move in the United States if You're Trans," which are especially pertinent to the 34% of Black transgender people who are extremely poor or the 41% of Black transgender people who have experienced homelessness (Forestiere 2020).

THE ROLE OF PUBLIC HEALTH

Social and epidemiological research focused on new models of health promotion is pivotal to the public health paradigm addressing the sexual and reproductive health of Black women. Race- and gender-specific programs must tackle this multimodal approach at the individual level (e.g., self-esteem resilience), interpersonal level (e.g., reducing stigma), community level (e.g., reducing residential segregation), and systems level (e.g., reducing unemployment), all of which are needed for long-term, sustainable efforts for the overall health of Black women (Prather et al. 2018). Public health strategies to address the crisis of sexual violence against Black women and girls include centering their voices in narratives and descriptions of their lived experiences (including those often left out, such as Black women with disabilities and LGBTQ+ Black women), becoming an educated and informed ally in obtaining knowledge about the history of colonialism and sexual violence (not only limited to the American context but throughout the world), and, finally, supporting frontline organizations that directly support, elevate, and amplify the voices of Black women in communities.

Federal policies such as the Violence Against Women Act have contributed to a revolution in the national culture around IPV and increasing protections, but we need a critical mass willing to enforce more support, resources, and protections for Black women. Health care policies that support routine screenings and readily available culturally specific counseling and referral resources can also help improve health outcomes. To have effective sexual assault services, public health entities must call out bias, discrimination, and institutionalized gendered racism. Indeed, sexualized racism and violence is a pervasive public health crisis (Barlow 2020). Furthermore, extending protections to sex workers (or completely decriminalizing sex work), enacting stronger police brutality laws (or defunding the institution of policing), and allowing incarcerated people to live in housing that matches their gender identity (or eliminating prisons entirely) are all additional steps that the law could take to keep Black transgender women, in particular, safe (Forestiere 2020).

CONCLUSION

An understanding of the deep-rooted sociocultural and historical framework of sexual violence, mechanisms shaping how Black girls and women cope, and nuances of Black survivors' lives must be realized to move us toward a culture of consent, harm reduction, and healing. Forty to sixty percent of Black women report being subjected to coercive sexual contact by age 18 (Barlow 2020). Black women should not be forgotten survivors in the fight to end sexual violence.

REFERENCES

Barlow JN. Black women, the forgotten survivors of sexual assault. American Psychological Association. 2020. Available at: https://www.apa.org/pi/about/newsletter/2020/02/black-women-sexual-assault

Blackburn Center. Black women and domestic violence. 2020. Available at: https://www.blackburncenter.org/post/2020/02/26/black-women-domestic-violence

Brown HL, Small MJ, Clare CA, Hill WC. Black women health inequity: the origin of perinatal health disparity. *J Natl Med Assoc*. 2021;113(1):105–113. https://doi.org/10.1016/j.jnma.2020.11.008

Burke T. What "Me Too" made possible. *Time Magazine*. October 18, 2022. Available at: https://time.com/6221110/tarana-burke-me-too-anniversary

Centers for Disease Control and Prevention. Preventing intimate partner violence. 2022. Available at: https://www.cdc.gov/violenceprevention/pdf/ipv/IPV-factsheet_2022.pdf

Clare CA. #MeToo in medical education. In: Coffin S, ed. *Higher Education's Looming Collapse: Using New Ways of Doing Business and Social Justice to Avoid Bankruptcy*. Lanham, MD: Rowman & Littlefield Publishers; 2020: 195.

Clare CA, Velasquez G, Mujica Martorell GM, Fernandez D, Dinh J, Montague A. Risk factors for male perpetration of intimate partner violence: a review. *Aggress Violent Behav*. 2021;56:101532. https://doi.org/10.1016/j.avb.2020.101532

Collins PH, Bilge S. *Intersectionality*. 2nd ed. Cambridge, UK: Polity Press; 2020.

Crenshaw KW, Ocen P, Nanda J. Black girls matter: pushed out, overpoliced, and underprotected. African American Policy Forum and Center for Intersectionality and Social Policy Studies. 2015. Available at: https://www.law.columbia.edu/sites/default/files/legacy/files/public_affairs/2015/february_2015/black_girls_matter_report_2.4.15.pdf

Flores AR, Meyer IH, Langton L, Herman JL. Gender identity disparities in criminal victimization: National Crime Victimization Survey, 2017-2018. *Am J Public Health*. 2021;111(4):726–729. https://doi.org/10.2105/AJPH.2020.306099

Forestiere A. America's war on Black trans women. *Harv Civ Rights-Civ Lib Law Rev*. 2020. Available at: https://harvardcrcl.org/americas-war-on-black-trans-women

Futures Without Violence. Black women's maternal health and intimate partner violence. 2019. Available at: https://www.futureswithoutviolence.org/wp-content/uploads/Black-Womens-Maternal-Health_Futures-Without-Violence_2019.pdf

Grace KT, Anderson JC. Reproductive coercion: a systematic review. *Trauma Violence Abuse*. 2018;19(4):371–390. https://doi.org/10.1177/1524838016663935

Greenberg MS, Ruback RB. A model of crime victim decision making. *Victimology*. 1985;10 (1–4):600–616.

Hargrove S. Intimate partner violence in the Black community. National Center on Violence Against Women in the Black Community. 2018. Available at: https://ujimacommunity.org/wp-content/uploads/2018/12/Intimate-Partner-Violence-IPV-v9.4.pdf

Howard M. (Sara) Saartjie Baartman (1789-1815). BlackPast. 2018. Available at: https://www.blackpast.org/global-african-history/baartman-sara-saartjie-1789-1815

Jones-DeWeever A. Black girls in New York City: untold strength & resilience. Washington DC: Institute for Women's Policy Research; 2009. Available at: https://iwpr.org/iwpr-general/black-girls-in-new-york-city-untold-strength-and-resilience

Lindsay-Dennis L, Williams LM, Pomeroy JJ. #MeToo: sexual violence, race, and Black Girls Matter. *Rejoinder*. New Brunswick, NJ: Institute for Research on Women at Rutgers University; 2019.

Maule R. Not just a movement for famous white cisgendered women: #MeToo and intersectionality. *Gend Womens Stud*. 2020;2(3):4. https://doi.org/https://doi.org/10.31532/gendwomensstud.2.3.004

McBride B, Goldenberg SM, Murphy A, et al. Protection or police harassment? Impacts of punitive policing, discrimination, and racial profiling under end-demand laws among im/migrant sex workers in Metro Vancouver. *SSM Qual Res Health*. 2022;2:100048. https://doi.org/10.1016/j.ssmqr.2022.100048

McGuire DL. *At the Dark End of the Street: Black Women Rape and Resistance—a New History of the Civil Rights Movement From Rosa Parks to the Rise of Black Power*. 1st ed. New York, NY: Alfred A. Knopf; 2010.

Morabito MS, Williams LM, Pattavina A. Decision making in sexual assault cases: replication research on sexual violence case attrition in the US: final technical report. NCJRS doc 252689. Washington, DC: US Department of Justice; 2019.

Morris, M. Race, gender, and the school-to-prison pipeline: expanding out discussion to include Black girls. African American Policy Forum. 2012. Available at: https://schottfoundation.org/wp-content/uploads/Morris-Race-Gender-and-the-School-to-Prison-Pipeline.pdf

Moses H. Oversexualization of Black girls, women must stop. *Marquette Wire*. October 20, 2020. Available at: https://marquettewire.org/4041391/featured/moses-oversexualization-of-black-girls-women-must-stop

Penn Carey Law. Prof. Dorothy Roberts traces the history of race and the regulation of Black women's bodies in chapter for the 1619 Project. March 24, 2022. Available at: https://www.law.upenn.edu/live/news/14612-prof-dorothy-roberts-traces-the-history-of-race

Prather C, Fuller TR, Jeffries WL, et al. Racism, African American women, and their sexual and reproductive health: a review of historical and contemporary evidence and implications for health equity. *Health Equity.* 2018:249–259. http://doi.org/10.1089/heq.2017.0045

Roberts DE. *Killing the Black Body: Race, Reproduction, and the Meaning of Liberty.* New York, NY: Random House/Pantheon; 1997:2776.

Ross LJ, Solinger R. *Reproductive Justice.* Oakland, CA: The Regents of the University of California, University of California Press; 2017:12-13.

Sawicki DA, Meffert BN, Read K, Heinz AJ. Culturally competent health care for sex workers: an examination of myths that stigmatize sex-work and hinder access to care. *Sex Relation Ther.* 2019;34(3):355–371. https://doi.org/10.1080/14681994.2019.1574970

Stacey M, Martin KH, Brick BT. Victim and suspect race and the police clearance of sexual assault. *Race Justice.* 2017;7(3):226–255. https://doi.org/10.1177/2153368716643137

Stephens D. Selling sexy: hip hop's commodification of Black female sexuality. Available at: https://africana.fiu.edu/people/faculty-grad-presentations/stephens_mainstream_hip_hop.pdf

Wellesley Centers for Women. Research & action midyear brief 2019. 2019. Available at: https://www.wcwonline.org/Research-Action-Midyear-Brief-2019/does-metoo-represent-black-girls-experiences-with-sexual-violence

West CM. Black women and intimate partner violence: new directions for research. *J Interpers Violence.* 2004;19(12):1487–1493. https://doi.org/10.1177/0886260504269700

Williams LM, Pattavina A, Morabito MS. Victim characteristics and case attrition: how who gets raped impacts sexual assault. Presented at: the American Society of Criminology 73rd Annual Meeting; Philadelphia, PA; November 2017.

Wurth MH, Schleifer R, McLemore M, Todrys KW, Amon JJ. Condoms as evidence of prostitution in the United States and the criminalization of sex work. *J Int AIDS Soc.* 2013;16(1):18626. https://doi.org/10.7448/IAS.16.1.18626

Xaymaca Z. Sex work as resistance to marginalization—lessons from Black feminist theory, disability justice, and Black-led sex worker organizing. *Disability Stud Q.* 2022;42(2). Available at: https://dsq-sds.org/index.php/dsq/article/view/9116/7733.

11

The Liberation Health Framework as a Strategy to Advance Birth Control Access

Kimberly A. Baker, DrPH, MPH, and Kenya Johnson, PhD, MSW

Ruby did not want any more children, but she could not convince a doctor to help her. "The only way you could get birth control in that time was for your doctor to prescribe it," she says. "And all the doctors I knew were Catholic. They sure weren't going to give us any. And we ourselves didn't know too much about birth control."…Ruby took matters into her own hands. "I'm not leaving the hospital until you do something to keep me from having babies," she told the obstetrician.

–Storming Caesar's Palace (Orleck 2005)

This opening passage chronicles a story told by Ruby Duncan, a civil rights activist who, along with other community organizers, shut down the Las Vegas Strip to demand health care and human rights for working-class Black mothers living in the state of Nevada in 1971. A central part of Mrs. Duncan's advocacy was the ability to control her own body and the decision to not bear more children. She also spoke of the desire of other women in similar circumstances that, due to the beliefs of health care providers, the beliefs of their families, state policies, and/or limited information, access to birth control was fleeting, and that would take groundswell activism to change.

It was during this same time period that the first Black woman elected to Congress, Shirley Chisolm, championed reproductive freedom for Black women with her fervent support of birth control and abortion rights despite opposition from many leaders in the Black freedom movement who felt birth control contributed to genocide within the Black community. Although not apparent, the experiences of Ruby and Shirley similarly capture the intersectionality of being Black, female, and working class in the fight for bodily autonomy in the United States. And now, some 50 years later, the historic fight and gains made toward birth control require immediate and consistent attention to ensure the protection of health and safety for Black females, especially those living in economically distressed communities and states with increasingly restrictive policies.

Policies and programs that ensure quality access to birth control are critical to the future of Black women's health and safety. In alignment with the reproductive justice framework, ensuring that women have the right to healthy birthing experiences as well as to parent their children in safe environments must be met with equal resolve in supporting the right to universal birth control for women who do not want children. Equitable and quality contraceptive access free from shame, stigma, and restrictive policies is not yet a reality for many Black women, particularly those living in more oppressive southern states. This gap in access is due in part to the complicated relationship between birth control, historical and current power structures, and the collective history of Black women and girls. Race, gender, and class discrimination have impacted institutional, community, and cultural responses to the birth control needs and desires of Black women and girls. The desire and need to use birth control dates back to enslavement and carries forward to present day, with challenges stemming from diminished reproductive rights to weakened access.

Conversely, Black women have also had to resist systematic reproductive coercion through government-supported initiatives of forced birth control and sterilization. This dichotomy continues to complicate the issue of birth control access for Black women and girls who, in many aspects, are in critical need of broader access and expanded rights. Black women have lived in this dualism for generations, and it is this experience that perpetuates the topic of birth control access as a stigmatized issue, particularly for those living in the southern United States. This chapter explores the application of the liberation health framework as a strategy to transform external and internalized oppressive messages, ideologies, and institutions that continue to limit birth control access for Black women.

THE DUALITY OF BIRTH CONTROL FOR BLACK WOMEN

The history of birth control in the United States involves a dichotomous relationship with Black women resulting in failed policies and programs that consistently limit reproductive freedom. For thousands of years, women have used different items, techniques, and strategies to manage their fertility (Riddle 1992). Enslaved Black women and their foremothers were no different and went to great lengths to circumvent the brutality of forced breeding and birth (Roberts 2000), many of them relying on traditions brought over from their African homelands (Perin 2001). During slavery, women used various methods including ingesting cotton root, spacing births, and extending lactation (Perin 2001; Webster 2021) to prevent unwanted pregnancies. Although these methods varied greatly in their success and failure rates, women effectively used whatever methods were available to them in an effort to maintain control over what little bodily autonomy they held.

After the emancipation of slavery, worries regarding the number of free Black people, particularly those now living in the South amongst the white ruling class, increased, coupled with fears of an increase in white women using methods for contraception and therefore limiting the growth of the white population. This prompted the passage of the Federal Comstock Act of 1873, banning the delivery of contraceptive devices and information. As the movement for women's suffrage expanded in the early 20th century, birth control access became synonymous with the fight for women's rights, for white women exclusively (Prescott and Thompson 2020).

For Black women, the history of birth control in the early to mid-20th century commonly centers around policies of forced birth control use, sterilization, the eugenics movement, and Margaret Sanger, the founding president of the Birth Control Federation of America, now known as Planned Parenthood Federation of America. Less is known about the needs and desires of Black women themselves regarding birth control during this time. Educator and women's rights activist Mary McLeod Bethune, founder of the National Council for Negro Women (NCNW), championed the issue of birth control access in a 1941 NCNW resolution on family planning, which urged

> every Negro organization throughout the country, the inclusion of all public health programs, especially the less familiar one of family planning, which aims to aid each family to have ALL the children it can support and afford, but no more - in order to insure better health greater security and happiness for all. (McLeod Bethune 1941)

This resolution was cemented by Dorothy Boulding Ferebee, the second president of NCNW and an obstetrician, who led several health initiatives in Washington, DC, and Mississippi that included expanding access to family planning for Black women. Black women in leadership saw access to birth control as critical for Black women, especially those living in the southern United States, and petitioned for white birth control movement leaders to consider the lived experiences of the Black women that NCNW and its partnering organizations served (Figure 11-1; McLeod Bethune 1941). Unfortunately, this national movement led by Black women to ensure quality programming and access to birth control for the communities they served was co-opted by policies and practices of white supremacy, which continues to have an impact on the relationship between the topic of birth control and Black women's autonomy and liberty today.

As modern contraception became available to women in the United States, several policies were enacted that further diminished the autonomy of Black women; these included state-sanctioned forced sterilization, mass dissemination of untested methods, and coerced birth control usage (Roberts 2000), leaving many in the African American community distrustful of initiatives focused on increased access to birth control, even when facilitated by Black leadership. Even more so, the rights of Black women pertaining to birth control and similarly situated issues including access to abortion, quality child care, and intimate partner violence became less of a priority during the Civil Rights Movement as the experience of misogynoir and gender discrimination permeated in national leadership and throughout the Black community.

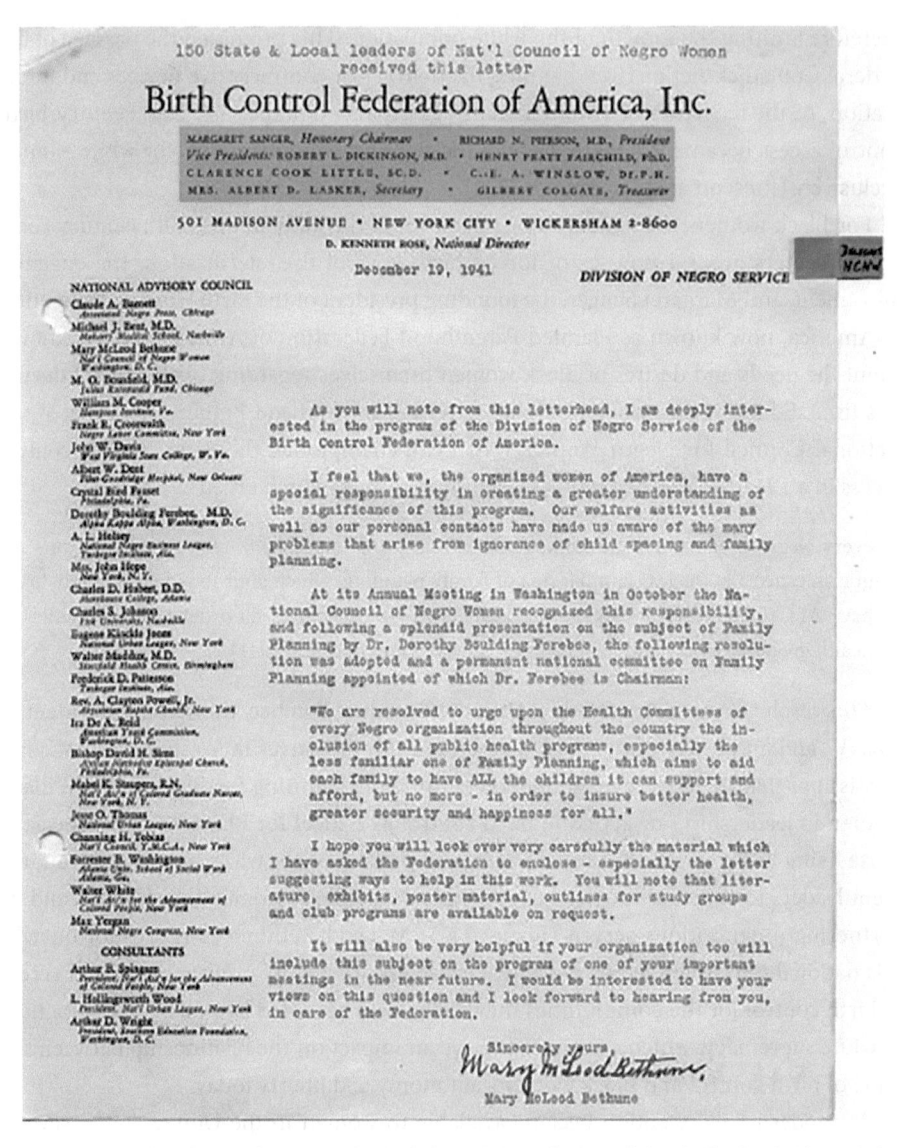

Source: Courtesy of the Bethune-Cookman University Archives, Bethune-Cookman University. Reprinted with permission.
Figure 11-1. Letter by Mary McLeod Bethune, 1941

Black women have had to fight against racist control of their reproduction all while simultaneously fighting against sexism and the freedom to exercise their autonomy within their own families and communities. At the core of this duality exists the salience of white supremacy, further complicating the relationship with birth control within the context of structural racism and its operationalization in the lives of Black women.

Institutional Oppression

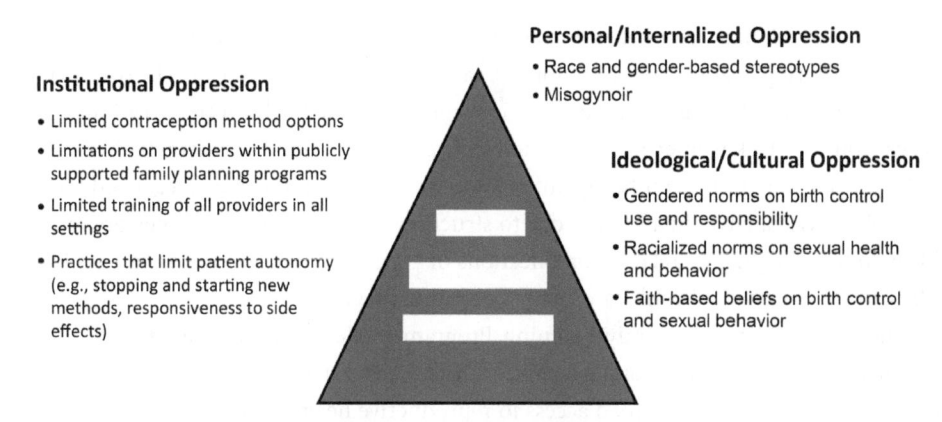

- Limited contraception method options
- Limitations on providers within publicly supported family planning programs
- Limited training of all providers in all settings
- Practices that limit patient autonomy (e.g., stopping and starting new methods, responsiveness to side effects)

Personal/Internalized Oppression

- Race and gender-based stereotypes
- Misogynoir

Ideological/Cultural Oppression

- Gendered norms on birth control use and responsibility
- Racialized norms on sexual health and behavior
- Faith-based beliefs on birth control and sexual behavior

Source: Courtesy of Dawn Belkin Martinez, PhD, LICSW (Belkin Martinez 2014). Adapted with permission.

Figure 11-2. The Liberation Framework and Birth Control Access

UNIVERSAL BIRTH CONTROL ACCESS AS A STRATEGY FOR LIBERATION

Increasingly, calls for free birth control, over-the-counter birth control reform (Sundstrom et al. 2020), and less-restrictive birth control policies overall have gained traction in direct response to the election of President Donald Trump and the rise of religious objections to birth control coverage. Under the leadership of President Barack Obama, the passage of the Affordable Care Act (ACA) in 2010 followed by the birth control coverage mandate in 2011 rapidly improved access to birth control for women in the United States, particularly for those women living in the 31 states that expanded coverage for Medicaid.

This experience was not the same for Black women, as Black women living in the South were less likely to be insured under ACA compared to other groups (Artiga et al. 2021). Overall, the number of women with out-of-pocket expenses related to birth control fell from 21% in 2012 to just 3% in 2016, and fewer women reported delays in health care services in 2015 as compared to those in 2011 (Ranji et al. 2012). Unfortunately, this increased access would soon diminish due to a series of judicial decisions and executive orders in 2014 (*Burwell v. Hobby Lobby*), 2017 (Executive Order Promoting Free Speech and Religious Liberty), and 2020 (*Little Sisters of the Poor v. Pennsylvania*) that expanded religious objection to birth control coverage on the basis of religious freedom. Further restrictions came in the form of state-level policies that defunded clinical sites providing abortion care, further disrupting contraception choice for women who rely on state-funded family planning facilities for care (Kavanaugh et al. 2022b).

Religious restrictions and state regulations, combined with the overturning of *Roe v. Wade* has placed access to birth control in further peril for the most marginalized women, particularly Black women. Access to contraception was disrupted during the COVID-19 pandemic, which had a significant impact on those unstably employed (Kavanaugh et al. 2022a), requiring a substantial need for increased access to birth control. The overturning of *Roe v. Wade* has significant implications on the state of birth control access among Black women. Black women are more likely to live in contraception deserts (Barber et al. 2019), specifically in the southern United States where abortion is now illegal and birth control is less available. In addition, due to structural inequities, Black women are more likely to have pregnancy-related complications or pregnancy-related deaths and are less likely to receive quality health care before becoming pregnant.

The Title X National Family Planning Program (Title X), administered by the US Department of Health and Human Services, Office of Population Affairs, is the only federal program that provides broad access to reproductive health services. Of the 3.1 million family planning users served through Title X in 2019, 24% self-identified as Black (Fowler et al. 2020). Among females served in the Title X program, 77% were using or had adopted a contraceptive method at their last encounter, and 8% of all female users exited their last encounter with no contraceptive method because they were either pregnant or seeking pregnancy (Fowler et al. 2020).

The percentage of those who are uninsured in the Title X program (41%) is much higher than the national rate (11%) for those uninsured (Fowler et al. 2020). Out of the 10 regions in the United States served by Title X, the southern region (Region IV) serves the largest percentage of Black clients at 40% and includes the following states: Kentucky, Tennessee, North Carolina, South Carolina, Florida, Georgia, Alabama, and Mississippi (Fowler et al. 2020). During the Trump administration, the number of clients served through Title X dropped from 3.9 million to 1.5 million (Frederiksen, Gomez, and Salganicoff 2021). The impact of the COVID-19 pandemic further diminished the Title X program in the subsequent years since the Trump administration cuts. In addition to these cuts, Title X has been underfunded since its inception. Current funding for the program has been maintained at $286.5 million since 2014; however, if funding for Title X was adjusted for inflation, the level would be at $1.1 billion (Dawson 2021).

Funding Title X at appropriate levels and significantly improving the quality of contraceptive care delivery that is culturally appropriate and responsive will help to improve access gaps severely impacting Black women. Broad access to birth control allows those marginalized by racism, ageism, sexism, classism, and geography an opportunity to practice bodily autonomy, freeing themselves from both external and internal oppressive practices. However, the holistic experience of Black women and birth control needs deeper exploration. Namely, how traditional (health care, education, housing, and the criminal justice systems) and cultural (religion, families, community spaces) institutions hold power over women directly limiting their autonomy must be explored.

For example, contraception service delivery must significantly transform to meet the full reproductive health needs of Black women and girls. The experiences that Black women have had with reproductive health providers have been disempowering and resulted in silenced interactions around sex, limited patient decision-making, and medical mistrust (Logan et al. 2021). Furthermore, Black women are less likely than white and Hispanic women to be satisfied with their birth control (Hirth et al. 2021). Much of this dissatisfaction could be attributed to contraception initiatives over the past decade focusing solely on birth control uptake rather than centering the unique needs of Black women.

Initiatives committed to ensuring Black women have equitable access to quality contraception services must ensure the full range of reproductive health care services are available, including patient-centered counseling and the removal of long-acting reversible contraception (Bryson, Koyama, and Hassan 2021; Holt et al. 2020). Black women feel that access to over-the-counter birth control would improve their own autonomy, be more convenient, and reduce barriers related to cost, stigma, embarrassment, and provider bias (Sundstrom et al. 2020). Clinical practice and structural changes that elevate patient control, holistic and inclusive services, and autonomy in reproductive health care may help to dismantle the effects of racism, as well as eliminate inequities in reproductive health (Treder et al. 2020).

THE LIBERATION HEALTH FRAMEWORK AND BIRTH CONTROL ACCESS

Given the complicated history of Black women and birth control in the United States, prescribing birth control as a means of liberation seems simplistic, negligent even. However, this same history requires the dismantling of multiple oppressive systems that limit the reproductive autonomy of Black women, and birth control is at the center of body ownership for women seeking to manage and control their reproduction. The authors of this chapter posit that the liberation health framework (Belkin-Martinez and Fleck-Henderson 2014), a clinically based, individualized, client-level social work framework, could be applied to birth control access initiatives, especially in a climate of increased abortion restrictions, contraceptive technologies, and criminal investigations (Figure 11-2).

The liberation health framework is an orientation to clinical social work practice born out of the socio-political crisis over the past two decades, with the goal of transforming both society and those living within it (Belkin-Martinez and Fleck-Henderson 2014). Based in liberation psychology, this framework grounds itself in the lived experiences of groups impacted by multiple oppressive systems to ensure interventions are within the context of that particular group's needs, wants, and desires (Belkin-Martinez and Fleck-Henderson 2014). For both social and individual change to occur, the liberation health framework operates on the following three levels: (1) transforming patterns of internalized oppression and building strengths, (2) enabling community connections, and (3) organizing social and political action to bring about collective shifts in power. It acknowledges that for socio-political change to occur, individuals must first be free from internalized oppression; only then can systemic change be addressed.

Internalized racism or internalized oppression, as the term is used interchangeably, includes the acceptance of socially constructed negative stereotypes and norms. Black women can be impacted by internalized racism in a number of ways, including disengagement from the reproductive health care system and difficulty making reproductive health decisions due to fear of conforming to stereotypes and receiving judgment (Treder et al. 2020). In patient-provider interactions, Black women are more likely to report stereotype-related gendered racism than white women, resulting in greater birth control-related mistrust than white women. This experience was also found to be related to pregnancy-related stress (Mehra et al. 2020; Rosenthal and Lobel 2020; Chinn, Martin, and Redmond 2021). Furthermore, women who reported perceived discrimination from a provider were at risk for contraception nonuse (Loder et al. 2021). And, for some women, it is the lived experience of gender-based racism that influences them to perform self-protective actions when interacting with the health care system and seeking same-race providers (Treder et al. 2022; Mehra et al. 2020; Thompson et al. 2022). Justice-informed, patient-centered care models are needed especially in areas that face the most restrictive state laws (Chinn, Martin, and Redmond 2021).

Applying a micro-level framework to a macro-level issue such as birth control access requires a shift from focusing on an individual's lived experience to a community's collective experience with reproductive health. It should be a point for critical examination that the liberation of Black women would allow for the liberation of all people who desire full reproductive rights and agency. Within this process, creating a plan of action would include meaningful engagement and co-creation with Black women to fully understand their common truths, desires, and needs for quality contraception service.

As young Black women navigate their own reproductive health service needs, familial and intergenerational influences play a critical role. Mothers and grandmothers of young Black women provide education, guidance, and support that are embedded in their lived experiences as they themselves had to navigate. Embedded in this guidance are values and beliefs that span a broad spectrum, ranging from stifling respectability standards and conservatism, to the open sharing of progressive values based in their own experiences with reproductive health decision-making. These interpersonal relationships serve as cultural exchanges that help to inform reproductive health decision-making and health-seeking behaviors among young Black women (Harris 2013).

Public health professionals interested in applying the liberation health framework must consider values and experiences present in the familial and social networks of Black women that may reflect internalized racist norms and stereotypes, then work alongside women to dismantle these beliefs. In addition to families, cultural institutions in the Black community such as national and local nonprofits, faith communities, and Historically Black Colleges and Universities must reclaim access to birth control as a priority issue as we face forced pregnancy and birth throughout the South and within the Midwest, regions where substantial Black communities reside. Public health professionals will also need to actively work with leadership across cultural institutions to dismantle ideologies, messages, and practices that are steeped in racialized gender-based stereotypes.

REFERENCES

Artiga S, Hill L, Orgera K, Damico A. Health coverage by race and ethnicity, 2010-2019. San Francisco, CA: Kaiser Family Foundation; 2021.

Barber JS, Ela E, Gatny H, et al. Contraceptive desert? Black-white differences in characteristics of nearby pharmacies. *J Racial Ethn Health Disparities.* 2019;6(4):719-732. https://doi.org/10.1007/s40615-019-00570-3

Belkin Martinez D, Fleck-Henderson A, eds. *Social Justice in Clinical Practice: A Liberation Health Framework for Social Work.* 1st ed. London, UK: Routledge; 2014. https://doi.org/10.4324/9781315813073

Bryson A, Koyama A, Hassan A. Addressing long-acting reversible contraception access, bias, and coercion: supporting adolescent and young adult reproductive autonomy. *Curr Opin Pediatr.* 2021;33(4):345–353. https://doi.org/10.1097/MOP.0000000000001008

Chinn J, Martin IK, Redmond N. Health equity among Black women in the United States. *J Womens Health (Larchmt).* 2021;30(2):212–219. http://doi.org/10.1089/jwh.2020.8868

Dawson R. What federal policymakers must do to restore and strengthen a Title X family planning program that serves all. *Guttmacher Policy Review.* 2021;24.

Fowler CI, Gable J, Lasater B, Asman K. Family planning annual report: 2019 national summary. Washington, DC: Office of Population Affairs, Office of the Assistant Secretary for Health, Department of Health and Human Services; September 2020.

Frederiksen B, Gomez I, Salganicoff A. Rebuilding Title X: new regulations for the federal family planning program. San Francisco, CA: Kaiser Family Foundation; 2021.

Harris A. "I got caught up in the game": generational influences on contraceptive decision making in African-American women. *J Am Assoc Nurse Pract.* 2013;25(3):156–165. https://doi.org/10.1111/j.1745-7599.2012.00772.x.

Hirth J. Dinehart EE, Lin Y-L, Kuo Y-F, Patel PR. Reasons why young women in the United States choose their contraceptive method. *J Womens Health (Larchmt).* 2021;30(1):64–72. https://doi.org/10.1089/jwh.2019.8182

Holt K, Reed R, Crear-Perry J, Scott C, Wulf S, Dehlendorf C. Beyond same-day long-acting reversible contraceptive access: a person-centered framework for advancing high-quality, equitable contraceptive care. *Am J Obstet Gynecol.* 2020;222(4 suppl):S878.e1–S878.e6. https://doi.org/10.1016/j.ajog.2019.11.1279

Kavanaugh M, Pleasure ZH, Pliskin E, Zolna M, MacFarlane K. Financial instability and delays in access to sexual and reproductive health care due to COVID-19. *J Womens Health (Larchmt).* 2022a;31(4):469–479. https://doi.org/10.1089/jwh.2021.0493

Kavanaugh ML, Zolna M., Pliskin E, et al. A prospective cohort study of changes in access to contraceptive care and use two years after Iowa Medicaid coverage restrictions at abortion-providing facilities went into effect. *Popul Res Policy Rev.* 2022b;41(6):2555–2583. https://doi.org/10.1007/s11113-022-09740-4

Loder C, Hall K, Kusunoki Y, Hope Harris L, Dalton V. Associations between perceived discrimination and contraceptive method use: why we need better measures of discrimination in reproductive healthcare. *Women Health*. 2021;61(5):461–469. https://doi.org/10.1080/03630 242.2021.1919816

Logan RG, Daley EM, Vamos CA, Louis-Jacques A, Marhefka SL. "When is health care actually going to be care?" The lived experience of family planning care among young Black women. *Qual Health Res*. 2021;31(6):1169–1182. https://doi.org/10.1177/1049732321993094

McLeod Bethune M. Letter by Mary McLeod Bethune, December 19, 1941. Smith Libraries Exhibits. Available at: https://libex.smith.edu/omeka/items/show/445

Mehra R, Boyd LM, Magriples A, Kershaw TS, Ickovics JR, Keene DE. Black pregnant women "get the most judgment": a qualitative study of the experiences of Black women at the intersection of race, gender, and pregnancy. *Womens Health Issues*. 2020;30(6):484–492. https://doi.org/10.1016/j.whi.2020.08.001

Orleck A. *Storming Caesars Palace: How Black Mothers Fought Their Own War on Poverty*. Boston, MA: Beacon; 2005:71

Perin L. Resisting reproduction: reconsidering slave contraception in the Old South. *J Am Stud*. 2001;35(2):255–274. https://doi.org/10.1017/S0021875801006612

Prescott H, Thompson L. A right to ourselves: women's suffrage and the birth control movement. *J Gilded Age Progress Era*. 2020;19(4):542–558. https://doi.org/10.1017/S1537781420000304

Ranji U, Salganicoff A, Sobel L, Rosenzweig C. Ten ways that the House American Health Care Act could affect women. Issue Brief. San Francisco, CA: Kaiser Family Foundation; 2017.

Riddle JM. *Contraception and abortion from the ancient world to the Renaissance*. Cambridge, MA: Harvard University Press; 1992. Available at: http://hdl.handle.net/2027/heb.01463.0001.001

Roberts D. *Killing the Black Body*. New York, NY: Vintage Books; 2000.

Rosenthal L, Lobel M. Gendered racism and the sexual and reproductive health of Black and Latina women. *Ethn Health*. 2020;25:3:367–392. https://doi.org/10.1080/13557858.2018.1439896

Sundstrom B, Smith E, Vyge K, et al. Moving oral contraceptives over the counter: theory-based formative research to design communication strategy. *J Health Commun*. 2020;25(4):313–322. https://doi.org/10.1080/10810730.2020.1752334

Thompson TM, Young Y-Y, Bass TM, et al. Racism runs through it: examining the sexual and reproductive health experience of Black women in the South. *Health Aff (Millwood)*. 2022;41(2):195–202. https://doi.org/10.1377/hlthaff.2021.01422

Treder K, White K, Woodhams E, Pancholi R, Yinusa-Nyahkoon L. Racism and the reproductive health experiences of US-born Black women. *Obstet Gynecol*. 2022;139(3):407–416. https://doi.org/10.1097/AOG.0000000000004675

Treder KE, Woodhams E, Pancholi R, Yinusa-Nyahkoon L, White KO. A qualitative exploration of the impact of racism on the reproductive health of US Black women. *Contraception*. 2020;102(4):274. https://doi.org/10.1016/j.contraception.2020.07.011

Webster C. Enslaved women's sexual health: reproductive rights as resistance. Black perspectives. Pittsburgh, PA: African American Intellectual History Society; 2021.

White K, Vizcarra E, Palomares L, et al. Initial impacts of Texas' Senate Bill 8 on abortion in Texas and at out-of-state facilities. Austin, TX: Texas Policy Evaluation Project; October 2021.

12

The Black Maternal Health Momnibus Act: A Labor of Love Led by Black Women

Jamila K. Taylor, PhD, MPA

The Black Maternal Health Momnibus Act is trailblazing legislation that was developed by Black women leaders. The historic legislative package aims to address almost every dimension of America's maternal health crisis, which disproportionately impacts Black women and families. Nationwide, Black women are more likely to die of pregnancy-related causes when compared to white women (Hoyert 2022). The root cause is racism, which shows up in almost every corner of American society and institutions, including the health care system. Black women have affirmed that, because of this, it is imperative to develop a comprehensive set of solutions.

This chapter will provide an overview of the process to develop key policy solutions included in the Black Maternal Health Momnibus Act, centering the critical role of Black women. Black women leaders have been stewards not only in developing the legislation but also in its advancement through the legislative process and usage as a national organizing tool for change.

VAST RACIAL DISPARITIES IN MATERNAL HEALTH SOUND THE ALARM

The United States has a maternal mortality rate that far outstrips that of other industrialized nations. The statistics not only show the continuation in the United States' poor standing as a global leader of maternal deaths but also show a continuation of another disturbing trend—a trend that shows a maternal mortality rate that continues to grow especially among Black and Hispanic women. Black women are three times as likely to die from pregnancy-related causes as white women (Figure 12-1). The maternal mortality rate among Hispanic women increased by a disturbing 44% in just one year (Hoyert 2022).

In the backdrop of the COVID-19 pandemic, which also had a disproportionate impact on Black and Hispanic pregnant women and birthing people, it is no surprise that the United States maternal mortality rates grew to the extent that they did (Ellington et al. 2020). However, the trend had been in an upward trajectory for decades.

Black Women Face Three Times the Maternal Mortality Risk as White Women

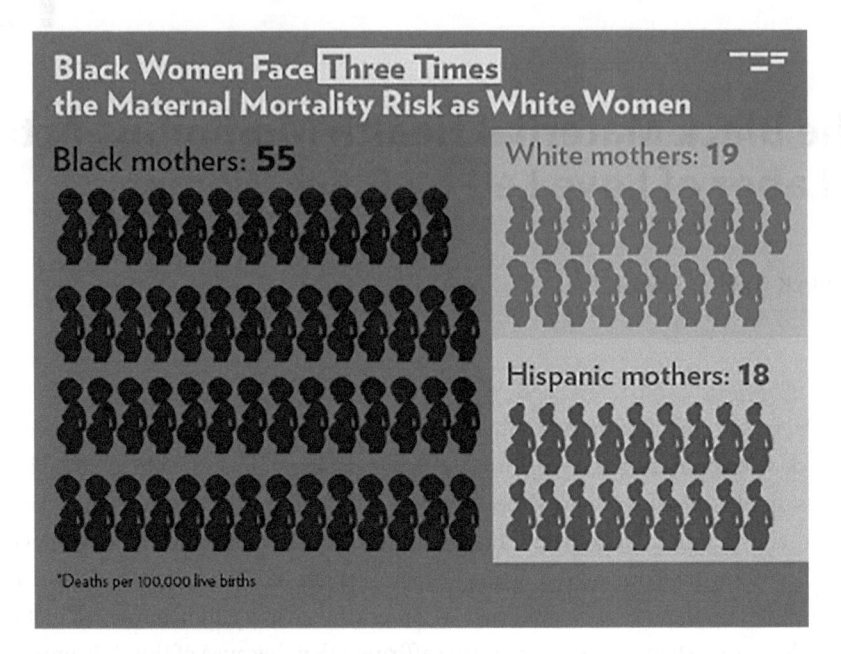

Black mothers: 55

White mothers: 19

Hispanic mothers: 18

*Deaths per 100,000 live births

Source: Reprinted with permission from The Century Foundation (2022).

Figure 12-1. Black Women Face Three Times the Maternal Mortality Risk as White Women

While there is certainly a multitude of factors that contribute to it, systemic racism is the root cause underlying the maternal mortality crisis among Black women.

The history of reproductive oppression in the United States has implications for how racism has been engrained within the structures of society. Egregious practices such as sexual exploitation, forced mating, and family separation were just some of the forms of subjugation Black people had to endure as part of the institution of slavery. The American health care system is no exception. Black women's bodies have been used against their will in the development of the study of obstetrics and gynecology—a clear manifestation of medical racism well before more high-profile incidences like the Tuskegee syphilis study (Centers for Disease Control and Prevention 2021).

The scientific advancements made during this time were then used to subsequently heal white women of their reproductive injuries and illnesses. Unfortunately, practices such as these have endured over time. It can be argued that the medical legacy of mistreatment, racism, and reproductive oppression linger on in Black women's interactions with the American health care system today. The vast racial disparities in maternal health between Black women and white women provide a window into the phenomenon.

The Aspen Institute defines structural racism as a system where public policies, institutional practices, and cultural representations work to reinforce and perpetuate racial inequity (Aspen Institute 2016). Under this definition, dimensions of American history

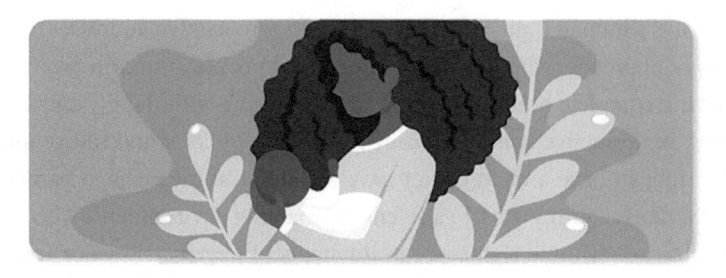

Source: Reprinted with permission from The Century Foundation (n.d.).

Figure 12-2. Black Maternal Health Momnibus Act of 2021

and culture, which have allowed privileges associated with "whiteness" and disadvantages associated with "color," are connected in ways that have adapted and endured over time (Taylor 2020). According to Thompson et al. (2022), both structural and individual racism have been identified as risk factors for poor maternal health outcomes, diminished and coercive contraceptive experiences, and delayed reproductive health screenings. Not only is structural racism seen in health care but also in policies and practices related to other social issues such as housing and residential segregation, access to nutrition, employment, pay equity, and others. It is because of regressive policies that Black women are disproportionately represented in publicly funded health care programs such as Title X and Medicaid.

The experience of racism can also impact a Black woman's ability to have a healthy pregnancy and birth. Because of this, there has been more discussion in recent years about racism as a social determinant of health. The social determinants of health are defined as health care conditions that affect the health and quality of life of people in a given environment, including where a person works, lives, or plays (Artiga and Hinton 2018). The Black maternal health crisis cannot be adequately addressed without taking into account how racism manifests in the health care system in a way that impacts the quality of care Black women receive or how experiencing it in broader society impacts their ability to be healthy. These concepts were foundational in the development of policy solutions included in the Black Maternal Health Momnibus Act (Figure 12-2).

LEVERAGING THE REPRODUCTIVE JUSTICE FRAMEWORK TO DEVELOP POLICY SOLUTIONS

The reproductive justice framework has been critical in ensuring the proper framing and contextualization of the issues that intersect when it comes to Black women's maternal health. Developed by a group of Black women in 1994 (e-mail communication, Toni M. Bond, PhD, May 31, 2023), the reproductive justice framework analyzes the ability of any woman to determine her reproductive destiny as linked to the conditions in her community. It is a human rights–based, structured approach that addresses the intersecting systems of oppression that prevent marginalized people, primarily women of color, from achieving complete bodily autonomy and parenting with dignity. Furthermore, as a movement, reproductive issues advocacy for women of color and Indigenous women centers the right to have a child or not have a child, and the right to parent the children we have. This requires work to also ensure enabling environments with society that support realization of these rights—central tenants of any social justice framework or accompanying movement. The reproductive justice framework has been used by Black women leaders as the basis for developing solutions to address the Black maternal health crisis in the United States.

In 2018, Black Mamas Matter Alliance (BMMA) developed recommendations for holistic care and set the standard for Black women's pregnancy and birthing experiences. The organization is a Black women-led cross-sectoral alliance that centers Black mamas and birthing people to advocate, drive research, build power, and shift culture for Black maternal health, rights, and justice (BMMA 2020). The recommendations developed by BMMA were grounded in reproductive justice and human rights frameworks, and included imperatives such as the following:

- listening to Black women,
- recognizing the historical experiences and expertise of Black women and families,
- providing care through a reproductive justice framework,
- disentangling care practices from the racist beliefs in modern medicine,
- replacing white supremacy and patriarchy with a new model of care,
- empowering all patients with health literacy and autonomy,
- empowering and investing in paraprofessionals, and
- recognizing that access does not equal quality care (Muse et al. 2018).

This holistic care manifesto, though not specific to policy goals, was essential in developing key aspects of the Black Maternal Health Momnibus Act that pertained to the quality of care Black women must be afforded to adequately address poor maternal health outcomes. Some of these aspects include bills such as the Kira Johnson Act, which establishes a grant program through the US Department of Health and Human Services specifically for community-based programs working to improve maternal health outcomes among Black pregnant and postpartum women (Taylor and Bernstein 2022). This Momnibus bill would also set up a training program aimed at ensuring respectful maternity care and preventing racism, bias, and discrimination in health care for all providers and others working in maternity care settings.

The Perinatal Workforce Act is another Momnibus bill grounded in recommendations from BMMA's holistic care work. It would establish grants for eligible education programs to grow and diversify the perinatal workforce, including nurses, physician assistants, and other specified health workers (Taylor and Bernstein 2022). Under this bill, the US Department of Health and Human Services must disseminate guidance on respectful maternity care delivery, including recruiting and retaining maternity care providers from diverse backgrounds and incorporating midwives and other perinatal health care workers into maternity care teams.

Later in the year 2018, BMMA released another report—this time, focused on advancing holistic maternal care for Black women specifically through policy. The policy priorities set forth by BMMA were identifying and ensuring mechanisms for engagement and prioritization of Black women and Black women-led entities in policy and program development and implementation; establishing equitable systems of care to address racism, obstetric violence, and neglect and abuse; and expanding and protecting meaningful access to quality, affordable, and comprehensive health care coverage, which includes the full spectrum of reproductive and maternal health care services for Black women (Lipscomb et al. 2018). The policy solutions outlined in the report served as an appropriate follow-up and went on to inform development not only of the Momnibus but also of other policy efforts.

The Center for American Progress became the first organization to publish a comprehensive policy framework to eliminate racial disparities in both maternal and infant mortality in May of 2019 (Taylor et al. 2019). Development of the framework was a cross-team effort, led by the Black women leaders of the Women's Health and Rights team of the national think tank. The authors outlined policy strategies in five areas and made recommendations to address maternal and infant health threats, which disproportionately impact Black mothers and their infants. The five buckets were as follows:

- improving access to critical services,
- improving quality of care provided to pregnant women,
- addressing maternal and infant mental health,
- enhancing supports for families before and after birth, and
- improving data collection (Taylor et al. 2019).

After publication of BMMA's reports and this comprehensive policy blueprint, policymakers, advocates, researchers, and the press started to cite the materials widely, and conversations with policymakers started to galvanize around what a comprehensive legislative package could look like to adequately address America's Black maternal health crisis.

BUILDING A COALITION OF BLACK WOMEN LEADERS TO ADVANCE MATERNAL HEALTH EQUITY

The BMMA began as a partnership between the Center for Reproductive Rights and SisterSong Women of Color Reproductive Justice Collective in 2013 (BMMA 2020). The groups commenced their work by collaborating on a story collection project that chronicled the obstacles Black women in the South were facing in accessing maternal health care. This, in turn, led to the discovery of the coordinated challenges of poor maternal health outcomes and persistent racial disparities. Their findings were shared in a joint report submitted to the United Nations Committee on the Elimination of Racial Discrimination titled, "Reproductive Injustice: Gender and Racial Discrimination in US Health Care" (Center for Reproductive Rights 2014).

Since its founding, BMMA has continued to serve as the driving force behind the national movement to advance maternal health, rights, and justice. BMMA's co-founding executive director, Angela D. Aina, asserts that Alliance members had a key role in developing solutions that would, in turn, become part of the Momnibus during a policy convening held in Washington, DC, in 2018 (A.D. Aina, MPH, oral communication, May 24, 2022). Shortly thereafter, the group connected with key players on Capitol Hill. One of the first members of Congress to approach BMMA about involvement in developing Momnibus legislation was Congresswoman Alma Adams (D-NC). Congresswoman Adams also introduced the first-ever Black Maternal Health Week resolution in 2018, alongside then-Senator Kamala Harris (D-CA).

Black women at all levels of government and across advocacy and policy spaces have been instrumental in developing and advancing the Black Maternal Health Momnibus Act. Breana Lipscomb, senior advisor for maternal health and rights at the Center for Reproductive Rights and co-chair of the BMMA Board of Directors, reflects on how introduction of the Momnibus gave Black women a platform to talk about the intersections of Black maternal health: "The Momnibus has provided an opportunity for Black women to have a platform to talk about all of these issues together, and not silo our issues—including things like environmental justice, the social determinants of health, and others" (videoconference interview, May 12, 2022). Lipscomb goes on to say that the Momnibus has helped open doors to conversations about how racism and discrimination impact maternal health and acknowledges its introduction as also elevating her own profile.

Congresswoman Lauren Underwood (D-IL), lead sponsor of the Momnibus, was motivated to start work on Black maternal health after the death of her friend Dr. Shalon Irving. Dr. Irving was a Centers for Disease Control and Prevention (CDC) epidemiologist and lieutenant commander in the US Public Health Service Commissioned Corps (Purnell 2022). She died of complications shortly after giving birth to her daughter. Congresswoman Underwood asserts that Black women's leadership in advancing the Momnibus has been essential. While she is credited for being the lead policymaker on the bill, Congresswoman Underwood gives credit and praise to the Black women-led initiatives that were doing the work well before government action. The Congresswoman states, "Everything that has happened, it was because of Black women's leadership. You can see the love and attention of Black women in the bill. Black women know how to create change." (oral communication, May 19, 2022). The Momnibus has sparked a wave of advocacy efforts across the country, and Black women continue to organize around it and build advocacy initiatives to gain support.

The Black Maternal Health Federal Policy Collective, a new coalition brought together in response to the prioritization of the Momnibus and other Black maternal health initiatives by the Biden-Harris administration and the 117th Congress, brings together dynamic Black women leaders from across the policy sector to develop strategies and solutions to tackle America's maternal health crisis (The Century Foundation 2022). The Collective has positioned itself as the go-to resource for policymakers, advocates, the press, and the public.

On April 9, 2019, Congresswomen Adams and Underwood launched the Black Maternal Health Caucus. This bipartisan Congressional caucus has a total of 115 members and is organized around the goals of "elevating the Black maternal health crisis within Congress and advancing policy solutions to improve maternal health outcomes and end disparities" (Black Maternal Health Caucus n.d.). According to Congresswoman Underwood, "it became very clear that there was bipartisan interest from the beginning" (oral communication, May 19, 2022). She goes on to say that soon after she and Congresswoman Adams filed paperwork to start the Caucus, they began to receive an overwhelming response from Congressional members from both sides of the aisle with interest in working on maternal health.

The Caucus's work continues to evolve—when President Joe Biden and Vice President Kamala Harris took office in 2021, the Caucus encouraged executive action on Black maternal health and worked closely with the administration to advance maternal health investments and policy solutions within the executive branch. The Caucus has also worked in lock-step with Black women leaders across the reproductive justice and maternal health fields, and was instrumental in the development of the Black Maternal Health Momnibus Act.

The Black Maternal Health Momnibus Act of 2021 was introduced during the 117th Congress on February 8, 2021. The first iteration of the Momnibus was introduced on March 9, 2020, in the 116th Congress. The critical package of legislation includes 12 individual bills and aims to address almost every dimension of the maternal health crisis in the United States. With this comprehensive set of solutions, the Momnibus addresses a range of issues, including the following:

- the social determinants of health,
- maternal mental health,
- perinatal workforce development,
- the effects of climate change,
- the unique circumstances facing incarcerated pregnant women and veterans,
- implementing quality measures in data collection,
- integrating telehealth models in maternity care settings,

- ensuring better maternal health data collection and surveillance during the COVID-19 public health emergency, and
- increasing equity and awareness of maternal vaccinations (Black Maternal Health Momnibus Act 2021a).

The House of Representatives version of the package has 189 cosponsors. It was also introduced in the Senate with lead sponsor Senator Cory Booker (D-NJ) and has a total of 32 cosponsors (Black Maternal Health Momnibus Act 2021b). The Black Maternal Health Momnibus Act of 2023 was introduced on May 15, 2023. This iteration includes 13 bills, with the newest addition being legislation focused on extending postpartum eligibility under the Supplemental Nutrition Program for Women, Infants and Children (WIC; Black Maternal Health Momnibus Act 2023).

The federal Black Maternal Health Momnibus Act has sparked localized efforts to introduce state Momnibus legislation. The California Momnibus legislation (S.B. 65) focuses on addressing maternal health equity in the state by increasing access to midwifery training programs, providing full-spectrum doula care to pregnant and postpartum Medicaid enrollees, and extending postpartum Medicaid coverage from 60 days to one year (Mun and Morcelle 2021).

The North Carolina Momnibus Act (S.B. 632) establishes two taskforces—one to develop recommendations in addressing the social determinants of health for Black mothers and ensuring the provision of respectful maternity care during public health emergencies and a second to study access issues and maternal mortality outcomes among pregnant and postpartum veterans. The bill goes further by establishing a grant program for community-based organizations serving Black mothers and families, earmarking funding for data collection and research and establishing specific rights of perinatal care patients, and developing implicit bias trainings in partnership with Black-led organizations, including community-based organizations and Historically Black Colleges and Universities (Mun and Morcelle 2021).

Illinois also introduced a Momnibus bill (H.B. 158). It aims to address structural racism by instituting health care reforms, such as Medicaid coverage of doula care and home visiting (Mun and Morcelle 2021). The legislation also establishes a task force aimed at implementing holistic review of state programs and departments and developing recommendations for improving maternal health in the state.

SEIZING THE MOMENT

During the 117th Congress, 58 maternal health bills were introduced (US Congress n.d.). This number has increased steadily over the last several congressional sessions. There continues to be traction and interest in developing new legislation to address poor maternal health outcomes, yet the political will to secure passage of a legislative package as comprehensive as the Momnibus has been lacking. In 2021, Congress embarked on an effort to develop a comprehensive budget bill to address various aspects of social and economic supports for individuals and families as a response to the COVID-19 pandemic—the Build Back Better Act. Reproductive justice advocates worked with Representative Underwood and other members of Congress in the Black Maternal Health Caucus to ensure that maternal health investments from the Black Maternal Health Momnibus Act were included. According to research conducted by The Century Foundation, the maternal health investments included in the Build Back Better Act would be life-saving if implemented:

- About 1.2 million uninsured mothers would be able to continue their postpartum Medicaid coverage for one year.
- About 92,000 nurses and perinatal nursing students would receive loans, scholarships, and programmatic support.
- About 30,000 doulas would receive loans, scholarships, and programmatic support.
- About 46,000 maternal mental health and substance abuse professionals would receive loans, scholarships, and programmatic support (Taylor and Bernstein 2021).

The impact could stretch even more as investments in the social determinants of health, implicit bias training, technology, and diversifying the perinatal work force are also included. Through the package, also referred to as a social infrastructure package, policymakers and advocates also set their sights on expanding a number of other social supports including health care coverage, economic relief, child care, climate justice, and more (Taylor 2021). The goal was to pass the package through a special Senate process known as reconciliation, whereby a simple majority is required as opposed to 60 votes. While the package did pass in the House of Representatives on November 19, 2021 (Build Back Better Act 2021), it did not secure the support needed to pass in the Senate. As a result of many months of negotiations, the Build Back Better Act was replaced by the Inflation Reduction Act, which did not include the aforementioned historic investments in Black maternal health.

The Biden-Harris Administration has not waited for Congress to act in advancing maternal health equity through legislation. On December 7, 2021, Vice President Harris hosted the first-ever White House Maternal Health Day of Action Summit. In her remarks at the event, she stated, "On this Day of Action, may the women of our nation know: I hear you. We hear you. And we are here to take action" (The White House 2021). Vice President Harris has long championed the issue of Black maternal health—serving as a leader of the Black Maternal Health Caucus while she was a US Senator and introducing key maternal health legislation including the Maternal CARE Act, the first Black Maternal Health Week Resolution, and the Senate version of the Black Maternal Health Momnibus Act in 2020 (Black Maternal Health Momnibus Act 2020).

The White House Summit featured esteemed advocates and experts from across the country, as well as celebrities with their own stories to tell as related to challenges experienced in birth and delivery. Allyson Felix, US Olympian in track and field, shared her story in an armchair discussion with Vice President Harris. Allyson was diagnosed with severe preeclampsia when she was 32 weeks pregnant (CDC 2022). Allyson's physician acted quickly, and she was admitted to the hospital for an emergency cesarean delivery after close monitoring. Since then, Allyson has offered her voice to advocating for better maternal health care among Black women.

For Serena Williams, another prominent Black woman, her birthing and postpartum experience was quite different. Williams's husband, Alexis Ohanian, participated in the White House Maternal Health Day of Action Summit on a panel moderated by Senator Cory Booker. The panel centered the role of men as advocates for mothers during moments of distress in birth and delivery, as well as during the postpartum period. Serena and her husband have spoken candidly about the challenges she faced after expressing discomfort shortly after the birth of their daughter. Serena had warned her providers that she may be undergoing complications due to a pre-existing pulmonary embolism condition and was initially ignored (Lockhart 2018). This is a clear example of how medical racism shows up in Black women's health care experiences, regardless of socioeconomic status. After some back and forth, Serena's health care team was responsive to her needs. Unfortunately, many women are not afforded the same attention and have died needlessly because their health concerns were discounted.

The Biden-Harris administration also issued the first ever Presidential Proclamation in recognition of Black Maternal Health Week, approved Section 1115 waivers submitted by states to extend postpartum Medicaid coverage to one year, awarded funding to increase maternity care among rural populations and address substance use disorders among pregnant and postpartum women, and championed the need to address bias and discrimination in maternity care. Increased investments in maternal health and efforts to eliminate racial disparities continue to be announced by key federal agencies such as the Department of Health and Human Services and the Centers for Medicare and Medicaid Services. Furthermore, the federal government has released a national maternal health equity strategy outlining a whole-of-government approach to the Black maternal health crisis.

CONCLUSION

Black women at all levels of government and throughout the reproductive justice and maternal health fields have led national efforts to develop and advance the Black Maternal Health Momnibus Act. This leadership has been essential in shifting the policy landscape, which has progressed in a way that is doing more to center Black women's experiences in maternal health care as well as the thought leadership of Black women that has propelled the work forward. Black women will continue to be the stewards of our reproductive destinies. The question is, will the political will to address the burgeoning maternal health crisis that is rooted in racism and inequality follow suit? One thing is certain—Black women will not stop fighting until the battle for maternal health equity is won.

REFERENCES

Artiga S, Hinton E. Beyond health care: the role of social determinants in promoting health and health equity. Kaiser Family Foundation. May 10, 2018. Available at: https://www.kff.org/racial-equity-and-health-policy/issue-brief/beyond-health-care-the-role-of-social-determinants-in-promoting-health-and-health-equity

Aspen Institute. 11 terms you should know to better understand structural racism. July 11, 2016. Available at: https://www.aspeninstitute.org/blog-posts/structural-racism-definition

Black Mamas Matter Alliance. About us. 2020. Available at: https://blackmamasmatter.org/about

Black Maternal Health Caucus. About the Caucus. Available at: https://blackmaternalhealthcaucus-underwood.house.gov/about

Black Maternal Health Momnibus Act. HR 959, 117th Cong (2021-2022). February 8, 2021a. Available at: https://www.congress.gov/bill/117th-congress/house-bill/959/text

Black Maternal Health Momnibus Act. S 346, 117th Cong (2021-2022). February 22, 2021b. Available at: https://www.congress.gov/bill/117th-congress/senate-bill/346

Black Maternal Health Momnibus Act. S 1606, 118th Cong (2023-2024). May 15, 2023. Available at: https://www.congress.gov/bill/118th-congress/senate-bill/1606

Black Maternal Health Momnibus Act. S 3424, 116th Cong (2019-2020). 2020. Available at: https://www.congress.gov/bill/116th-congress/senate-bill/3424

Build Back Better Act. HR 5376, 117th Cong (2021-2022). September 27, 2021. Available at: https://www.congress.gov/bill/117th-congress/house-bill/5376?r=1&s=4

Center for Reproductive Rights. Reproductive injustice: racial and gender discrimination in US health care. 2014:6–40. Available at: https://www.reproductiverights.org/sites/crr.civicactions.net/files/documents/CERD_Shadow_US_6.30.14_Web.pdf

Centers for Disease Control and Prevention. The Syphilis Study at Tuskegee timeline. April 22, 2021. Available at: https://www.cdc.gov/tuskegee/timeline.htm

Centers for Disease Control and Prevention. Unexpected pregnancy complications: Allyson Felix's story. February 16, 2022. Available at: https://www.cdc.gov/hearher/allysonfelix/index.html

The Century Foundation. Black Maternal Health Federal Policy Collective. Available at: https://tcf.org/black-maternal-health-federal-policy-collective

The Century Foundation. The worsening US maternal health crisis in three graphs. March 2, 2022. Available at: https://tcf.org/content/commentary/worsening-u-s-maternal-health-crisis-three-graphs

Ellington S, Strid P, Tong VT, et al. Characteristics of women of reproductive age with laboratory-confirmed SARS-CoV-2 infection by pregnancy status—United States, January 22-June 7, 2020. *MMWR Morb Mortal Wkly Rep.* 2020;69(25):769–775. https://doi.org/10.15585/mmwr.mm6925a1

Hoyert DL. Maternal mortality rates in the United States, 2020. Centers for Disease Control and Prevention. February 23, 2022. Available at: https://www.cdc.gov/nchs/data/hestat/maternal-mortality/2020/maternal-mortality-rates-2020.htm

Lipscomb BN, Taylor JK, Dawes Gay E, et al. Advancing holistic maternal care for Black women through policy. Black Mamas Matter Alliance. December 2018:1–8. Available at: https://blackmamasmatter.org/wp-content/uploads/2018/12/BMMA-PolicyAgenda-Digital.pdf

Lockhart PR. What Serena Williams's scary childbirth story says about medical treatment of Black women. *Vox*. January 11, 2018. Available at: https://www.vox.com/identities/2018/1/11/16879984/serena-williams-childbirth-scare-black-women

Mun H, Morcelle M. State Momnibus bills take aim at the Black maternal mortality epidemic. National Health Law Program. May 6, 2021. Available at: https://healthlaw.org/state-momnibus-bills-take-aim-at-the-black-maternal-mortality-epidemic

Muse S, Dawes Gay E, Aina AD, et al. Setting the standard for holistic care of and for Black women. Black Mamas Matter Alliance. 2018:3–27. Available at: https://blackmamasmatter.org/wp-content/uploads/2018/04/BMMA_BlackPaper_April-2018.pdf

Purnell TS, Irving W, Irving S, et al. Honoring Dr. Shalon Irving, a champion for health equity. *Health Aff (Millwood)*. 2022;41(2):304–308. https://doi.org/10.1377/hlthaff.2021.01447

Ross L. What is reproductive justice? In: *Reproductive Justice Briefing Book: A Primer on Reproductive Justice and Social Change*. Berkeley Law. 2007: 4–5. Available at: https://www.law.berkeley.edu/php-programs/courses/fileDL.php?fID=4051

Taylor J. Advancing maternal health equity in the next reconciliation package. The Century Foundation. September 10, 2021. Available at: https://tcf.org/content/commentary/advancing-maternal-health-equity-next-reconciliation-package

Taylor J, Bernstein A. Four ways the Build Back Better Act could improve Black maternal health. The Century Foundation. October 20, 2021. Available at: https://tcf.org/content/commentary/four-ways-build-back-better-act-improve-black-maternal-health

Taylor J, Bernstein A. Tracking progress of the Black Maternal Health Momnibus. The Century Foundation. January 24, 2022. Available at: https://tcf.org/content/data/black-maternal-health-momnibus-tracker

Taylor J, Novoa C, Hamm K, Phadke S. Eliminating racial disparities in maternal and infant mortality. Center for American Progress. May 2, 2019. Available at: https://www.americanprogress.org/article/eliminating-racial-disparities-maternal-infant-mortality

Taylor JK. Structural racism and maternal health among Black Women. *J Law Med Ethics*. 2020;48(3):506–517. https://doi.org/10.1177/1073110520958875

Thompson TM, Young Y, Bass TM, et al. Racism runs through it: examining the sexual and reproductive health experience of Black women in the South. *Health Aff (Millwood)*. 2022;42(2):195–202. https://www.healthaffairs.org/doi/10.1377/hlthaff.2021.01422

US Congress. Maternal health. Available at: https://www.congress.gov/search?q=%7B%22source%22%3A%22legislation%22%2C%22search%22%3A%22maternal%22%7D&pageSize=100&page=1

The White House. Remarks by Vice President Harris at the Maternal Day of Action Summit. December 7, 2021. Available at: https://www.whitehouse.gov/briefing-room/statements-releases/2021/12/07/remarks-by-vice-president-harris-at-the-maternal-day-of-action-summit

Appendix III: From the Archives

- Ross L, Solinger R. *Reproductive Justice: An Introduction.* Oakland, CA: University of California Press; 2017. https://www.ucpress.edu/book/9780520288201/reproductive-justice

    The reproductive justice framework provided a radically different way to place reproductive health and rights in the context of the experiences of women of color and the struggle for equality, social justice, and human rights.... [Reproductive justice's] centering of women of color, social justice, and human rights provides a galvanizing moral reason for radical change and a concrete basis for building coalitions among organizations working toward a more humane society.... The world needs radical reproductive justice.

    –Dorothy Roberts (Ross 2017)

- Crenshaw K. Demarginalizing the intersection of race and sex: a Black feminist critique of antidiscrimination doctrine, feminist theory and antiracist politics. *Univ Chic Leg Forum.* 1989;1(8). https://chicagounbound.uchicago.edu/cgi/viewcontent.cgi?article=1052&context=uclf

In this landmark essay, Kimberlé Crenshaw introduced the term "intersectionality" to address the marginalization of Black women not only within antidiscrimination law but also within feminist and antiracist theory and politics. Intersectionality is an analytical framework that illuminates how systems of race, economic class, gender, sexuality, ethnicity, and age often operate together and exacerbate each other. These mutually constructing features of social organizations shape Black women's experiences and, in turn, are shaped by Black women.

- Roberts DE. *Killing the Black Body: Race, Reproduction, and the Meaning of Liberty.* New York, NY: Penguin Random House; 1997.

Dorothy Roberts analyzes the reproductive rights of Black women throughout US history. The book combines historical, sociological, and legal frameworks to examine how federal and state governments have infringed on Black women's bodies from slavery to the 1990s.

- Avery B, Barrow W, and Brazile D, et al. We remember: African American women for reproductive freedom. The National Council of Negro Women, Inc; 1989. https://birthequity.org/wp-content/uploads/2022/01/WeRememberBrochure-1.pdf

In the summer of 1989, a group of 16 Black women advocating for equal access to abortion made history by publishing this brochure. The collective statement laid out an 11-point definition of reproductive freedom, which originated from the belief that women should be empowered to make informed reproductive decisions and should be able to access affordable, high-quality contraceptive options and health care.

- Women of African Descent for Reproductive Justice. "Black Women on Health Care Reform." *Washington Post.* August 16, 1994. https://www.washingtonpost.com/nation/2019/08/16/reproductive-justice-how-women-color-asserted-their-voice-abortion-rights-movement

On August 16, 1994, Women of African Descent for Reproductive Justice published a historic full-page ad with more than 800 signatures in *The Washington Post* and *Roll Call*. The statement, addressed to Members of Congress, called for "the full range of reproductive services," including prenatal care; contraception; and screening and treatment for cancer, sexually transmitted diseases, and HIV/AIDS. The statement also asserted that health care reform "must include strong anti-discriminatory provisions to ensure the protection of all women of color, the elderly, the poor and those with disabilities. In addition, the plan must not discriminate on the basis of sexual orientation."

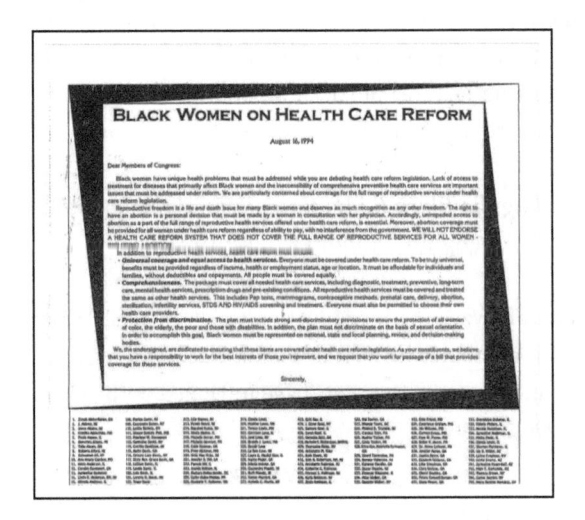

Source: Courtesy of Women of African Descent for Reproductive Justice. Reprinted with permission of Loretta Ross.

IV. RE-CENTERING HEALTH AND WELL-BEING: SETTING THE STANDARD FOR HOLISTIC SOLUTIONS

13

A Holistic Public Health Solution Approach to Reducing Maternal Mortality

Wendy C. Wilcox, MD, MPH, MBA, Maria J. Small, MD, MPH, and Sascha James-Conterelli, DNP

The United States has the worst maternal mortality rate among economically advantaged countries. According to the Centers for Disease Control and Prevention (CDC), the US maternal mortality ratio in 2020 was 23.8 per 100,000 live births (Hoyert 2022). The United States has more than twice the maternal mortality rates of France and Canada (those with the next highest maternal mortality rates of industrialized countries) and nearly eight times that of New Zealand, the nation with the lowest maternal mortality rate (Hoyert 2022). Further definition of maternal mortality rates and ratios will be discussed later in this chapter. The maternal mortality ratio in the United States has increased since 2005 to 2007. In 2018, the maternal mortality ratio in New York State was 18.2 deaths per 100,000 live births (New York City Department of Health and Mental Hygiene [NYC DOHMH] 2018).

Even more disturbing is the inequity in maternal deaths among Black women and American Indian or Alaska Native women, as compared to other racial groups. In the United States, Black women are about three times more likely to die during pregnancy than their white counterparts (New York State Department of Health [NYSDOH] 2022). In some communities, this inequity is even more stark. For example, in New York City, based on 2018 data, Black women were eight times more likely to die of a pregnancy-related death than white women (Petersen et al. 2019). In New York State during this same period of time, the disparity was five times more likely (NYC DOHMH 2018). One curious fact is that this disparity persists whether the state has a high overall maternal mortality rate or a low overall maternal mortality rate (Petersen et al. 2019).

The pregnancy-related maternal mortality ratio (PRMR) is the pregnancy-related maternal mortality rate, divided by the general fertility rate and expressed per 100,000 live births. In a study conducted by CDC, states were anonymously classified by PRMR and divided into three groups. One group contained those states with the lowest PRMR, next were those with a mid-range PRMR, and last were those with the highest PRMR. States with a low PRMR are considered high-performing (have the lowest number of maternal deaths) and states with a high PRMR are considered low performers (have the highest number of maternal deaths). The PRMR was then calculated by race/ethnicity (by the low, mid-range, and high groups) and the disparity ratios (comparisons of PRMR between two racial/ethnic groups) were calculated for each of the groups of states. The study findings showed that a disparity existed in each of the groupings. Even in states with a low pregnancy-related maternal mortality ratio (a.k.a. "high-performing states"), Black women had a PRMR three times higher than white women. This disparity was consistent across all three groupings (Petersen et al. 2019).

OUR STORY

The authors of this chapter are an obstetrician-gynecologist, a maternal fetal medicine (MFM) specialist, and a doctor of nursing practice in midwifery. As African American women, our interest in this subject represents more than a scientific or professional one. The women who have died during the pregnancy and postpartum period could be our sisters, daughters, friends, and patients. We acknowledge that all people who give birth do not identify as women, and, for the purposes of our discussion, we will use the words woman/women to signify all persons capable of giving birth. We are deeply committed, experienced senior leaders in maternal health, and we have a profound personal and professional commitment to solving this problem. In this chapter, we strive to get to the roots of the complex and multifactorial causes of the awful maternal mortality problem that persists in the United States. We propose solutions to address the racial inequities within our current health care system to enable a more affirming, patient-centered, racially and culturally centered approach.

ACKNOWLEDGMENT OF THE IMPACT OF THE LOSS

When discussing maternal mortality, it is important for the conversation not to become a discussion about rates and ratios. We must remember the pregnant women who have lost their lives during childbirth and preserve their stories. It is fundamentally important to stop and recognize the women who have died during childbirth and the pregnancy and postpartum periods. These women represent mothers, daughters, sisters, wives, aunts, and cousins. These women are members of our community and they are our patients. They leave behind grieving children, husbands, partners, and parents. Their loss is personal for us.

There is an intangible burden and a tangible burden to maternal mortality. The intangible burden is each woman's loss of participation in their families, community, and society. These women who have died are no longer able to sing in church, take their children to school, or care for elderly parents. There is no way to measure the profound impact of the loss of a mother on the lifetime of an orphaned child.

Additional individuals who are sometimes overlooked include the health care teams. These teams may have cared for the woman during her pregnancy, or they may encounter the woman when brought in for a sentinel event. Even when the team has no prior relationship with the woman, experiencing the loss of a reproductive-aged woman is often more than health care personnel can bear and can lead to long-term psychological trauma (Rivera-Chiauzzi et al. 2022).

Losing a woman of reproductive age has devastating consequences. There is also an economic burden of maternal mortality. Economic measures associated with maternal mortality increased by an estimated 30%, from 32,824 years of potential life lost and value of statistical life of $7.9 billion in 2018 to 43,131 years and $10.4 billion in 2020 (White et al. 2022).

DEFINITIONS OF MORTALITY DURING PREGNANCY

Maternal mortality as defined by the World Health Organization (WHO) is the death of woman during pregnancy or within 42 days of the termination of a pregnancy, irrespective of the duration or site of the pregnancy, from any cause related to or aggravated by the pregnancy or its management, but not from accidental or incidental causes. This same definition is used by the CDC National Vital Statistics system (NVSS). The NVSS was established in 1986 and reports the national mortality ratio, the number of maternal deaths per 100,000 live births. NVSS uses the number of maternal deaths while pregnant or within 42 days of the end of a pregnancy, from any cause related to or aggravated by the pregnancy or its management, but not from accidental or incidental causes (Hoyert 2022). This definition and timeframe are consistent with that used by WHO. The NVSS is what is used for international comparisons.

The WHO definition of maternal mortality allows for calculation of a maternal mortality rate and comparison to other countries (CDC 2023).

In 1986, CDC launched another system called the Pregnancy Mortality Surveillance System (PMSS) in collaboration with the American College of Obstetricians and Gynecologists (ACOG). The PMSS uses data collected for all women who died during a pregnancy or within one year of pregnancy from all 50 states; Washington, DC; and New York City. All of the information is summarized, and medically trained epidemiologists determine the cause of death and whether the death was pregnancy-related. *International Classification of Diseases,* Tenth Revision (ICD-10) codes are used to code cause of death. The data from PMSS help scientists and public health professionals understand trends and clinical causes of pregnancy-related deaths and propose actions to prevent them (Callaghan 2012).

A more intensive review of maternal deaths is the process that is used by maternal mortality review committees (MMRCs; CDC 2023). MMRCs use the following definitions when evaluating maternal deaths: Pregnancy-associated deaths are defined as all deaths that have a temporal relationship to pregnancy, but not necessarily causally related to pregnancy (CDC Foundation 2017). Pregnancy-associated deaths are further categorized based on whether they are a result of a pregnancy or not. Pregnancy-related death is death of a woman during pregnancy or within one year of the end of a pregnancy, due to a pregnancy complication or a chain of events initiated by a pregnancy. Pregnancy-associated but not related death is a death of a woman within one year of the end of a pregnancy due to a cause not related to the pregnancy (e.g., accidents, homicides; CDC Foundation 2017).

Similar to the PMSS, MMRCs allow for a more in-depth analysis of the cause of death, analysis of circumstances surrounding the death, and determination of cause, specifically whether the death is pregnancy-related or not. This is determined by a multidisciplinary group that includes clinical providers, community members, and patients or patient-care advocates, such as doulas (CDC Foundation 2017). It is a common misperception that the data curated by the MMRCs falsely elevates the reported maternal mortality rate for comparison purposes. This does not happen because, as stated earlier, the WHO definition is used for uniformity when comparing nations.

THE NEW YORK EXPERIENCE

In 2010, New York ranked 46th out of 50 states for maternal mortality (NYSDOH 2017). By 2018, New York ranked 23rd with a rate of 20.6 deaths per 100,000 births (NYSDOH 2022). Since 2010, a great deal of work has been done within the state by multiple stakeholders. During this period of time, ACOG District 2 launched two Safe Motherhood Initiatives (SMIs; ACOG, District 2 n.d.). The first SMI involved a small group of physicians performing maternal mortality reviews on a small number of maternal deaths. The second involved a greater number of clinicians from across New York State and over the course of a few years developed three clinical bundles focused on addressing the top causes of maternal mortality at that time. The three bundles addressed obstetric hemorrhage, severe hypertensive disorders of pregnancy, and thromboembolic disorders.

The New York State Department of Health was also active in this endeavor. It launched a committee on maternal mortality, which was focused on developing guidance to address severe hypertension in pregnancy, statewide guidelines for severe hypertension in pregnancy (with particular focus on educating emergency department providers), and reduction of non-medically indicated deliveries before 39 weeks gestation. New York City Department of Health and Mental Hygiene published two maternal mortality reports (NYC DOHMH n.d.-a; NYC DOHMH n.d.-b) and one report on severe maternal morbidity (NYC DOHMH 2018). Major hospital associations were also involved.

Despite improvement in overall maternal mortality, the Black-white disparity persisted. Black women are four times more likely to die of a pregnancy-related death than white, non-Hispanic women in New York State (NYSDOH 2022). In 2018, the New York State governor established the New York State Taskforce on Maternal Mortality and Disparate Racial Outcomes (New York State Taskforce on Maternal Mortality and Disparate Racial Outcomes 2019). The task force was comprised of obstetrics-gynecology and midwifery leaders, hospital representatives, government representatives, and other stakeholders who provided expert policy advice on improving maternal outcomes, addressing racial and economic disparities, and reducing the frequency of maternal mortality and morbidity in New York State. One of the primary recommendations of the task force was to establish a maternal mortality review board (NYC DOHMH 2018). In 2019, Public Health Law Section 2509 was enacted, establishing a state maternal mortality review board to review each pregnancy-associated death and issue a biennial report to the Commissioner of Health (NYSDOH 2022). Public Health Law Section 2509 also allows the city of New York to establish its own board. In New York State, pregnancy-associated death reviews are performed by two boards (a.k.a. committees), a New York State and New York City committee (NYSDOH 2022).

In 2022, New York State released its first report based on the 2018 cohort. Top-level findings from this report showed that more than half of pregnancy-associated deaths occurred between 43 days and 1 year after completion of a pregnancy. The leading causes of pregnancy-related deaths were thromboembolic events, hemorrhage, and mental health conditions. The top causes of pregnancy-associated events were mental health conditions, cardiovascular causes, and cancer (NYSDOH 2022). This differs from the US data, which showed that the top causes of pregnancy-related deaths in 2018 were other cardiovascular conditions, infection or sepsis, cardiomyopathy, and hemorrhage (CDC 2023).

CAUSAL FACTORS

In New York State, the early efforts to address maternal mortality focused on addressing the top clinical causes of maternal mortality, especially pregnancy-related maternal mortality. After these were addressed, maternal mortality was decreased in the state, but not the racial disparity. It soon became apparent that the state needed to investigate other potential causes of the maternal mortality disparity. For this reason, the Taskforce on Maternal Mortality and Disparate Racial Outcomes was created.

In this chapter, we examine the root causes that have led to the US crisis of maternal mortality. This includes both extrinsic and intrinsic causes. Extrinsic causes include anything external to the patient, including lack of quality care and the US history of racism and white supremacy influencing government and economic policy, which molded the origin story of the American medical system. Structural racism has continued to influence health care for Black and Brown people in America. Extrinsic causes also include interpersonal biases and conflict between the patient and her caretaker, which may lead to inadequate or incorrect care. Intrinsic causes include factors within the patient, and for that we apply the theory of weathering.

Lastly, we examine some of the efforts that have been made to respond to this problem, including clinical quality improvement, targeting the top causes of maternal mortality, programs to address racism and implicit bias, and focusing on increasing the diversity of clinical disciplines, such as increasing the number and racial/ethnic diversity of midwives in America. Efforts targeted directly to the patient including the maternal home, companion support (including doula support), and postpartum support utilizing community resources, such as support groups, community health workers, and nurse home visiting, are also examined. Last, we review efforts re-examining the composition of the health care team and the role of learners within health care, such as targeting teaching institutions to improve racial and ethnic diversity and utilizing teaching institutions as vessels to target curricula on respectful care, cultural humility, trauma-informed and resilient systems, and anti-racism.

Some Deep-Seated Truths

The United States was founded on the economic and cultural backbone of slavery (Sublette and Sublette 2017). Starting in 1619, Blacks were brought to the Americas on slave ships to work in death camps (Schwartz 2010). The African diaspora included North, Central, and South America and the Caribbean. As the United States came into being, the concept of "whiteness" was born out of Anglo-Saxon Protestantism and as other immigrants moved to the states. Whiteness became a means to consolidate power and subjugate slaves. Certainly, health care was rendered only so far as it protected the property and financial investment of the slave owner. On December 14, 1711, a law was passed by the New York Common Council that made Wall Street the city's first official slave market for the sale and rental of enslaved Africans and Native Americans (Sublette and Sublette 2017). The bond market also grew from the sale of slaves.

Women and children were especially vulnerable under the conditions of slavery. As a consequence, during slavery, infant mortality reached as high as 50% (Steckel 1986). After the African slave trade was banned in 1808, breeding of slaves became lucrative. In fact, some would argue that one of the reasons why African slavery was banned was to make the existing slaves in America a more valued commodity. Breeding of slaves became an industry unto itself. For instance, the economies of Maryland and Virginia depended on breeding slaves (Beckert and Rockman 2016).

As breeding plantations grew, the profession of obstetrics and gynecology became more refined. James Marion Sims, once touted as the "father of gynecology," performed experiments in an especially grotesque fashion on enslaved women who could not say "no." One such patient contracted blood poisoning, and another who had more than 30 operations for vaginal fistula repair eventually died of complications. During his operations, Sims did not use anesthesia, and the surgeries were conducted with the women being naked on their knees, bent forward over on their elbows with an onslaught of onlookers. Sims acknowledged the advantage of being able to operate on people who were his property: "There was never a time that I could not, at any day, have had a subject for operation" (Sims 1884).

François Marie Prevost, a slave-holding surgeon, pioneered cesarean section surgeries using enslaved women's bodies to perfect the technique (Owens and Fett 2019). Samuel Cartwright, a southern physician, claimed to have found a disease called "drapetomania," a "mental illness" that causes enslaved Africans to run away from their confinement. He argued that it could be prevented by keeping Black people in submission and could be cured by whippings. Cartwright also described "dysaesthesia aethiopica," a "disease" in Black people characterized by reduced intellectual ability, laziness, and partial insensitivity of the skin (Willoughby 2018).

There are many other examples of cruel and inhumane treatment of enslaved people and/or Blacks during the Jim Crow Era at the hands of white doctors. Until the 1960s, racial segregation was common. Separate was not equal, and segregation took on many forms. There was discrimination in all facets of health care, including in nursing, medical, and midwifery schools. There was also discrimination in professional societies, including the American Medical Association, American Nursing Association, and the American College of Nurse Midwives.

It is little wonder how the aforementioned experimentation and treatment may still have influence on the present-day medical system and why racism is determined to be a root cause of the disparity we see today in maternal mortality. According to Bassett (2022), "Racism is not simply the result of private prejudices held by individuals, but is also produced and reproduced by laws, rules, and practices, sanctioned and even implemented by various levels of government, and embedded in the economic system as well as in cultural and societal norms." An ongoing count by the *Washington Post* estimates 1,800 Congressmen once enslaved Black people (Bailey, Feldman, and Bassett 2021).

Systemic racist policies, such as the 1933 federal government-founded Home Owners Loan Corporation, which drew red lines around communities with large Black populations and flagged them as hazardous areas where Blacks would not receive loans, influence the health disparity maps we see today. Black communities were deemed unworthy of investment. Decreased property taxes (the way schools and other municipal projects are often funded) in communities where Black people live further drive the lack of investment in infrastructure, hospitals, schools, parks, and grocery stores or investment in the wrong kinds of influences, such as pollution-driving entities including bus depots, sanitation depots, sewage treatment plants, and landfills. Social determinants of health (SDOH), such as economic stability, physical environment, food, housing, education, and the health care system, are driven by economic and public policy developed over time and have lasting effects that remain evident (Bailey, Feldman, and Bassett 2021).

Another way in which racism has impacted the health of African Americans can be explained by a process called weathering. First introduced in a study by Geronimus in 1992 to investigate infant outcomes, the weathering hypothesis proposed that the health of African American women may begin to deteriorate in early adulthood as a physical consequence to socioeconomic disadvantage.

One such study that has examined and supported the weathering hypothesis is the Coronary Artery Risk Development in Young Adults (CARDIA) study (Forrester 2018). This large, population-based, observational, multicenter study was extended to 30 years and enrolled 5,114 Black and white individuals from four cities across the United States. The study began enrolling individuals between 1985 and 1986 and enrolled participants who were free from disease. The study participants were stratified almost equally between Black and white individuals, men and women, ages 18 to 23 years and 24 to 30 years, higher socioeconomic status and lower socioeconomic status. The hypothesis of the CARDIA study is that biologic age (BA) is a construct that captures accelerated biological aging attributable to "wear and tear" from various exposures. Weathering, by definition, is the difference between BA and chronological age, and these variables' associations with race and psychosocial factors were studied in a middle-aged biracial cohort.

Assessments occurred at years 2, 5, 7, and 10 and then at five-year intervals. The study examined seven different biomarkers, health behaviors such as alcohol and tobacco consumption, socioeconomic status, symptoms of depression, discrimination, and social participation. The findings from the CARDIA study were nothing less than profound. Blacks weathered by approximately six years more than whites. Blacks had a mean BA of 57.1 years while whites had a mean BA of 52.3 years. Mean weathering for Blacks was 2.6 years and −3.5 years for whites. At year 30, Blacks had a mean BA that was older than their mean chronological age, whereas the opposite was seen in whites. The weathering hypothesis has a larger implication than that originally proposed by Geronimus and provides a partial explanation for the increased rate of Black maternal deaths. The trend of maternal mortality rates increases sharply with age. In the United States in 2019, the rate for women aged 40 years and older was 7.8 times higher than the rate for women aged younger than 25 years (Hoyert 2022).

A MULTISOLUTION APPROACH

Due to the multifactorial nature of maternal mortality and the reasons why Black women are more severely impacted, a multisolution approach is also in order. The solutions will need to be patient-centric, racially conscious, and culturally humble.

Legislation

Federal and state legislation is needed to help promote a healthy pregnancy and postnatal care. Bills such as the Black Maternal Health Momnibus Act (2021) would direct multiagency efforts to improve maternal health, particularly among racial and ethnic minority groups, veterans, and other vulnerable populations. In addition, the United States is in a very unique minority of countries in that it does not offer or mandate states to offer paid pregnancy benefits. Access to paid maternity leave is particularly salient because, just as a woman is recuperating from the childbirth process and possibly initiating breastfeeding, she must think about when to return to work. Paid pregnancy benefits can help women meet their personal and family health care needs while also fulfilling work responsibilities.

Integrated Care

Medical care can be very siloed, placing an extra strain on the person seeking care, as well as unconducive to improved communication among members of the health care team. There are innovative programs that seek to offer integrated care, which means bringing together multiple disciplines in one place to provide care to pregnant persons in a centralized fashion. One such program is the maternal home.

The maternal home incorporates two important frameworks: the socio-ecological model, which illustrates a patient's interaction with their environment through enhanced resources and self-efficacy, and the sociocultural model, which encourages effective use of and accessibility to resources through a social justice and equity lens (Salihu 2015; Chirkov 2020). The maternal home models the care principles of the patient-centered medical home that provide comprehensive services to birthing persons without insurance restrictions or any medical or mental health qualifiers. Eliminating eligibility barriers provides an equitable foundation for any birthing person to receive the support they need—a distinguishing factor from the few other similar prenatal care coordination programs across the country (Institute for Healthcare Improvement 2016).

The maternal home uses maternal care coordinators and social workers to provide enhanced, wrap-around services for individuals who have any medical, behavioral, or SDOH needs that may lead to adverse pregnancy outcomes. Medical interventions may include assistance with managing pregnancy-related complications such as gestational diabetes or adherence to medication. Behavioral interventions may include providing interim supportive counseling while a patient awaits a mental health appointment or reviewing stress management strategies. SDOH interventions include providing social support to a patient who has little to no local support or using evidence-based tools to screen for intimate partner violence, alcohol or drug use, and trauma. Additional SDOH interventions include arranging transportation and connecting patients with housing programs, English-learning programs, childbirth education and resources, and parenting support.

New York City Health + Hospitals has implemented a maternal home in its 11 acute care facilities (NYC Health + Hospitals 2021). Patients who seek prenatal care are screened using standardized, evidence-based questionnaires and assigned a risk tier. Patients at moderate to high risk are kept in the maternal home where they receive coordination of care, extra support, and follow-up, as well as referrals to care, such as the Special Supplemental Nutrition Program for Women, Infants, and Children (WIC); the Supplemental Nutrition Assistance Program (SNAP); housing; doula services; mental health services; nurse-family partnership; and lactation services. There are other examples of medical homes across the United States, some of which have a particular aim, such as preventing preterm delivery or treating patients with substance abuse.

Another approach to using an integrated care model is one that addresses two-generation care for the mother and child. The 3-2-1 Integrated Model for Parents and Children Together (IMPACT) is a program pilot offered by NYC Health + Hospitals and aims to prevent two-generational trauma by providing enhanced support during the prenatal period, addressing any mental health concerns, and then continuing to provide these supports, in addition to using evidence-based parenting skills, throughout pediatric care to the entire family (NYC Health + Hospitals 2020). The 3-2-1 IMPACT program integrates three disciplines—mental health, pediatrics, and women's health—to deliver a two-generation approach that treats children and parents with one goal: to improve the long-term health trajectory for each family unit. Support that is started in the prenatal period transitions from prenatal to postpartum care for both the mother and child to ensure the new parent continues to have the support they need to safely care for the infant and to encourage the best environment in which to raise a child.

Midwifery Care

Midwifery has existed since early documented times: "And so it was, as she had a very hard time in her childbearing, that the *midwife* was saying to her, 'Do not be afraid, because this one is also a son for you [emphasis added]'" (Gen. 35:16-18). Although there is significant documentation of the works of midwives, midwives were first documented in America in 1619. Early American settlers bought their own midwives, and birth practices passed down through ancestors and seniors within the community. The majority of midwives were enslaved Africans providing primary, prenatal, postpartum, and pediatric care to families regardless of race or religion. The majority of births were attended by a midwife. By the late 20th century, the profession of obstetrics and gynecology was introduced to the United States by white privileged males seeking to move birth from the community to the hospital setting. "The Midwife Problem" was published and initiated a campaign to eliminate Black midwives, resulting in a steady decline in midwifery presence in the United States (Bowdoin 1928). Four nurses, Carolyn Conant van Blarcom, Lillian Wald, Mary Beard, and Mary Breckenridge actively joined the campaign to eliminate immigrant midwives in hopes of decreasing maternal and infant mortality and combining public health nursing with midwifery to establish a new profession of "nurse-midwifery."

After the elimination of the majority of Black, Indigenous, and immigrant midwives, white nurses took over the profession (American College of Nurse-Midwives [ACNM] 2021). Midwifery was re-envisioned through nursing and explicitly excluded Black midwives. Today, only 2% of the recorded midwives in the United States identify as Black. Recently, ACNM published a statement acknowledging the dark history of the profession and the continued devastating effects (ACNM 2021). Currently, midwives provide the majority of care for birthing families globally (Sandall et al. 2016). For example, in Japan, Finland, Germany, and the United Kingdom, all women and birthing people have access to midwifery care. Interestingly, all of these countries also have very low maternal mortality rates. Unfortunately, the majority of Americans do not have access to midwifery care despite the US having the highest rate of maternal mortality among all developed nations. In 2020, midwives attended roughly 10% of births in the United States (ACNM 2022).

The inclusion of midwifery care has been well documented to improve birth outcomes. In the 2014 *Lancet* Series on Midwifery, midwifery care demonstrated an improvement in birth outcomes and an increase in patient satisfaction (ten Hoope-Bender 2014). The traditional holistic approach that defines midwifery care naturally addresses SDOH, identifying each person as an individual as well as a member of a larger community. ACOG and the ACNM developed a joint statement on practice relationships. It states, "Ob-gyns and CNMs/CMs are experts in their respective fields of practice and are educated, trained, and licensed independent clinicians who collaborate depending on the needs of their patients" (ACOG and ACNM 2011). The physician-midwife collaborative care model enhances the care for women and birthing people throughout the lifespan. As nationally certified independent practitioners with expertise in normal physiologic development and care for women and birthing people, midwives are an essential contribution in all settings of patient care. Homer et al. estimate that more than 80% of maternal deaths in the United States may be avoided with an increase in midwifery (Homer et al. 2014). Midwives are frequently cited as key to addressing the US maternal mortality crisis (White House 2022). While an increase in the midwifery workforce will increase client access to midwifery care in the United States, what is truly needed to address the inequities in health care is an increase in Black providers, including Black midwives.

Specialty Obstetric Care

It is important for individuals with higher-risk pregnancy conditions to deliver in the appropriate level of care facility, with providers that have a team-based approach to care. This care team should include a full spectrum of health care providers, inclusive of a maternal fetal medicine specialist, high-risk obstetrics provider, and other subspecialists required to reduce the risk for maternal morbidity and mortality (American Association of Birth Centers et al. 2019). In the United States, states with higher densities of MFM providers have lower statewide maternal mortality ratios (Sullivan 2005). MFM providers are known to practice in systems of care with hospitals and teams of other specialists. Recognition of the appropriate level of hospital for maternity care for women, as well as reducing barriers to accessing those institutions, is a key component of best practice.

The regionalization of these specialty care facilities, clear identification of appropriate levels of maternal care, and policies that facilitate access to them is essential to enabling individuals to remain in or close to their communities and social supports (American Association of Birth Centers et al. 2019). Recommendations for optimal maternal cardiac care highlight the necessity for comprehensive, specialty obstetric care models. In the United States, cardiovascular disease (CVD) is the leading cause of pregnancy-related deaths, with death occurring either during the pregnancy or in the postpartum period (CDC 2023). Acquired heart disease is the driver of the increase in CVD-related maternal deaths (ACOG's Presidential Task Force on Pregnancy and Heart Disease and Committee on Practice Bulletins 2019). Black women have a 3.4-times higher risk for CVD-related death compared to non-Hispanic white women. Key recommendations include screening women before pregnancy for high-risk cardiac disease (when possible), as well as forming care teams that include MFM, cardiology, primary care, and social work, including care navigators to ensure individuals are able to access regional health centers.

Another key component of the model is paying particular attention to the postpartum period when care should focus on ongoing, multidisciplinary support for future pregnancy goals and reduction of risk related to cardiac disease including weight and stress management (Mehta et al. 2021). Survivors of preeclampsia experience a two-fold increased risk for CVD within three to five years of delivery. It is known that the cardiac changes from preeclampsia may persist and contribute to future cardiac dysfunction for several months postpartum and beyond (Johnson and Louis 2022). Attendance for the traditional postpartum visit is typically low. Understanding that while mothers may not have time for traditional self-care visits, they do not miss pediatric visits; this prompts initiatives to support maternal/child care in the pediatrician visit by adding care coordination (such as that in the maternal home) or coupling the postpartum and newborn visits so that mom and baby may both receive clinical attention. Also, home care follow-up, providing blood pressure cuffs, and access to telehealth visits and text messages are other ways to ensure maternal health needs are attended to during this critical period.

The cardiac model clearly demonstrates the key association between structural racism, health outcomes such as preeclampsia (Johnson and Louis 2022), and the need for comprehensive care. Food deserts and neighborhoods devoid of safe and clean air, water, and exercise space has been associated with communities populated by Black and Brown people, and the systemic lack of investment in these communities has led to a direct correlation with health disparities (Bassett 2022). Similarly, the lack of investment in these communities correlates with unequal access to mental health and health care facilities (Bailey et al. 2021). There are also increased rates of smoking, substance abuse, asthma, hypertension, cardiac disease, obesity, and other health inequities. Hypertensive disorders of pregnancy, such as severe preeclampsia, occur more frequently in the setting of obesity. These pregnancy-related conditions result in vascular remodeling that may lead to long-term cardiovascular disease. This cycle of adverse maternal health outcomes is directly related to structural inequities and is further exacerbated by mental health stressors, a known mediator of cardiovascular disease (National Academies of Sciences, Engineering, and Medicine 2022).

Partner Support

A high-quality, supportive partner relationship may also contribute to improved maternal and infant well-being postpartum, indicating a potential role for partner relationships in mental health interventions, with possible benefits for infants as well (Stapleton et al. 2012). Pregnant women with involved partners have been found to be more likely to receive early and more regular prenatal care and reduce cigarette smoking (Padilla and Reichman 2001; Teitler 2001). Fathers have also been found to reduce maternal stress (Ghosh et al. 2010). A qualitative study of Black mothers and fathers participating in a National Healthy Start conference acknowledged the importance of engaging fathers no matter the pattern of family formation (Alio et al. 2013). Interventions should take advantage of the prenatal period during which expectant partners, like mothers, are particularly open to advice, support, and information (Bond et al. 2010). Health care providers can play a greater role in promoting more "father-friendly" practices in preconception, prenatal, intrapartum, and postpartum/interconception care (Bond et al. 2010).

CONCLUSION

In this chapter, we have examined US history and how that has impacted the current state of maternal mortality in the United States, as well as the higher rate of maternal mortality for Black women. We explored multiple factors that led to inequity, including structural racism and environmental factors, such as a lifetime of stress and interpersonal factors that may manifest in intrinsic factors causing accelerated aging and other health-related disorders: the weathering hypothesis. We have also explored how weathering may affect maternal health and maternal mortality. We have proposed a few examples of holistic, patient-centered approaches, some of which involve breaking health silos and introducing integrated care strategies to improve care models. We have also discussed multidisciplinary care, including nurse-midwives and MFM specialists. It is our belief that it will take all of these types of strategies and more, as well as significant investment of resources, to combat and overcome the centuries of subjugation and mistreatment that have caused the outcomes that we see in maternal health today.

REFERENCES

Alio AP, Lewis CA, Scarborough K, Harris K, Fiscella K. A community perspective on the role of fathers during pregnancy: a qualitative study. *BMC Pregnancy Childbirth*. 2013;13(1):60. https://doi.org/10.1186/1471-2393-13-60

American Association of Birth Centers; American College of Nurse-Midwives; Association of Women's Health, Obstetric and Neonatal Nurses; et al. Obstetric care consensus #9: levels of maternal care (replaces obstetric care consensus number 2, February 2015). *Am J Obstet Gynecol*. 2019;221(6):B19–B30. https://doi.org/10.1016/j.ajog.2019.05.046

American College of Nurse-Midwives. Essential facts about midwives. April 2022. Available at: https://www.midwife.org/acnm/files/cclibraryfiles/filename/000000008273/EssentialFactsAboutMidwives_Final_2022.pdf

American College of Nurse-Midwives. Truth and reconciliation resolution from the American College of Nurse-Midwives. March 2021. Available at: https://www.midwife.org/acnm/files/cclibraryfiles/filename/000000008214/ACNM_Truth_and_Reconciliation_Resolution-2021.pdf

American College of Obstetricians and Gynecologists, American College of Nurse-Midwives. Joint statement of practice relations between obstetrician-gynecologists and certified nurse-midwives/certified midwives. February 2011. Available at: https://midwife.org/ACNM/files/ACNMLibraryData/UPLOADFILENAME/000000000224/ACNM-College-Policy-Statement-(June-2018).pdf

American College of Obstetricians and Gynecologists, District 2. Safe motherhood initiative. n.d. Available at: https://www.acog.org/community/districts-and-sections/district-ii/programs-and-resources/safe-motherhood-initiative

American College of Obstetricians and Gynecologists' Presidential Task Force on Pregnancy and Heart Disease and Committee on Practice Bulletins—Obstetrics. ACOG practice bulletin no. 212: pregnancy and heart disease. *Obstet Gynecol*. 2019;133(5):e320–e356. https://doi.org/10.1097/AOG.0000000000003243

Bailey ZD, Feldman JM, Bassett MT. How structural racism works—racist policies as a root cause of US racial health inequities. *N Engl J Med*. 2021;384(8):768–773. https://doi.org/10.1056/NEJMms2025396

Bassett MT. Tackling structural racism. *J Public Health Manag Pract*. 2022;28(suppl 1):S1–S2. https://doi.org/10.1097/PHH.0000000000001457

Beckert S, Rockman S. *Slavery's Capitalism: A New History of American Economic Development*. Philadelphia, PA: University of Pennsylvania Press; 2016.

Black Maternal Health Momnibus Act of 2021, HR 959, 117th Congress. Library of Congress. April 23, 2021. Available at: https://www.congress.gov/bill/117th-congress/house-bill/959

Bond MJ, Heidelbaugh JJ, Robertson A, Alio PA, Parker WJ. Improving research, policy and practice to promote paternal involvement in pregnancy outcomes: the roles of obstetricians–gynecologists. *Curr Opin Obstet Gynecol.* 2010;22(6):525–529. https://doi.org/10.1097/GCO.0b013e3283404e1e

Bowdoin J. The midwife problem. *JAMA.* 1928;91:460–462.

Callaghan WM. Overview of maternal mortality in the United States. *Semin Perinatol.* 2012;36(1):2–6. https://doi.org/10.1053/j.semperi.2011.09.002

Centers for Disease Control and Prevention. Pregnancy Mortality Surveillance System. US Department of Health and Human Services. 2023. Available at: https://www.cdc.gov/reproductivehealth/maternal-mortality/pregnancy-mortality-surveillance-system.htm#about-pmss

Centers for Disease Control and Prevention Foundation. Report from maternal mortality review committees: a view into their critical role. 2017. Available at: https://www.cdcfoundation.org/sites/default/files/upload/pdf/MMRIAReport.pdf

Chirkov V. An introduction to the theory of sociocultural models. *Asian J Soc Psychol.* 2020;23(2):143–162. https://doi.org/10.1111/ajsp.12381

Forrester S, Jacobs D, Zmora R, Schreiner P, Roger V, Kiefe CI. Racial differences in weathering and its associations with psychosocial stress: the CARDIA study. *SSM Popul Health.* 2018;7:003–3. https://doi.org/10.1016/j.ssmph.2018.11.003

Geronimus AT. The weathering hypothesis and the health of African-American women and infants: evidence and speculations. *Ethn Dis.* 1992;2(3):207–221.

Ghosh JK, Wilhelm MH, Dunkel-Schetter C, Lombardi CA, Ritz BR. Paternal support and preterm birth, and the moderation of effects of chronic stress: a study in Los Angeles County mothers. *Arch Womens Ment Health.* 2010;13(4):327–338. https://doi.org/10.1007/s00737-009-0135-9

Homer CS, Friberg IK, Dias MA, et al. The projected effect of scaling up midwifery [erratum in: Lancet. 2014;384(9948):1098]. *Lancet.* 2014;384(9948):1146–1157. https://doi.org/10.1016/S0140-6736(14)60790-X

Hoyert DL. Maternal mortality rates in the United States, 2020. NCHS Health E-Stats. Centers for Disease Control and Prevention. February 22, 2022. Available at: https://www.cdc.gov/nchs/data/hestat/maternal-mortality/2020/maternal-mortality-rates-2020.htm

Institute for Healthcare Improvement. The maternity medical home: the chassis for a more holistic model of pregnancy care? 2016. Available at: https://www.ihi.org/communities/blogs/_layouts/15/ihi/community/blog/itemview.aspx?List=7d1126ec-8f63-4a3b-9926-c44ea3036813&ID=222

Johnson JD, Louis JM. Does race or ethnicity play a role in the origin, pathophysiology and outcomes of preeclampsia? An expert review of literature. *Am J Obstet Gynecol.* 2022;226(2):S876–S885. https://doi.org/10.1016/j.ajog.2020.07.038

Mehta L, Sharma G, Creanga A, et al. Call to action: maternal health and saving mothers: a policy statement from the American Heart Association. *Circulation.* 2021;144(15):e251–e269. https://doi.org/10.1161/CIR.0000000000001000

National Academies of Sciences, Engineering, and Medicine; Health and Medicine Division; Food and Nutrition Board; Roundtable on Obesity Solutions. *Addressing Structural Racism, Bias and Health Communication as Foundational Drivers of Obesity: Proceedings of a Workshop Series.* Washington, DC: The National Academies Press; 2022. https://doi.org/10.17226/26437

New York City Department of Health and Mental Hygiene. New York City, 2008-2012, severe maternal morbidity. 2018. Available at: https://www.nyc.gov/assets/doh/downloads/pdf/data/maternal-morbidity-report-08-12.pdf

New York City Department of Health and Mental Hygiene. Pregnancy associated mortality New York City 2001-2005. n.d.-a. Available at: https://www.cmqcc.org/resource/2178/download

New York City Department of Health and Mental Hygiene. Pregnancy associated mortality New York City 2006-2010. n.d.-b. https://www1.nyc.gov/assets/doh/downloads/pdf/ms/pregnancy-associated-mortality-report.pdf

New York City Department of Health and Mental Hygiene. The state of doula care in New York City 2019. City of New York. November 19, 2018. Available at: https://www1.nyc.gov/assets/doh/downloads/pdf/csi/doula-report-2019.pdf

New York State Department of Health. New York State maternal mortality review report. 2017. Available at: https://www.health.ny.gov/community/adults/women/docs/maternal_mortality_review_2012-2013.pdf

New York State Department of Health. New York State maternal mortality review report on pregnancy-associated deaths in 2018. 2022. Available at: https://www.health.ny.gov/community/adults/women/docs/maternal_mortality_review_2018.pdf

New York State Taskforce on Maternal Mortality and Disparate Racial Outcomes. Recommendations to the governor to reduce maternal mortality and racial disparities. 2019. Available at: https://www.health.ny.gov/community/adults/women/task_force_maternal_mortality/docs/maternal_mortality_report.pdf

NYC Health + Hospitals. NYC Health + Hospitals announces Maternal Medical Home program. May 10, 2021. Available at: https://www.nychealthandhospitals.org/pressrelease/maternal-medical-home-program-provides-wraparound-care-services-to-pregnant-patients

NYC Health + Hospitals. System launches 3-2-1 IMPACT program; provides early intervention services to families. December 9, 2020. Available at: https://www.nychealthandhospitals.org/pressrelease/system-launches-3-2-1-impact-program-provides-early-intervention-services-to-families

Owens DC, Fett SM. Black maternal and infant health: historical legacies of slavery. *Am J Public Health*. 2019;109(10):1342–1345. https://doi.org/10.2105/ajph.2019.305243

Padilla YC, Reichman NE. Low birthweight: do unwed fathers help? *Child Youth Serv Rev*. 2001;23(4-5):427–452. https://doi.org/10.1016/S0190-7409(01)00136-0

Petersen EE, Davis NL, Goodman D, et al. Racial/ethnic disparities in pregnancy-related deaths—United States, 2007–2016. *MMWR Morb Mortal Wkly Rep*. 2019;68(35):762–765. https://dx.doi.org/10.15585/mmwr.mm6835a3

Rivera-Chiauzzi E, Finney RE, Riggan KA, et al. Understanding the second victim experience among multidisciplinary providers in obstetrics and gynecology. *J Patient Saf*. 2022;18(2):e463–e469. https://doi.org/10.1097/PTS.0000000000000850

Salihu HM, Wilson RE, King LM, Marty PJ, Whiteman VE. Socio-ecological model as a framework for overcoming barriers and challenges in randomized control trials in minority and underserved communities. *Int J MCH AIDS*. 2015;3(1):85–95.

Sandall J, Soltani H, Gates S, Shennan A, Devane D. Midwife-led continuity models versus other models of care for childbearing women. *Cochrane Database Syst Rev.* 2016;4(4):CD004667. https://doi.org/10.1002/14651858.CD004667.pub5

Schwartz MJ. *Birthing a Slave: Motherhood and Medicine in the Antebellum South.* 1st ed. Cambridge, MA: Harvard University Press; 2010.

Sims JM. *The Story of My Life.* New York, NY: D. Appleton and Co; 1884.

Stapleton LR, Schetter CD, Westling E, et al. Perceived partner support in pregnancy predicts lower maternal and infant distress. *J Fam Psychol.* 2012;26(3):453–463. https://doi.org/10.1037/a0028332

Steckel RH. A dreadful childhood: the excess mortality of American slaves. *Soc Sci Hist.* 1986;10(4):427–465. https://doi.org/10.2307/1171026

Sublette N, Sublette C. *The American Slave Coast: A History of the Slave-Breeding Industry.* Reprinted. Chicago, IL: Lawrence Hill Books; 2017.

Sullivan SA, Hill EG, Newman RB, Menard MK. Maternal-fetal medicine specialist density is inversely associated with maternal mortality ratios. *Am J Obstet Gynecol.* 2005;193(3 pt 2):1083–1088. https://doi.org/10.1016/j.ajog.2005.05.085

Teitler JO. Father involvement, child health and maternal health behavior. *Child Youth Serv Rev.* 2001;23(4/5):403–425. https://doi.org/10.1016/S0190-7409(01)00137-2

ten Hoope-Bender P, de Bernis L, Campbell J, et al. Improvement of maternal and newborn health through midwifery. *Lancet.* 2014;384(9949):1226–1235. https://doi.org/10.1016/S0140-6736(14)60930-2

The White House. White House blueprint for addressing the maternal health crisis. June 2022. Available at: https://www.whitehouse.gov/wp-content/uploads/2022/06/Maternal-Health-Blueprint.pdf

White RS, Lui B, Bryant-Huppert J, Chaturvedi R, Hoyler M, Aaronson J. Economic burden of maternal mortality in the USA, 2018–2020. *J Comp Eff Res.* 2022;11(13):927–933. https://doi.org/10.2217/cer-2022-0056

Willoughby CD. Running away from drapetomania: Samuel A. Cartwright, medicine, and race in the antebellum South. *J South Hist.* 2018;84(3):579–614. https://doi.org/10.1353/soh.2018.0164

14

Perinatal Safety, Midwifery Model Care, and Public Health: Delivering Optimal Outcomes at the Intersection

Jennie Joseph, LM, Claudia Tillman, PhD, MA, Kendra Ippel, MS, Aurora Sullivan, MPH, and Deanna J. Wathington, MD, MPH

Midwifery was the standard of perinatal care during the 19th century and the unfailing backbone of the community birth infrastructure. Due to "medical advances" and emerging predominance of the medical/surgical approach, a shift occurred from the midwifery model to the medical model (Brodsky 2008; Rooks 2014). This resulted in more interventions; more surgery; eventually rising, not falling, mortality and morbidity rates; and a distinct increase in disparate outcomes that remain in the 21st century, particularly by race/ethnicity. This plight is ostensibly and consistently noticeable in the United States, given many other countries still utilize a midwifery or community-based perinatal care approach.

In the United States, the most developed nation in the world, women and babies are dying from pregnancy-related causes. Although many of these deaths are preventable, the overall maternal mortality rate continues to rise and clearly underscores the persistent and historical reality that deep racial disparities remain. The Centers for Disease Control and Prevention (CDC) reported that the 2018 maternal mortality rate was 17.4 per 100,000 live births in the United States. According to the most recent CDC Pregnancy Mortality Surveillance System data, pregnancy-related mortality from 2014 to 2017 shows "wide racial and ethnic gaps exist between Black (47.1 deaths per 100,000 live births), white (13.4), and Hispanic (11.6) women" (CDC 2022).

Nearly 3 million women live in counties with no hospitals offering obstetric care, and 6.9 million women live in counties with limited access to perinatal care or services. Furthermore, a correlation between higher rates of positive birth outcomes such as vaginal delivery, and lower rates of undesirable outcomes including cesarean deliveries, preterm birth, low birth weight, and neonatal death have been found in areas where perinatal health workers (e.g., midwives, doulas, community health workers) provide care (March of Dimes 2022). Given these facts, we posit the following questions: Could it be possible that creating a **culture** and **environment** that supports *all* pregnant people could make the difference in health, safety, gestational age, birth weight, and breastfeeding rates in women at risk for poor maternal health outcomes in the United States? How can we achieve this public health priority within our current maternal-child health system? And, above all, who do we need to help achieve this goal?

Public health and midwifery care have had a long, yet perhaps unacknowledged, negative relationship in the United States when it comes to the safety of childbearing people, particularly those of color. Historically, women of African descent, Indigenous and immigrant women, and those who depended on and have thrived due to the protective practice of midwifery have been left behind as the uncompromising and purposeful eradication of midwives in the United States began in the early 20th century (Dawley 2000). Led by a new public health mandate that was monetized and organized by the federal government (the Sheppard-Towner Act of 1921) and women's new-found voting power, the slow, intentional decimation of community-based midwifery and the community birth infrastructure that had upheld public safety for centuries was endorsed (American College of Nurse-Midwives 2021).

This chapter addresses a "new" application of the midwifery model of care, one that embraces public health and social justice while also scaling the utilization of community-based perinatal providers. We call for rebuilding and re-investment in the community birth infrastructure comprising midwives, perinatal doulas, maternal-child health (MCH) community health workers, perinatal health educators, and other allied perinatal care providers including mental health professionals. Through our programs, we operationalize perinatal safety and invest in perinatal equity by creating Perinatal Safe Spots in what we have termed **materno-toxic zones** throughout the United States. These areas are geographical yet may also pop up anywhere that a Black, Brown, Indigenous, or marginalized person's perinatal well-being is being impacted or they are being harmed.

MIDWIFERY MODEL CARE

Commonsense Childbirth (CSC) began in Central Florida as a midwifery-led practice providing clinical and support services during the perinatal period and has grown into a nonprofit organization with national and international reach. CSC works to inspire and effect change in maternal-child health care systems, to improve birth outcomes, and to create perinatal safety for at-risk populations and community providers through three main strategic approaches—advocacy, direct care, and education. This includes policy development and optimizing community impact and funding via a National Perinatal Task Force; national scaling of direct services within the JJ Way Framework, and provision of professional and community education and workforce development.

CSC programs holistically embrace clinical, educational, and psychosocial supports, provide culturally safe and respectful care, and ensure that patient-centered choice and decision-making remains paramount as the organization guides, connects, and helps navigate parents through interdisciplinary collaborators and complicated maternity care systems.

CSC utilizes the JJ Way—a midwifery model of care and the codified methodology supporting all CSC Initiatives. The model was created by Jennie Joseph, a British-trained midwife, who founded CSC in 1998. Today, she remains committed to and impassioned about reducing MCH inequities and believes there are solutions to achieving birth justice. The model of care is centered around supporting healthy births for everyone and is composed of four pillars:

- Immediate unrestricted **access** to quality care, support, and triage—regardless of ability to pay;
- Fostering and facilitating **connections** among women to their baby, family, community, trustworthy care providers, resources, and support systems;
- Shared **knowledge** of safe, skillful, evidence-based care and support; leading to
- **Empowerment** of women, care providers, agencies, organizations, and systems.

The innovative midwifery model is built on a human rights and justice framework of compassionate, person-centered maternity care that reaches populations that do not typically receive such services or support. It deploys certified and/or licensed providers to deliver community-based and culturally congruent clinical care, health education, nonclinical care, health navigation, and wrap-around support while building strong collaborative relationships with all stakeholders.

JJ Way-accredited providers create safe, accessible, and professional environments to ensure all clients are treated with mutual respect and dignity. No client is turned away, thereby providing unimpeded and dependable access to support, triage, resources, and referrals, and the providers are trusted by our community to fulfill those promises every time.

The overarching goal is to eliminate racial and class disparities in perinatal health and improve birth outcomes for all by providing access to community-based maternity support centers known as Perinatal Safe Spots that are owned, organized, and operated by community-embedded, trusted providers whose practice aligns with the four tenets of the JJ Way model—access, connections, knowledge, and empowerment.

Perinatal Safe Spots are part of the access and support strategy for pregnant and postpartum people and families in materno-toxic zones. Licensed and certified perinatal providers, paraprofessionals, perinatal educators, MCH community health workers, and perinatal mental health professionals work to increase access and safety for women to quality prenatal, postpartum, and inter-conceptional health care and support services. These services can also be coordinated and connected via telehealth.

WHAT DOES MATERNO-TOXIC MEAN?

Materno-toxic areas are zones or counties, often located in disenfranchised urban neighborhoods or low-resource rural areas, where women and babies are particularly at risk of a poor birth outcome because it is not safe to be pregnant, breastfeeding, or parenting in those areas. In the United States today, many zip codes, both urban and rural, are not conducive to raising families or protecting their health (Commonsense Childbirth National Perinatal Task Force n.d.). In addition, the toxicity of **implicit and explicit biases, racism, classism,** and **sexism** is created wherever a pregnant woman of color may be. As such, the materno-toxic status is not always because of a specific geographic location or economic status but may simply surround them because of discrimination. Thus, even a Black woman living in an affluent area, with a high income and health insurance and "the best" gynecologist in the area, still could be exposed to such toxicity and be equally unsafe.

> The toxicity of implicit and explicit biases, racism, classism, and sexism is created wherever a pregnant woman of color may be.

Where a person lives, works, plays or worships may negatively affect their health, but the social determinants of health also include the **structural** effects of racism, classism, sexism, and conscious and unconscious biases, perpetrated personally or institutionally to the point of ill health, or even death. Essentially, mothers can suffer and experience the effects of being in a living, breathing, materno-toxic zone all their own, based on other people's response or reaction to their race, socioeconomic status, citizenship, or being othered while pregnant, delivering their baby or during the postpartum year, regardless of location.

In fact, recent research has confirmed that one in six women experience mistreatment during childbirth and that Black, Hispanic, and Indigenous women experience more mistreatment than whites (Vedam et al. 2019).

A ROADMAP TO EQUITY

A roadmap to equity, improved outcomes, and sustainability must include a plan to support, coordinate, and operate outpatient and community-based perinatal health care services expressly to mitigate and eliminate racial disparities among Black and Indigenous people of color (BIPOC) in all materno-toxic environments in the United States. To that end, the roadmap must include **safety**, **quality**, and **workforce development**.

Safety

Safety for the community-at-large, birthing people, and their families, as well as safer systems for stakeholders, providers, agencies, and institutions charged with their care, must be the driving force for equity in perinatal health (Commonsense Childbirth n.d.).

This is achievable if we embrace and invest in proven and protective solutions that have been historically and traditionally led by BIPOC and which improve perinatal outcomes for all groups. An investment in systemic safety therefore must be through connections with community-centric programs—meaning those that are community-owned or community-led and delivering care by community-embedded, community-vetted, and acceptable providers. These programs must be welcomed and incorporated into the larger systems as bona fide and essential members of maternity care teams. This will help to ensure safety, trust, and cultural congruence and that we preserve respect and dignity for people while providing equitable perinatal health services to the communities most impacted by historical and structural racism, violence, and harm.

Quality

Quality of the services is maintained by the hospital systems' and public health systems' joint commitment to financial support, strategic partnerships, and strong collaborative protocols with all the community-based perinatal actors and agencies who serve BIPOC and/or marginalized childbearing people (Commonsense Childbirth n.d.). The economic parity, sustainability, and capacity of the community-based programs must be factored in, fully supported from inception, and integrated smoothly into an interdisciplinary continuum that is endorsed, and thereby allows the health care systems to publicly acknowledge their mutual relationships (i.e., designation as a community-friendly hospital status or similar language). Quality improvement and assurance measures are based on the incorporation and execution of successful, cross-sectoral, and equitable partnerships and structural community supports, rather than siloed clinical protocols and hospital-based policies alone.

Workforce Development

Growing and diversifying the pipeline for future perinatal careers is key. Educating the current workforce on how to replicate models and clinical behaviors that are protective and/or how to support and begin the integration of structural changes for the long-term benefit of all childbearing people must be paramount (Commonsense Childbirth n.d.).

It is necessary to ensure the following:

- Training, certification, and accreditation for perinatal providers in evidence-based practices that work for their profession or license and place of service.
- Certification for nonlicensed perinatal providers that provides a National Provider Identifier (NPI) number and ability to bill and be reimbursed for services.
- Equitable Medicaid and commercial insurance reimbursement for all community perinatal providers, both licensed and nonlicensed, if serving areas of critical need,

health care provider shortage areas, medically underserved areas, urban or rural maternity care deserts, marginalized populations, or BIPOC populations—including telehealth services.
- Public, private, and philanthropic investments and commitments for financial stability and economic justice for all community-based and -serving perinatal health and perinatal support providers.
- Access to financial and equitable support for all health care career institutions and programs training and certifying providers from traditionally underserved populations.
- Access to financial and equitable support for all health care career students from traditionally underserved populations.
- Business incubator, entrepreneurship, and development training for individual and group perinatal practices and services.
- Small business financial support, investment, and services for individual and group perinatal practices and services.
- Equitable compensation for jobs that integrate and recognize the contributions of entry-level perinatal health providers as part of the interdisciplinary care team.

EASY ACCESS CLINIC

Interdisciplinary perinatal teams need real support, education, and facilitation on how to work collectively and professionally together to address and redress the inequities and moral injury they themselves experience inside the structural, bureaucratic, and financial constraints of the current medical care and public health systems. One such example is the Easy Access Clinic—a midwifery-led outpatient maternity clinic developed by CSC founder Jennie Joseph, which collaborates with interdisciplinary perinatal professionals and has proven the ease with which intractable racial disparities can be reduced and intersectional issues mitigated. Statistics demonstrate how a small Central Florida Easy Access Clinic consistently achieves the triple aim of better outcomes, better experience, and lower costs—while maintaining equity even throughout the first year of the COVID-19 pandemic (Association of Maternal and Child Health Programs 2020).

The simplest, most time-efficient and cost-effective way to arrive at equity is to organize, mobilize, and support the community-based, community-embedded perinatal providers who are active and established right now. At the same time, we can grow and nurture the currently frustrated and shut-out pipeline of perinatal workers who are trapped along the perimeters of this "crisis" and unable to find an entry point to share their talents and expertise.

Facilitating and incentivizing relationships between the large hospital and public health systems and on-the-ground community stakeholders and individuals will operationalize a pathway to improved perinatal outcomes for all. Incorporating financial and structural supports along with collaborative agreements will ensure capacity and sustainability are built in and maintained.

Facilitating, supporting, growing, and empowering a sustainable, community-based, community-led perinatal workforce is a safe, efficient, and just route to operationalizing equitable outcomes at scale.

PERINATAL WORKFORCE AND COMMUNITY HEALTH WORKERS: A VITAL PARTNERSHIP

CSC's decades of experience in meeting the needs of the most vulnerable and disenfranchised maternity patients has demonstrated that access to dignified and connected community-based care makes economic sense and, most importantly, saves lives. More broadly, there is increasing evidence that programs that utilize community health workers (CHWs) and other community-embedded providers improve many health outcomes (Center for Health Worker Innovation 2021; Marill 2021). There is no question that it is crucial for community MCH infrastructure to utilize the many trained and dedicated individuals who are already on the ground working with target populations alongside the larger system of perinatal health services provision.

MCH CHW training for the perinatal specialty must include the following essential topics to address health disparities effectively and mitigate obstetric racism, classism, and other discrimination:

- Safety and quality in maternal health care and support,
- Characteristics of health models and health systems,
- Barriers to health care services,
- Health system navigation and collaboration,
- Reproductive and maternal justice, and
- Related community resources.

BENEFITS OF PERINATAL SAFE SPOTS AND EASY ACCESS CLINICS

The goal is for the Perinatal Safe Spots and accredited Easy Access Clinics to derive the same benefits as the JJ Way:

- **Access** to planning and support for the pre-implementation phase, during implementation, and ongoing through training. Access to technical support, collective care, mentoring, and the community of practice is key to maintaining sustainability and is embedded continually throughout the process while accreditation is earned and remains in place.

- **Connection** to the collective and the community of practice, which engenders trust and transparency between Perinatal Safe Spots and Easy Access Clinic providers and local MCH providers, institutions, and agencies. This, in turn, promotes safer and better-quality interdisciplinary collaborations and smoother health navigation. The business planning and incubation aspects of accreditation lead to sustainable community-embedded practices that solidify the safety net for longer-term mitigation of MCH health disparities.
- **Knowledge** and understanding of unwieldy and bureaucratic health systems that allow Perinatal Safe Spots and Easy Access Clinics to customize and adapt their solutions on a local level and in culturally congruent ways. By listening to and incorporating the knowledge and shared lived experiences of clients and providers in their communities, larger institutions, systems, and agencies learn about collaborative opportunities to improve **safety** and **quality** for clients and providers while achieving their own goals toward reducing disparities. The shared knowledge supports everyone toward creating sustainable partnerships and equitable, transparent financial relationships.
- **Empowerment** for all actors and funders in the MCH ecosystem in the United States. Accreditation for Perinatal Safe Spots and Easy Access Clinic practices empowers people from the grassroots community through the pipeline of community-embedded perinatal health workers, the clinician and institutional providers and systems, and ultimately through the government and insurance payors.

EVIDENCE, OUTRAGE, OUTCOMES

Evidence of CSC's strategies and approaches in reducing MCH health disparities has been consistent. As Eichelberger et al. (2016) asked, "Where, then, is the space for evidence-based outrage in medicine? What P value would be necessary to conclude that persistent health disparities are unacceptable?" (p. 1771). As community-based perinatal providers and birth workers, we have long recognized and concur that data demonstrate "the significant disparities Black women face across their reproductive lives and conclude that these outcomes are not only statistically significant, but morally significant and fundamentally unjust" (p. 1771).

While documentation and discussion of persistent, heart-wrenching disparities in MCH is necessary and ongoing, it is just as vital to provide and disseminate evidence of successes and the reduction or erasure of such disparities. In 2007, CSC engaged in an evaluation study in which 100 of the highest-risk patients were enrolled prospectively and followed through their pregnancies and deliveries (Figure 14-1). When compared to the county and state percentages of that same year, CSC had eliminated the racial disparity. It is worth noting that in the same year, 2007, African American women were at a

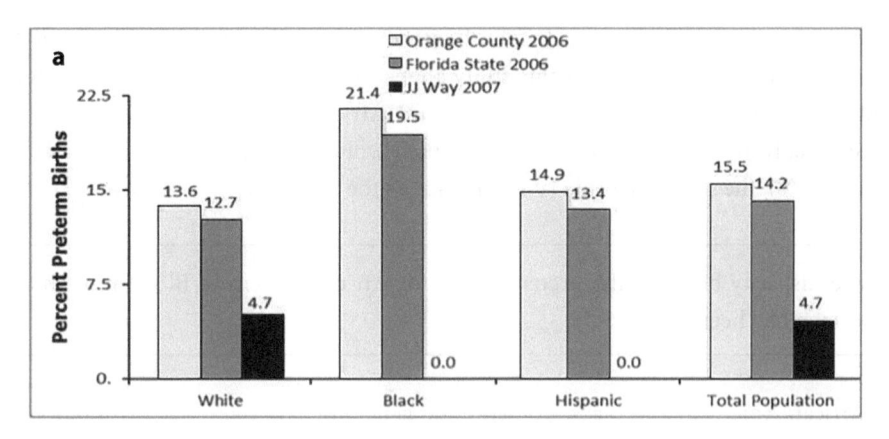

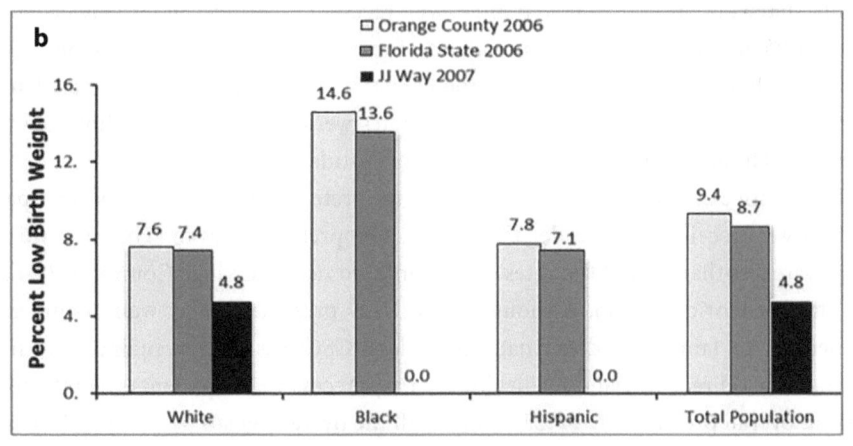

Figure 14-1. Preterm Birth (a) and Low Birth Weight (b) by Race: Health Council Study, 2006–2007

Source: Reprinted with permission of Commonsense Childbirth (https://commonsensechildbirth.org).

one in five risk of having a preterm birth in Florida (Association of Maternal and Child Health Programs 2009).

In 2014, CSC participated in a study specifically investigating the effects of utilizing the JJ Way model to reduce perinatal health disparities. The findings of this study matched women with the same age, race, and zip code from the Florida Vital Statistics database and revealed statistically significant longer gestational periods and lower preterm birth rates for women of color who were cared for within the model in 2014 (Cole, Rojas, and Joseph 2018).

> There were no premature or low birth weight babies born among the African American and Hispanic women in the cohort.

A more recent research study before the pandemic was completed in 2017 with 256 women included. The results of this study aligned with the previous two (Cole, Rojas, and Joseph 2018). The preterm birth rates for African American and Black women were actually lower (8.6%) than the rates of their white counterparts in Orange County, Florida (9%), the state of Florida (9%), and across the nation (9%).

> The disparity between the preterm rates for African American/Black and white women had been erased.

African American and Black women (who generally have the worse birth outcomes locally, statewide, and across the country) who received care under the JJ Way had lower preterm birth rates (8.6%) than individuals of the same race in Orange County (13%), the state of Florida (13.3%), and the nation (13%). White women who participated in the JJ Way also fared well as their preterm birth rates were lower (5%) than those of white women in Orange County (9%) and the state of Florida (9%).

The positive outcomes are also reflected in the preterm rate comparisons of Hispanic women who received care under the JJ Way. The preterm rates for Hispanic women (4%) were less than half of the rates of Hispanic women in Orange County (9.3%) and the state of Florida (8.9%). Although COVID-19 presented many well-documented challenges for families and perinatal providers, CSC was able to maintain positive outcomes via direct care and telehealth for Easy Access Clinic patients (>4,000 visits) with an overall preterm rate of .21%, although the overall census of patients decreased during the pandemic.

EQUITABLE OUTCOMES AT SCALE

CSC is fully engaged in a revolutionary approach to eliminating health disparities in perinatal care and has already begun scaling this place-based, person-centered approach to maternal and infant health. The life-saving model of Perinatal Safe Spots is transforming maternal health in historically underresourced communities and materno-toxic zones, regardless of the prevailing conditions, by placing trusted, unbiased, and culturally safe providers back into the heart of their communities. Of course, this also demands that those community providers are recognized and receive equitable reimbursement from federal, state, and private insurers.

CSC has dedicated its resources to providing accessible care to communities. The mission is "equitable outcomes at scale," and the best way to achieve this mission is through replication and training of care providers. Currently, more than 170 Perinatal Safe Spots are providing service across the nation. Recently, Perinatal Safe Zones were launched in two states in conjunction with community partners (including, to its credit,

Figure 14-2. Equitable Outcomes at Scale Conceptual Map

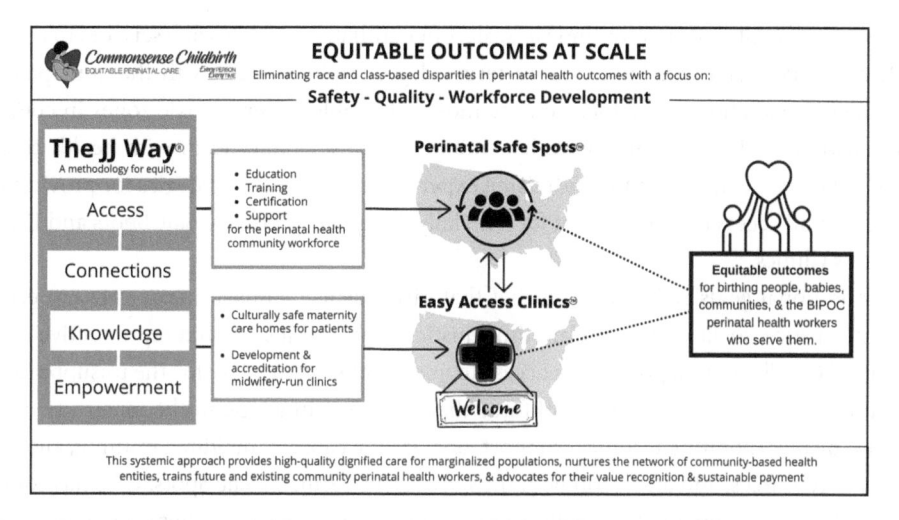

Source: Reprinted with permission of Commonsense Childbirth (https://commonsensechildbirth.org).
Note: BIPOC = Black, Indigenous, person of color.

an outstanding hospital system). These zones contain multiple Perinatal Safe Spots that engage in communication, collaboration, and collective care to provide effective, equitable, and safe care to the families within their communities.

CSC works side-by-side with local health care leaders and practitioners to plan, implement, and sustain this proven model. The deliverables (assessments, training, resources, and data collection) are tailored to each community's needs and the local dynamics in which the Perinatal Safe Spot operates. CSC is creating a community maternal health advisory group, developing materials, connecting local communities to other partners, offering "best-practices" training and continuing education, training local practitioners to implement and evaluate the JJ Way, and linking neighborhood and health care facilities' assessment tools to determine strategic plans. CSC is also providing seed grant funding to help identified Perinatal Safe Spots build sustainable infrastructure (technical, business, educational) and to connect to and strengthen services through our national community of practice.

CSC believes these investments in the midwifery model of care and the community birth infrastructure provide for the development and incubation of an entrepreneurial workforce willing to create and sustain community-based, community-owned businesses that provide dependable perinatal support and clinical services to members of their community (Figure 14-2). In addition, the investment helps grow and diversify the health care workforce, creating a career and entrepreneurial pipeline, models for ambulatory and retail health care clinics, collaborative maternity care and delivery systems, and perinatal safety hubs adjacent to and within materno-toxic areas.

CSC's overall goal is to continue to scale, offer affiliation, and provide services to more than 200 Perinatal Safe Spots within targeted geographical areas with the anticipated scaling of that effort and a focus on the most vulnerable materno-toxic zones in counties across the United States. CSC has built a multidisciplinary team with health care, technology, operational, and fundraising expertise to implement strategies for providing widespread access to, and support for, officially designated Perinatal Safe Spots and Easy Access Clinics.

Additional goals reflect CSC's belief that birth justice is linked inextricably to economic justice, social justice, racial/ethnic justice, maternal justice, and reproductive justice. CSC will continue to provide access to and build sustainability for the unsupported and uncompensated perinatal workforce that is already in action in the maternity care space by incorporating technical support, operational capacity building, training, allocation of resources, and affiliation with the network of Perinatal Safe Spots. CSC has committed to continuing to utilize collective data about outcomes and patient care to inform and drive policy and legislative decisions regarding perinatal care providers, reimbursement, and value. CSC leads a national network that brings together leaders and learners engaged in applying this model at the local levels. This community of practice is sharing best practices, resources, challenges, and lessons learned to elevate the entire community birth infrastructure.

CONCLUSION

We ask the question again: Could it be possible that creating a **culture** and **environment** that supports *all* pregnant people could make the difference in health, safety, gestational age, birth weight, and breastfeeding rates in women at risk for poor maternal health outcomes in the United States? We believe the answer is yes, provided we are willing to embrace this public health priority, invest in the rebuilding of our community-based perinatal and midwifery work force, and commit to fortifying our community birth infrastructure.

REFERENCES

American College of Nurse-Midwives Board of Directors. Truth and Reconciliation Resolution from the American College of Nurse-Midwives. March 2021. Available at: https://www.midwife.org/acnm/files/cclibraryfiles/filename/000000008234/ACNM_Truth_and_Reconciliation_Resolution-Apr2021.pdf

Association of Maternal and Child Health Programs. JJ-Way Model of Maternity Care – Easy Access Clinic. Innovation Station Practice Summary and Implementation Guidance. 2020. Available at: https://perinataltaskforce.com/wp-content/uploads/2021/06/JJ-Way-Model_Innovation-Station-Handout-min.pdf

Association of Maternal and Child Health Programs. JJ-Way Model of Maternity Care. Innovation Station Sharing Best Practices in Maternal and Child Health. June 2009. Available at: https://perinataltaskforce.com/wp-content/uploads/2021/06/JJ-way-AMCHP-Best-Practice-min.pdf

Brodsky PL. Where have all the midwives gone? *J Perinatal Educ*. 2008;17(4):48–51. https://doi.org/10.1624/105812408X324912

Center for Health Worker Innovation. Community health workers—an effective strategy to help address health disparities in marginalized populations. February 16, 2021. Available at: https://chwi.jnj.com/voices-from-the-front-line/community-health-workers-an-effective-strategy-to-help-address-health-disparities-in-marginalized-populations

Centers for Disease Control and Prevention. Pregnancy Mortality Surveillance System. April 13, 2022. Available at: https://www.cdc.gov/reproductivehealth/maternal-mortality/pregnancy-mortality-surveillance-system.htm#race-ethnicity

Cole HE, Rojas PX, Joseph J. Building a movement to birth a more just and loving world. National Perinatal Task Force. March 2018. Available at: https://www.pacesconnection.com/fileSendAction/fcType/0/fcOid/478556595873144043/filePointer/478556595873144064/fodoid/478556595873144055/Groundswell_Report_final_online%20March%202018%20National%20Perinatal%20Task%20Force%20.pdf

Commonsense Childbirth National Perinatal Task Force. What is a materno-toxic area? Available at: https://perinataltaskforce.com/faq/#:~:text=WHAT%20IS%20A%20MATERNO%2D-TOXIC,being%20pregnant%2C%20breastfeeding%20or%20parenting

Dawley K. The campaign to eliminate the midwife. *Am J Nurs*. 2000;100(10):50–66.

Eichelberger KY, Doll K, Ekpo GE, Zerden ML. Black lives matter: claiming a space for evidence-based outrage in obstetrics and gynecology. *Am J Public Health*. 2016;106(10):1771–1772. https://doi.org/10.2105/AJPH.2016.303313

March of Dimes. Nowhere to go: maternity care deserts across the US. 2022 report. 2022. Available at: https://www.marchofdimes.org/sites/default/files/2022-10/2022_Maternity_Care_Report.pdf

Marill MC. Community health workers, often overlooked, bring trust to the pandemic fight. Kaiser Health News. February 8, 2021. Available at: https://khn.org/news/article/community-health-workers-often-overlooked-bring-trust-to-the-pandemic-fight

Rooks J. The history of midwifery. May 22, 2014. Available at: https://www.ourbodiesourselves.org/book-excerpts/health-article/history-of-midwifery

Vedam S, Stoll K, Taiwo TK, et al. The Giving Voice to Mothers Study: inequity and mistreatment during pregnancy and childbirth in the United States. *Reprod Health*. 2019;16(1):1–18. https://doi.org/10.1186/s12978-019-0729-2

15

Community-Based Doulas: A Critical Part of the Paradigm Shift to Create Birth Equity

Kanika A. Harris, PhD, MPH, Mother Mother Binahkaye Joy, and Zainab Sulaiman, MSc

Before there were doulas and midwives, there were mothers who attended to their daughters, sisters who held space for their sisters, and bands of aunties and grandmothers who gathered around the birthing mother and centered on her needs. In fact, for most of the history of humanity, circles of womenfolk have practiced the art and intricacies of giving birth within their own communities among themselves and surrounded by family.
　—Mother Mother Binahkaye Joy (Black Women's Health Imperative 2022)

Doulas have gained traction in recent years as a foremost solution to ending inequities in maternal and infant health outcomes, especially for Black pregnant people. Community-based doulas, nonclinical trained birth workers who are often from the communities that they serve, provide a culturally informed model of care to advocate for and support families at minimal cost. Community-based doulas' role in supporting families with birth education, comfort measures, and navigating discriminatory and traumatic care experiences has been demonstrated to improve maternal and birth outcomes. This chapter illuminates the crucial role doulas play in improving outcomes and experiences for communities most affected by discrimination and disparities in health outcomes and highlights intervention approaches that are integrating community-based doulas within the context of midwifery care.

WHY WE NEED DOULAS: HISTORICAL CONTEXT
What Are Doulas?

"Doulas provide services at the intersections of our most essential human rights—the right to give birth, the right *not* to give birth, and the right to safely parent children—three cornerstones of reproductive justice" (Ross 2016, pp. xiv-xv). Doulas are birth support workers who provide nonclinical (informational, physical, emotional, and logistical) support during pregnancy, childbirth, and early postpartum (DONA 2022; International Childbirth Education Association 2021). Doulas are not medically trained, and, thus, they do not diagnose, perform any medical procedures, or prescribe medications (Dekker 2022).

Over time, the role of the doula has expanded to include a "full spectrum" of care, assistance in critical care services that include everything from fertility and preconception to antepartum, prison births, and guidance and support for abortions as well as death (Mahoney and Mitchell 2016). Although family members also provide support during these critical points of care, doulas are often brought in for additional support when needed.

The American College of Obstetricians and Gynecologists, Association of Women's Health Obstetrics and Neonatal Nurses, and March of Dimes, among others, all provide evidence that continuous support during pregnancy and labor is associated with improved overall satisfaction of the birth experience—including fewer cesarean deliveries, better pain management, an increase in breastfeeding rates, less medical interventions, a decrease in postpartum depression, and infants who are less likely to be born prematurely (International Childbirth Education Association 2022).

A Cochrane Review that included 26 trials worldwide with more than 15,000 people found statistically significant results that birthing people who had continuous support had better birth outcomes (Bohren et al. 2017). The study also concluded that no adverse effects had been connected to continuous support in birthing families (Bohren et al. 2017).

Doulas have become a critical part of the conversation to achieve birth equity and birth justice—"the assurance and conditions of optimal births for all people with a willingness to address racial and social inequities in a sustained effort" (National Birth Equity Collaborative 2022). Radical doulas and community-based doulas usually have a full-spectrum training and also root their practice in the reproductive justice movement to serve the most marginalized birthing people (Carathers 2019). Radical doula work has been essential for Black birthing families by disrupting high maternal mortality rates, unnecessary medical interventions, stress, abuse, violence, and discrimination they experience within the US medical system (Carathers 2019; Salinas, Salinas, and Kahn 2022).

Before the 1930s, women typically gave birth at home surrounded by relatives, friends, and midwives (Palley and Palley 2014). Cancelmo (2021) explains that as a result of the colonization of North America and medicalization of labor and delivery, birth drastically changed, and by the 1950s, 95% of births happened in hospital settings and were attended by men. This cultural shift led to significant gaps in care, support, the continuous flow of information, trust, control, and options for birthing families. It also led to very low breastfeeding rates due to the popularization of formulas.

Throughout most of the nation's history, women were cared for at home immediately after birth with intensive support for at least two weeks (Temkin 1999). Even Black enslaved women, who were forced to return to work immediately after giving birth, had the support and care they needed from enslaved midwives (Owens and Fett 2019).

Since the start of the 19th century, birth has been seen through a white patriarchal medical model that values the male body. Birth is treated like a stressor and sickness (Cancelmo 2021). Birthing people were taught that their bodies were simply vehicles to be sedated and controlled during childbirth. They were made to believe that their bodies were unnecessary or insufficient to nourish or feed their babies and convinced that formula was the optimal choice (Harris, Etienne, and Arrington 2022).

Recognizing that birth could be different, by the late 1960s and 1970s, predominantly white middle-class women led an effort to restore natural birthing practices and midwifery (Morton 2014). And, by the early 1990s, employing doulas from organizations such as the Doulas of North America (DONA) became popular. However, these services were predominately available only to white women with access to competent medical care who could afford the privileges of additional support teams in their health care (Carathers 2019).

For Black birthing people, this shift to the medicalization of birth came at a high cost by severing the bedrock of communities, erasing centuries of ancient wisdom and technology, and silencing sacred cultural practices that affirmed birthing parents and their families. Black people were forced to transition to giving birth in hospital settings, meaning they would be involuntarily submitting to white institutional spaces that upheld white racist normative practices—organizational structures, operations, and procedures that did not consider them in design or practice (Cancelmo 2021).

For Black and Brown people, the birth movement has long been a unique form of activism (Carathers 2019). But the racist narrative of single-parent households, adolescent pregnancy, poverty, and broken homes has distorted its rich history and disrupted the narrative of resistance. In an effort to fight decades of oppression and disinvestment in Black and Brown communities, community-based solutions, agency, and strategies have emerged to empower women and birthing people to thrive.

In a society where access to care could be denied at any time for any cause, as a matter of survival, Black families began using creative strategies to support mothers and babies during childbearing years (Mullings and Wali 2000). One example is multigenerational living. The practice of sharing a household ensures the hands-on presence of multiple caregivers for new babies and older siblings while protecting newly postpartum women from the deadly isolation that has claimed too many Black mothers' lives in recent times (Mullings and Wali 2000).

Care work is another lifeline for families and communities. When families work in community, a vital component of maternal and infant health and wellness forms. Caregivers can pick up on many important signs and nonverbal cues just by being in the same space as the birthing family. A person who has just given birth is going through tremendous recalibration in their body, and having another person with them who can notice whether or not they are dehydrated or showing signs of elevated blood pressure or excess bleeding signaling postpartum hemorrhage can make the difference between life and death.

In addition to access to clean water, a peaceful environment, nourishing food, and ample rest, birthing people and babies need an informed family surrounding them so that they may more easily recover. If birthing people exert too much effort trying to do everything themselves, they consequently delay the healing process or can even cause additional injury to their postpartum bodies.

Multigenerational families were a practical, life-affirming solution to many racially rooted health care disparities for Black women. The pressure to hold it all, manage it all, and care for everyone was somewhat alleviated by the real-time interventions of mothers, sisters, aunties, and grandmothers collaborating in the care of the birthing family. In addition, the parents, who, despite conceiving a child together, might not be ready to marry or become a single unit, were allowed the softer possibility of taking a breath and acclimating to their new roles as co-parents with the support of family.

According to Freire (2000), knowledge is not static or proprietary, and communities are the experts of their own reality and solutions. When multigenerational families cohabitated, knowledge was more readily transferred. A mother could see her own intelligence reflected back to her through the stories the women in her family told, as they took turns doing laundry, assisting the mama, or holding the baby. All the while, the mama would be able to take a moment to eat a meal with two whole hands.

When there is not already a strong family dynamic or positive multigenerational cohabitation, doulas are often called on to reduce the gap in essential caregiving for the birthing family. Doulas model mother-centered support and help families relearn the intuitive ways of supporting during pregnancy, birth, and postpartum. For many families, the resource of a doula sparks a cultural recovery of maternal memory. Doulas inspire other family members to reawaken ancestral knowledge and acquire tangible skills for how they can take positive actions to assist any birthing family to thrive.

Part of Our Work Is Returning to Our Birthing Practices and Decolonizing Birth Work

A return to centering birth as something families naturally experience together is a radical acknowledgment of the intuitive intelligence of Black family practices. Even in times of enslavement, Black people who did not share language, religion, geography, or bloodlines were able to cultivate life-saving care practices for one another, especially for birthing women and the babies born to them. Often babies were sold away from birth parents to places where surrogate mothers and aunties would assume their care, knowing that somewhere their own blood children were receiving the same care from another mother. Despite the brutality of chattel slavery, the legacy of maternal intelligence endured so much that slavery prevailed because of Black women's labor to keep their collective babies alive (Owens and Fett 2019).

Radical doulas serving Black communities in today's world are an echo forward of the same determination that inspired enslaved people to care for their young, even when they were not always blood relatives. This propensity to preserve the future as best as possible is embedded in Black cultural practices throughout the African diaspora. Even though gains have been made for some Black people in access to housing, education, and financial security, there remains a lasting imprint of racism for many Black mothers attempting to navigate maternal health care systems.

In a system that has largely profited on mothers' insecurities and fears of inadequacy, a doula's presence resets the energy of possibility. They symbolically represent a remembrance of cultural knowledge that Black people come from a people who know how to birth and care for their babies, even amid hard times. Doulas create space for the conscious, communal integration of organic birth behavior—birthing people and mothers birthing babies without interventions, laboring in their own time, holding infants to their chest, being surrounded by other mothers, and resting and being cared for.

All of these moments are revolutionary acts of reclamation, decolonizing birth one family at a time and liberating the internal family dynamics from the exploitative grip of capitalism. The more families can resource within themselves, the less dependent they are on systems that seek to harm them and disrupt their natural capacity to be together and care for themselves.

Using a holistic, multifaceted approach, this model of care provides a greater array of services to the community through ongoing relationships, shared experiences, and a shared culture and language. In a community-based doula program, community strengths are leveraged to implement programs, and this approach rejects the prevailing deficit-based approach used in most clinical settings for the support of underresourced Black communities.

CREATIVE WAYS TO MEET THE NEEDS OF COMMUNITIES: EXPANDING ON COMMUNITY-BASED DOULA MODELS

The community-based doula movement directly appeals to everyday people in everyday families to take an active role in improving birth outcomes in their communities. The community-based doula model can start early within the pregnancy, providing support through the early months of parenting (Abramson, Breedlove, and Isaacs 2006). Whereas some doula training models focus heavily on acquiring a fixed set of skills and meeting certain qualifications by a predetermined time, community-based doulas are encouraged to realize their potential to serve their community from where they are in the moment, while continuously increasing their skills as birth workers.

Community-based doulas are trained to study their communities through the lens of birth, compassion, and possibility. They are equipped with knowledge about pregnancy, birth, and postpartum and are taught how to engage a network of birth-related support services for the families they serve. From this initiation, they can develop a more nuanced sensitivity to their communities' unique challenges and opportunities. This approach leads to more mothers and families accessing the support they need (Abramson, Breedlove, and Isaacs 2006).

This is a critical shift in doula training models because community-based doulas have a greater understanding and ability to help their clients engage more meaningfully with the resources around them. Not only do doulas develop relationships with other doulas while going through training, but they also learn how to better collaborate with community health workers in their area. As doulas build more trust with the families they are serving, they become vital information bridges for families who might otherwise not have access to the available support.

Community health workers often have access to critical resources and can work together with doulas to deepen relationships and reduce burnout. In this way, the community-based doula creates more visibility for resource sharing and continuity of care for families who are birthing in the margins of society and may or may not have access to culturally sensitive care providers.

Community-based doula training models also prepare doulas for a kind of success that does not lead to chronic burnout. In an effort to reimagine the way families access support for birthing labors, community-based doula programs encourage all stakeholders to assess themselves as a resource first and to realize themselves as someone who can be a potential benefit to the family. Doing this shifts the paradigm of constantly outsourcing essential support needs to people and companies who are not emotionally, physically, or historically connected to the community. Rather, community-based doula programs normalize everyday citizens as people who have the power to positively impact the birthing culture in their families and communities. This expansion of knowledge sharing increases the number of pathways for people to learn what doulas do and how to build more capacity within their families to support birthing people.

Another way community-based doula programs create sustainability is that each class of doulas becomes another group of people in the community who can encourage and recruit the next cohort of future birth workers. Mobilized from within, community-based doulas activate a growing consciousness for people in their families and communities that there is a viable way for them to take greater responsibility for how mothers and families access support. Organizations such as Ancient Song Doula Services, Mama Glow, Harambee Village Doulas, Mamatoto Village, and Birth Detroit are Black female-led organizations creating a movement of liberation and healing to provide holistic care services to the needs of the communities they reside in.

The community-based doula model at HealthConnect One is an innovative replication-focused train-the-trainer model. Community-based trainers are prepared to train community members as doulas with the HealthConnect One curriculum.

In HealthConnect One's community-based doula model, doulas are carefully selected community members whose ethnicity, racial background, and socioeconomic status reflect that of the community they serve. Practitioners are chosen for their capacity to serve as nurturers, role models, and teachers.

In addition to didactic sessions on pregnancy, childbirth, adolescence, and breastfeeding, HealthConnect One's community-based doula training program emphasizes active learning through role-playing, bidirectional learning, and discussion. The model has five essential components:

1. Employ women who are trusted members of the community of focus.
2. Extend and intensify the role of a doula with families from early pregnancy through the first months postpartum.
3. Collaborate with community stakeholders/institutions and use a diverse team approach.
4. Facilitate experiential learning using popular education techniques and the HealthConnect One training curriculum.
5. Value doulas' work with salary, supervision, and support.

In partnership with community doula organizations, these five elements are essential for optimizing community support and ensuring that doulas are respected and valued in their work. Compared to the national average, HealthConnect One community-based doula partnerships produced 24.5% fewer low–birth weight babies, 23.4% fewer babies born by cesarean delivery, and 19.4% fewer preterm babies among Black birthing people on Medicaid between 2017 and 2021 (HealthConnect One 2022).

Organizations such as the Black Women's Health Imperative (BWHI) are filling the gaps to educate, liberate, and groom the next generation of reproductive health leaders. BWHI has developed a full-spectrum community doula program for college students titled NOURISH (New Opportunities to Uncover Our Resources, Intuition, Spirit, and Healing) to address maternal and child health. The NOURISH program is unique in that it is a preconception doula training model to educate and expose young women to the importance of preconception health while giving them hands-on training and knowledge as doulas and community birth workers.

BWHI hopes to re-engage communities in traditional frameworks of care and support that have protected Black birthing families for generations. Young doulas-in-training can provide support for birthing families and learn what it takes to show up to pregnancy healthy and whole. Their prevention model is that "knowing is by doing." Young Black women are suffering from fibroids and heavy menstrual cycles and hidden warning signs of chronic conditions such as high blood pressure and type 2 diabetes. BWHI also plans to expose students to careers in maternal and child health, such as midwifery, to invigorate a movement and address the disparities in maternal and child health training at Historically Black Colleges and Universities.

THE FUTURE OF DOULA WORK: MEDICAID REIMBURSEMENT—AT WHAT COST?

Doulas are not a "cure-all" to disparities in maternal mortality and reproductive injustices. The role of a doula is to bridge the gap between birthing families and health care systems to facilitate clients' access to care. The doula model has been viable and sustainable for predominantly white and affluent communities who can afford to pay the out-of-pocket costs of a doula or the expense of doula training and birth services (Salinas, Salinas, and Kahn 2022). Black birthing communities, including clinicians and hospitals, benefit significantly from their unique training and expertise, and these professionals should be adequately compensated for their contributions.

Doulas who provide community-based services may charge on a sliding scale and serve more clients, many of whom are Medicaid recipients. Even though they are committed to serving their communities, community-rooted doulas and the perinatal birth workforce cannot continue to work for free. Advocacy around sustainable billing practices that align with the work community-based doulas provide has been ongoing for nearly a decade.

Recognizing the benefits of doulas in closing gaps in care, we have reached a pivotal moment in history when policies around the United States are making doula costs reimbursable through insurance coverage. Prioritizing and centering community-based doulas in reimbursement structures will reduce inequities and enable all doulas—traditional, community-based, or private—to be covered for their support of birthing people. We must get ahead of the question of at what cost.

Attempting to integrate white racist medical frameworks of accreditation, reimbursable rates, and who has the right to receive doula care are at the center of the debate about accessible and affordable doula care. The current model of health care is antithetical to birth justice and equity. We have learned from history that if we integrate doulas into the same reimbursable medical models of care as traditional health workers, we may lose vital expertise, knowledge, resources, and time that help birthing families thrive. We have an opportunity to create equitable and culturally congruent care by collaborating with doulas, families, and policymakers to ensure this work is accessible and sustainable for everyone, no matter their economic status.

REFERENCES

Abramson R, Breedlove G, Isaacs B. *The Community Based Doula: Supporting Families Before, During, and After Childbirth*. Washington, DC: Zero to Three Press; 2006.

Black Women's Health Imperative. *NOURISH Full Spectrum Doula Training Curriculum*. 2022.

Bohren MA, Hofmeyr GJ, Sakala C, Fukuzawa RK, Cuthbert A. Continuous support for women during childbirth. *Cochrane Database Syst Rev.* 2017;7(7):CD003766. https://doi.org/10.1002/14651858.CD003766.pub6

Cancelmo CM. Protecting Black mothers: how the history of midwifery can inform doula activism. *Sociol Compass*. 2021;15:12867. https://doi.org/10.1111/soc4.12867

Carathers JY. *Radical Doulas Make "Caring a Political Act": Full-Spectrum Birth Work as Reproductive Justice Activism*. Doctoral dissertation. Portland State University; 2019.

Dekker R. Evidence on: doulas. Evidence Based Birth. 2022. Available at: https://evidencebasedbirth.com/wp-content/uploads/2018/01/Doula-Handout.pdf

DONA International. What is a doula? 2022. Available at: https://www.dona.org/what-is-a-doula

Freire P. *Pedagogy of the Oppressed*. 30th anniversary ed. New York, NY: Continuum; 2000.

Harris K, Etienne S, Arrington L. Postnatal unit care and safe transition home. *Clin Obstet Gynecol*. 2022;65(3):563–576. https://doi.org/10.1097/GRF.0000000000000732

HealthConnect One. The case for support: community-based doula replication. 2022. Available at: https://www.healthconnectone.org/wp-content/uploads/2020/10/CBD-Fact-Sheet-March20.pdf

International Childbirth Education Association. What is a doula? 2022. Available at: https://icea.org/resources/what-is-a-doula

Mohoney M, Mitchell L. *The Doulas: Radical Care for Pregnant People*. New York, NY: The Feminist Press; 2016.

Morton CH. *Birth Ambassadors: Doulas and the Re-emergence of Woman-Supported Birth in America*. Amarillo, TX: Praeclarus Press; 2014:51–101.

Mullings L, Wali A. *Stress and Resilience: The Social Context of Reproduction in Central Harlem*. New York, NY: Kluwer Academic/Plenum Publishers; 2000.

National Birth Equity Collaborative. Birth equity for all Black birthing people. 2022. Available at: https://birthequity.org

Owens DC, Fett SM. Black maternal and infant health: historical legacies of slavery. *Am J Public Health*. 2019;109(10):1342–1345. https://doi.org/10.2105/AJPH.2019.305243

Palley ML, Palley HA. *The Politics of Women's Health Care in the United States*. New York, NY: Palgrave MacMillan; 2014.

Ross L. Forward. In: Mohoney M, Mitchell L. *The Doulas: Radical Care for Pregnant People*. New York, NY: The Feminist Press; 2016:ix–xvi.

Salinas J, Salinas M, Kahn M. Doulas, racism, and whiteness: how birth support workers process advocacy toward women of color. *Societies*. 2022;12(1):10. https://doi.org/10.3390/soc12010019

Temkin E. Driving through: postpartum care during World War II. *Am J Public Health*. 1999;89(4):587–595. https://doi.org/10.2105/ajph.89.4.587

16

We Are Not a Monolith: Nativity, Racial Discrimination, and Maternal/Infant Health Across the Black Diaspora

Yanica F. Faustin, PhD, MPH, Kristin Z. Black, PhD, MPH, and Jon M. Hussey, PhD, MPH

Research focused on immigrants provides a valuable opportunity to advance our understanding of how living in the United States affects health within and between major groups. While studies have paid close attention to inequities in birth outcomes between Black and white birthing people and US-born and foreign-born Latinx populations (Collins and David 2009; Crump, Lipsky, and Mueller 1999; Hummer et al. 1999), not enough attention has been paid to inequities in adverse birth outcomes between US-born and foreign-born Black populations and the underlying factors contributing to these disparate outcomes.

While several studies have documented that foreign-born women, collectively, and Latinas and Asians, specifically, have lower rates of adverse birth outcomes than white women, there is less research on the smaller (but growing) population of Black foreign-born women giving birth in the United States. As foreign-born mothers continue to represent a growing fraction of all Black births in the United States (Anderson 2018), studying their outcomes has the potential to reveal new insights into the etiology of US racial/ethnic health inequities more broadly. The consideration of nativity in research may also inform more robust data collection and tailored interventions. This chapter highlights a parent study that concluded that while all Black birthing persons in New York City are at an increased risk of experiencing both general and pregnancy-related discrimination, the health impact of racial stress differs by nativity.

ASSOCIATION BETWEEN RACIAL STRESS AND PRETERM BIRTH WITHIN US BLACK WOMEN ACROSS THE DIASPORA

The persistent racial/ethnic disparities in preterm birth have yet to be fully explained. Potential risk factors worth further attention include exposure to and consequences of racial stress and systemic racism. Examining maternal health inequities across the African diaspora allows for an exploration of how differential exposure to racial stratification in the United States results in differing outcomes for Black birthing persons. Research attention to Black immigrant births has not kept pace with their growing numbers.

Our mixed-methods study investigated preterm birth disparities within the Black population across the diaspora. We asked the following questions: (1) What is the association between nativity and preterm birth for African-born, Caribbean-born, and US-born Black mothers? and (2) Are there differences in the descriptions of instances of racial discrimination within the Black population? This concurrent mixed-methods design utilized birth records, which we analyzed by using logistic regression to examine variation in preterm delivery, and semi-structured interviews. The quantitative strand (demonstrating the disparate preterm birth rates), coupled with the qualitative strand (focused on perceptions and processing of racial discrimination), works to improve our understanding of the connection between racism and adverse infant outcomes, and the variation in how racism, as a threat to health, influences Black birthing persons in different ways. Using a mixed-methods design provides a more nuanced understanding of preterm birth disparities and demonstrates the diversity in the lived experiences of Black birthing persons and their outcomes.

Stress, Racism, and Maternal Health

Racism is a system of oppression that operates at multiple levels, structuring opportunity and assigning value based on an individual's perceived race (Jones 2000; Slaughter-Acey et al. 2015). Research has shown that experiencing racial discrimination causes stress (Ong, Fuller-Rowell, and Burrow 2009), and stress adversely affects health (Pearlin et al. 1981). The dysregulation that occurs from increased exposure to racial stress is representative of bio-psycho-social mechanisms through which stress can operate over the life course, leading to poor health outcomes and racial health inequities (Gee, Walsemann, and Brondolo 2012; Ong, Fuller-Rowell, and Burrow 2009).

Given the differing orientations to Black identity, racial discrimination may be differentially internalized within the Black population, which leads to differential links between racial discrimination and physical health (Dominguez et al. 2009; Giscombe and Lobel 2005). We know that stress influences health outcomes (Pearlin et al. 1981). Understanding whether this race-based stress and reproductive health outcomes relationship operates differently for US-born and foreign-born Black populations is key to developing a better understanding of the persistent racial/ethnic health inequities in the United States.

Stressors that contribute to persistent inequities are typically those that extend across the life course (Ong, Fuller-Rowell, and Burrow 2009), influencing health trajectories and creating an elevated risk for adverse health outcomes, making it especially imperative to examine chronic stressors or accumulated stress. Cumulative exposure to the health-related impacts of racial/ethnic discrimination is generally lower among the foreign-born versus US-born. Foreign-born Black women may experience and perceive racism differently, especially if they belonged to the racial majority in their countries of origin (Arthur and Katkin 2006; Dominguez et al. 2009; Viruell-Fuentes, Miranda, and Abdulrahim 2012). Interestingly, reports of racial discrimination by US-born Black women are more similar to reports of Caribbean-born women than African-born women (Nuru-Jeter et al. 2009). This suggests perceptions and attributions about racism may differ by region of origin. Health disparities across these major groups of the Black population may therefore be attributable to differences in the way these groups conceptualize race and interpret racial discrimination (Deaux et al. 2007).

The exposure to risk factors, such as racial stress, for foreign-born Black women could vary depending on the duration of US residence and age at migration. The chronic stress of living in the inherently racially stratified United States could result in physiologic wear and tear (also known as allostatic load—a measure of the accumulation of stress over time) and erode the body's ability to regulate (Dominguez 2008; Hobel, Goldstein, and Barrett 2008). Perceived racial discrimination experiences are considered to be among the stressors that are chronically experienced over the life course (Ong, Fuller-Rowell, and Burrow 2009). Indeed, Lu and Halfon (2003) hypothesized that increased allostatic load, due to cumulative stress over the life course, can impact reproductive function (Hobel, Goldstein, and Barrett 2008). A life course approach suggests that examining the different societal contexts shaping the lives of US-born Black women, African-born women, and Caribbean-born women (Gee, Walsemann, and Brondolo 2012; Hogan et al. 2012) is vital toward an increased understanding of the varying health trajectories of the Black birthing population.

Black Nativity

The US Black immigrant population is growing. Foreign-born Black women, in particular, are continuing to make up a larger share of the overall Black population living in the United States (Anderson 2018). Since 1980, the Black immigrant population has more than quadrupled (Mederios-Kent 2007). The rising demographic prominence of Black immigrants in the United States makes it even more important to gain an increased understanding of the reproductive health differences between US-born and foreign-born Black women.

Research has suggested that there is variance in how US-born and foreign-born Black women perceive racial discrimination; differential exposure to self-reported racism over the life course may be a critically important factor that distinguishes US-born Black women from their foreign-born counterparts (Dominguez et al. 2009). Racial stress negatively influences reproductive health (Rosenthal and Lobel 2011; Rosenthal and Lobel 2018); therefore, improving our understanding of the different relationships between racism and nativity is essential for developing interventions to lessen the impact of racial stress on sexual and reproductive health for all Black birthing persons living in the United States. In addition, Black immigrants may face barriers related to being immigrants that may not present challenges for Black Americans, such as citizenship status affecting access to health-promoting factors and resources.

Concepts such as the weathering hypothesis (Geronimus 1996) and the life course health model (Lu and Halfon 2003) argue that exposure to racism deteriorates one's health over time and that the impact extends beyond that individual to influence future generations; this is how historical trauma is passed down from generation to generation (Brave Heart et al. 2011). The historical trauma passed down, although connected, differs across these three groups. The analysis of disparities within the Black population provides evidence that racism and racial stress harm the health of Black birthing persons in the United States and that nativity may serve as a buffer mitigating the magnitude of the effect of racism for those who are foreign-born.

There is still a great deal to learn about the birth outcomes of Black immigrants in the United States as compared to Black Americans or as compared to other immigrant groups. Black immigrants may have increased susceptibility to experiencing discrimination relative to other immigrant groups, which adversely impacts health. Often, research studies that do highlight differences by nativity conclude that there is a **healthy immigrant effect** at play for the foreign-born group, providing an advantage or buffer, resulting in lower rates of the adverse outcome. However, a report out of New York City (New York City Department of Health and Mental Hygiene 2016) indicated that Black immigrant mothers from the Caribbean and sub-Saharan Africa had higher rates of adverse maternal health outcomes as compared to Black Americans.

More studies are needed to gain further insight, considering this topic is currently underresearched, relative to Black-white health inequities. Black immigrants are prone to erasure in ways that Latinx and Asian immigrants are not. Hence, there is a much larger body of literature on the impact of migration on health for those immigrant populations in comparison to Black immigrants. Considering the differences in the lived experiences across the diaspora for Black birthing persons, it is essential to not treat this population as monolithic when creating interventions to tackle the maternal health inequity crisis in the United States. However, due to the invisibility of the Black migrant in the United States, there is relatively little data collection and research on Black immigrant reproductive health outcomes. The Black population living in the United States is diverse, the nuances regarding racism and how it influences health are dynamic, and the consideration of intersecting identities, such as race and nativity, are all vital to consider and understand as we work toward mitigating the health inequities experienced by Black birthing persons living in the United States.

INVESTIGATING WITHIN-BLACK DISPARITIES

Preterm Birth Risk Among Foreign-Born and US-Born Black Women in New York City—A Mixed-Methods Study

Objective

The purpose of this study was to take a mixed-methods approach toward investigating disparities in preterm delivery within the Black population living in the United States by nativity and regional origin (i.e., US-born Black women, African immigrants, and Caribbean immigrants).

Using a unique data set of New York City births, this is the first study, to our knowledge, to model how the duration of residence in the United States and age at arrival impact the odds of preterm delivery among US- and foreign-born Black women. This is also the first study, to our knowledge, to evaluate the extent to which maternal sociodemographic and health characteristics explain these duration and timing associations on preterm delivery among foreign-born Black women.

The goal of the study was to better understand the complex phenomena of racial disparities in birth outcomes within the Black population and provide evidence to support health equity efforts that consider the diversity within the Black birthing population. The innovative mixed-methods design of this research allowed for both a quantitative investigation along with a qualitative exploration of potential underlying mechanisms contributing to disparities in preterm delivery within the Black population.

Mixed-Methods Approach

This mixed-methods study on foreign-born and US-born Black women concurrently analyzed quantitative data to examine differences in preterm delivery by nativity and by duration and qualitative data to examine variations in identity and perceived discrimination by region of origin. We then interpreted these two strands of data alongside one another to elicit a richer, deeper, and more complete inquiry of how racism is impacting the health of Black birthing persons and their infants across the Black diaspora.

The quantitative study examined more than 167,000 births to Black foreign-born individuals from 2008 to 2016. This allowed for an examination of variation in prevalence and risk of adverse birth outcomes by region of origin within the Black population and an examination of the relationship between duration and birth outcomes within the Black foreign-born population (Africans and Caribbeans), increasing our understanding of how living in the United States can impact health over time. When analyzed alongside the qualitative strand, we can have an improved understanding of these quantitative associations.

The additional qualitative context not only serves as a vital complement to the quantitative strand, but it is also one of the first qualitative contributions to focus on racial identity and perceived discrimination across these three groups of Black birthing persons in one study. The analysis focused on the exploration of the narratives on Black identity and perceptions of race-based discriminatory experiences. We paid special attention to the discordant and concordant views by nativity and region to shed light on differential perceptions of racial discrimination and varying orientations toward identifying as Black in the United States.

This mixed-methods approach was vital to better document and understand the complex and nuanced relationship between racial stress and health for Black birthing persons and the role duration plays for the foreign-born Black population. Existing research on health inequities for Black birthing persons is primarily quantitative. There are also important qualitative contributions that have been made. There are little to no mixed-methods studies on inequities this population faces, and even less that consider nativity within the Black population. This mixed-methods study design allowed for the demonstration of patterns and connections between prevalence rates of adverse birth outcomes and orientations to Black identity and narratives of racial discrimination in a manner that a solely quantitative study or solely qualitative study would not be able to accomplish.

LESSONS LEARNED

Black birthing persons in the United States are typically treated as a monolithic population, but this is far from the truth. Unfortunately, this occurs at every stage, from data collection, to research, to practice and policy. It is a harmful practice with a real impact. It masks variability in Black-white inequities when all Black birthing persons are grouped. It contributes to the invisibility of the foreign-born Black population. It fails to capture the different needs of different groups who are all experiencing inequities, and, perhaps most importantly, it prevents us from accurately estimating the effect racism has on the sexual and reproductive health of Black birthing persons in this country. In addition, foreign-born Black women's rates of adverse outcomes also differ by region of origin and duration of US residence. This illustrates that the country-of-origin context matters as well as the length of exposure to the racially stratified US system. Improving our understanding of the relationship between racial stress and maternal health inequities for Black birthing persons across the diaspora can be translated to efficacious interventions and comprehensive policies.

Blanketed interventions focused on behavior change have been the norm for far too long. Immigrant rights are rarely discussed in the reproductive health field; however, there are oppressive migration policies that immigrants face when attempting to access reproductive health care in the United States, and Black migrant groups are often subject to discrimination by race in addition to discrimination by citizenship status. Even within the foreign-born Black population, there is variation in federal immigration policy in which countries are seen as preferred. This has been made evident by the practices enacted for Haitian immigrants, many of which include pregnant women and children fleeing poverty and violence in their homeland, who have been met with harsh punishment at the border and immediate, inhumane deportation flights (Human Rights Watch 2022).

This is indicative of the fact that the structural factors influencing the immigrant experience are not a monolith, either. The growing number of Black immigrants living in the United States has called further attention to the investigation of maternal health disparities by nativity within the Black population, just as research has been done for Latinx and Asian populations for decades. As research continues to demonstrate that there are different rates of adverse outcomes for US-born and foreign-born Black populations (Mason et al. 2010), practice and policy will need to adjust. The nativity lens, from data collection to policy, is vital for the development of innovative research, effective interventions, equitable practices, and overall comprehensive approaches toward the elimination of racial health inequities.

Data Justice

Data limitations have been a major barrier to realizing the potential insights about reproductive health inequities that the study of Black immigrant health promises. Specifically, there is a great need for data sets that contain adequate numbers of Black immigrant births, date of migration (not collected on the standard US birth record), and key maternal (e.g., health behaviors) and social (e.g., discrimination) factors implicated in prominent theories of immigrant health. For example, recent studies based on survey data have reported intriguing evidence that the association between duration of US residence and birth weight among infants born to US immigrants may be nonlinear and conditional on migration timing (i.e., during childhood vs. adulthood; Teitler, Martinson, and Reichman 2015; Teitler, Hutto, and Reichman 2012). However, while evidence of these associations was found within Latinx and Asian subgroups, sample size limitations prevented a parallel investigation among foreign-born Black women.

Data limitations have also hampered efforts to evaluate racial discrimination as a potential mechanism linking nativity to birth outcomes. Key migrant reproductive health studies by Elo, Vang, and Culhane (2014); Teitler, Martinson, and Reichman (2015); and Teitler, Hutto, and Reichman (2015) have suggested that future research investigate duration of US residence and perceived racial discrimination in the Black population, as they could be of great importance. Little is known about the role of racial discrimination in shaping the health outcomes of foreign-born Black women (Collins and David 2009). Currently, studies examining the effect of these important potential mechanisms for foreign-born Black birthing persons are limited. While virtually all births to Black immigrants are recorded in the US Vital Records system, research is hampered by the lack of data on key measures that would allow for an investigation of how racism and racial stress impact Black birthing persons across the diaspora.

The lack of research on the health of foreign-born Black women is a significant gap in the literature. This further perpetuates the invisibility of the Black migrant and hampers efforts to tackle inequities, considering how challenging it is to create change when it is not possible to accurately capture the magnitude of the disparity. It is hard to create interventions intended to serve people whom we are failing to include in typical data collection practices. If we fail to capture nativity, it will remain increasingly difficult to assess how and to what degree racism is impacting the birth of Black birthing persons in America if we are treating the Black populations as monolithic.

Tailored Approaches

Interventions aimed at lessening the high rates of adverse reproductive health outcomes experienced by all Black birthing populations will need to consider the varying needs that different nativity groups may have by region of origin.

One example of an organization that pivoted to add a program focused on the unique needs of the pregnant and postpartum immigrant community in Brooklyn, New York, is Life of Hope (Life of Hope 2021). Life of Hope is a nonprofit organization that serves immigrant families. The organization started a women's health initiative that targets immigrant mothers, primarily those who come from francophone countries and may or may not be comfortable with the English language upon arrival. One of the goals of the women's health initiative is to provide additional support services to these pregnant and postpartum mothers that consider their unique linguistic and cultural barriers.

There is a need for tailored community-based interventions that intentionally factor in the heterogeneous nature of the Black population living in the United States and do not obscure variation in their birth outcomes by lumping all Black births into one group. After all, we are not a monolith; therefore, cookie-cutter, individual-level, blanketed research approaches, policies, and practices targeted at eliminating racial health inequities will not suffice. Rather, a systemic, holistic approach that factors in the heterogeneity of the Black population living in the United States is vital.

WHERE WE ARE NOW, AND WHERE DO WE GO FROM HERE?

Currently, the practice and approach to addressing Black birthing inequities do not typically incorporate intersectional identities of Black birthing persons. Moving forward, understanding that the heterogeneity of the Black population exists and is a vital consideration for creating community-based approaches (informed by historical context and/or modern-day country-specific adversities) is needed to eliminate health inequities experienced by Black birthing persons across the diaspora in the United States. Addressing maternal health inequities requires a systemic, holistic approach rather than an individual approach.

There is vital context on the heterogeneous lived experiences of Black birthing persons in the United States. Conducting the work of tackling maternal health inequities requires an understanding and appreciation of this, that can inform data collection, interventions, and policies.

All Black birthing persons face oppressive systems in the United States that increase their risk of experiencing stress—stress due to racism in their everyday life and stress due to experiences with racism during their pregnancy, labor, and delivery care as well. However, there is great variation in the outcomes that result for these Black birthing persons across the diaspora, even among the foreign-born. The potential mechanisms at play here are rooted in intergenerational trauma, historical context, and intersectionality and how those three tenets interplay and influence a person or a community's perceptions and navigation of care. In short, the Black birthing population living in the United States is very diverse in several ways, nativity being one of them. It would be egregious to continue the use of blanketed approaches targeted toward eliminating racial/ethnic inequities in maternal and infant health outcomes.

REFERENCES

Anderson M. A rising share of the US Black population is foreign born; 9 percent are immigrants: and while most are from the Caribbean, Africans drive recent growth. Pew Research Center. 2018. https://doi.org/10.1016/j.jbankfin.2017.09.006

Arthur CM, Katkin, ES. Making a case for the examination of ethnicity of Blacks in United States Health Research. *J Health Care Poor Underserved*. 2006;17(1):25-36. https://doi.org/10.1353/hpu.2006.0017

Brave Heart MY, Chase J, Elkins J, Altschul DB. Historical trauma among Indigenous peoples of the Americas: concepts, research, and clinical considerations. *J Psychoactive Drugs*. 2011;43(4):282-290. https://doi.org/10.1080/02791072.2011.628913

Collins JW, David RJ. Racial disparity in low birth weight and infant mortality. *Clin Perinatol*. 2009;36(1):63-73. https://doi.org/10.1016/j.clp.2008.09.004

Crump C, Lipsky S, Mueller BA. Adverse birth outcomes among Mexican-Americans: are US-born women at greater risk than Mexico-born women? *Ethn Health*. 1999;4(1-2):29-34. https://doi.org/10.1080/13557859998164

Deaux K, Bikmen N, Gilkes A, et al. Becoming American: sterotype threat effects in Afro-Caribbean immigrant groups. *Soc Psychol Q*. 2007;70(4):384-404. https://psycnet.apa.org/doi/10.1177/019027250707000408

Dominguez TP. Race, racism, and racial disparities in adverse birth outcomes. *Clin Obstet Gynecol*. 2008;51(2):360-370. https://doi.org/10.1097/GRF.0b013e31816f28de

Dominguez TP, Strong EF, Krieger N, Gillman MW, Rich-Edwards JW. Differences in the self-reported racism experiences of US-born and foreign-born Black pregnant women. *Soc Sci Med.* 2009;69(2):258-265. https://doi.org/10.1016/j.socscimed.2009.03.022

Elo IT, Vang Z, Culhane JF. Variation in birth outcomes by mother's country of birth among non-Hispanic Black women in the United States. *Matern Child Health J.* 2014;18(10):2371-2381. https://doi.org/10.1007/s10995-014-1477-0

Gee GC, Walsemann KM, Brondolo E. A life course perspective on how racism may be related to health inequities. *Am J Public Health.* 2012;102(5):967-974. https://doi.org/10.2105/AJPH.2012.300666

Geronimus AT. Black/white differences in the relationship of maternal age to birthweight: a population-based test of the weathering hypothesis. *Soc Sci Med.* 1996;42(4):589-597. https://doi.org/10.1016/0277-9536(95)00159-X

Giscombe CL, Lobel M. Explaining disproportionately high rates of adverse birth outcomes among African Americans: the impact of stress, racism, and related factors in pregnancy. *Psychol Bull.* 2005;131:662-683. https://doi.org/10.1037/0033-2909.131.5.662

Hobel CJ, Goldstein A, Barrett ES. Psychosocial stress and pregnancy outcome. *Clin Obstet Gynecol.* 2008;51(2):333-348. https://doi.org/10.1097/GRF.0b013e31816f2709

Hogan VK, Rowley D, Bennett T, Taylor KD. Life course, social determinants, and health inequities: toward a national plan for achieving health equity for African American infants—a concept paper. *Matern Child Health J.* 2012;16(6):1143-1150. https://doi.org/10.1007/s10995-011-0847-0

Human Rights Watch. Haitians being returned to a country in chaos. March 24, 2022. Available at: https://www.hrw.org/news/2022/03/24/haitians-being-returned-country-chaos

Hummer R, Biegler M, De Turk P, et al. Race/ethnicity, nativity, and infant mortality in the United States. *Soc Forces.* 1999;77(3):1083-1117. https://doi.org/doi:10.2307/3005972

Jones CP. Levels of racism: a theoretic framework and a gardener's tale. *Am J Public Health.* 2000;90(8):1212-1215. https://doi.org/10.2105/AJPH.90.8.1212

Life of Hope. Haitian Women's Birth Equity Pregnancy & Postpartum Support Group. 2021. Available at: https://www.lohnyc.org/hwbe-support-group

Lu MC, Halfon N. Racial and ethnic disparities in birth outcomes: a life-course perspective. *Matern Child Health J.* 2003;7(1):13-30. https://doi.org/10.1023/A:1022537516969

Mason SM, Kaufman JS, Emch ME, Hogan VK, Savitz DA. Ethnic density and preterm birth in African-, Caribbean-, and US-born non-Hispanic Black populations in New York City. *Am J Epidemiol.* 2010;172(7):800-808. https://doi.org/10.1093/aje/kwq209

Mederios-Kent M. Immigration and America's Black population. *Popul Bull.* 2007;62(4):1-16.

New York City Department of Health and Mental Hygiene. Severe maternal morbidity in New York City, 2008-2012. 2016. Available at: https://www.nyc.gov/assets/doh/downloads/pdf/data/maternal-morbidity-report-08-12.pdf

Nuru-Jeter A, Dominguez TP, Hammond WP, et al. "It's the skin you're in": African-American women talk about their experiences of racism. An exploratory study to develop measures of racism for birth outcome studies. *Matern Child Health J.* 2009;13(1):29-39. https://doi.org/10.1007/s10995-008-0357-x

Ong AD, Fuller-Rowell T, Burrow AL. Racial discrimination and the stress process. *J Pers Soc Psychol.* 2009;96(6):1259-1271. https://doi.org/10.1037/a0015335

Pearlin L, Lieberman M, Menaghan E, Mullan J. The stress process. *J Health Soc Behav.* 1981;22(4):337-356.

Rosenthal L, Lobel M. Explaining racial disparities in adverse birth outcomes: unique sources of stress for Black American women. *Soc Sci Med.* 2011;72(6):977-983. https://doi.org/10.1016/j.socscimed.2011.01.013

Rosenthal L, Lobel M. Gendered racism and the sexual and reproductive health of Black and Latina women. *Ethn Health.* 2018;25(3):367-392. https://doi.org/10.1080/13557858.2018.1439896

Slaughter-Acey JC, Sealy-Jefferson S, Helmkamp L, et al. Racism in the form of microaggressions and the risk of preterm birth among Black women. *Ann Epidemiol.* 2015;26(1):7-13.e1. https://doi.org/10.1016/j.annepidem.2015.10.005

Teitler J, Martinson M, Reichman NE. Does life in the United States take a toll on health? Duration of residence and birthweight among six decades of immigrants. *Int Migr Rev.* 2015;51(1):37-66. https://doi.org/10.1111/imre.12207

Teitler JO, Hutto N, Reichman NE. Birthweight of children of immigrants by maternal duration of residence in the United States. *Soc Sci Med.* 2012;75(3):459-468. https://doi.org/10.1016/j.socscimed.2012.03.038

Viruell-Fuentes EA, Miranda PY, Abdulrahim S. More than culture: structural racism, intersectionality theory, and immigrant health. *Soc Sci M.* 2012;75(12):2099-2106. https://doi.org/10.1016/j.socscimed.2011.12.037

17

Reclaiming Black Breast Power: Breastfeeding and Chestfeeding Among Black Birthing Persons

Camille A. Clare, MD, MPH, and Nekisha Killings, MPH

Conversations around Black reproductive health, sexuality, and public health must include an exploration of infant feeding and its connection to the lived experiences of Black birthing people during the perinatal period. Black babies are less likely to receive human milk than their white counterparts. This is so, even in the face of well-documented health benefits of human milk feeding for both the baby and the birthing person. This chapter will discuss the historical context of Black breastfeeding and chestfeeding that contributes to the current state and illuminate the support services and resources currently in place as local and systemic solutions to the challenges faced.

YESTERDAY SHAPES TODAY: HISTORICAL CONTEXT OF BLACK BREASTFEEDING AND CHESTFEEDING

The historical context of Black breastfeeding in the United States is broad and storied. Dating back to the transatlantic slave trade, which ushered in an era of forced breeding and wet nursing, Black women's autonomy around birthing and infant feeding was systematically stripped from them, leaving a wake of trauma that still impacts infant feeding choices today. This issue is layered and multifaceted. Of course, lived experiences and personal health choices are unique to every individual. However, a shared history and ongoing collective trauma create a common landscape upon which Black birthing people navigate the perinatal period and make birthing and infant feeding decisions.

One of the chief responsibilities of enslaved pregnant persons was to bear children through breeding to expand their owner's working stock. The resulting pregnancies are directly responsible for the ballooning of the Black population from what is believed to have been somewhere around 400,000 African persons trafficked to the United States during the transatlantic slave trade to a population of nearly four million in 1860 (Hacker 2020), despite astronomical infant and maternal mortality rates (Steckel 1986; Owens and Fett 2019). The average enslaved birthing person bore 10 children, with many bearing more than 20 children in a lifetime.

Even when enslaved women were married, captors determined the level of prenatal care and work schedules they might enjoy. Some enslavers were concerned enough about the welfare of the infant (or, rather, the additional labor they would eventually become) that they allowed for reduced work in the latter parts of pregnancy and time off to nurse the newborn briefly after delivery. Many enslavers separated their enslaved into groups known as "gangs." Women with nurslings were often put into a "sucklers gang" who worked under special conditions to accommodate breastfeeding. Other enslavers made the enslaved mothers return to work immediately, carrying the infant with them or leaving them in the care of others and occasionally returning to breastfeed throughout the day. Some captors prepared detailed instructions for nursing mothers, accounting for every month of her breastfeeding journey and accommodating the nursing relationship relatively well within the parameters of slavery and the general understanding of breastfeeding science at the time (Heuman and Walvin 2003).

According to Tannenbaum (2012), when an enslaved baby was born, if it was viable, it likely suckled at the breast. After all, breastfeeding was the customary method of infant feeding for all humans at that time. However, the conditions and length of time an infant nursed would have greatly varied, depending upon factors including whether the parent was nursing other children, if the parent lived in the quarters with their children, and if their children remained on the same plantation or were sold away.

In one particularly gruesome detailed account in William Wells Brown's slave narratives (Brown 1847), a story is shared about a long, hot journey by foot led by human trafficker James Walker. In the caravan was a group of newly traded enslaved humans, including women and children. One mother had a fussy nursling who cried more than Walker preferred. At a stop at an inn, Mr. Walker ripped the infant from the mother's arms and gave it to the innkeeper. The mother, devastated, wailed and begged for her baby to be returned. Mr. Walker simply ignored her and barked for her to be chained to the other enslaved men, women, and children now that she was no longer carrying the child (as it was customary for those carrying children to not be bound to the chain gang). Along that same trip, a remarkably similar scene happened with a blind baby, and that child was sold for one dollar to another innkeeper. Understandably distraught, mothers often resisted but were forced to journey on without their children (Brown and Cashin 2016).

Practices such as this continued throughout enslavement to reconstruction. The Jim Crow Era brought with it its own set of horrors, deeply impacting families and thwarting any semblance of birthing and infant feeding in peace and safety. The deliberate erasure of granny midwives and medicalization of birth, systemic racism and discrimination, and the "War on Drugs" followed by mass incarceration all had documented and detrimental outcomes.

Meanwhile, there was money to be made in a new industry. Scientific advances around food sterilization and preservation shifted infant feeding norms from primarily human milk to primarily formula for white mothers over the first half of the 20th century. Black mothers, while not initially inclined to follow suit, eventually experienced the same transition as an expression of their independence and a march toward modernity. By the 1970s, the United States experienced its lowest breastfeeding rates among all groups. In the 1980s and 1990s, most white mothers returned to breastfeeding and chestfeeding as the benefits of human milk and the risks of formula feeding became more widely known and understood. However, Black parents did not switch back to human milk feeding en masse. Five decades later, racial disparity gaps are narrowing.

TODAY SHAPES TOMORROW: CURRENT STATES OF BLACK BREASTFEEDING AND CHESTFEEDING

The harm that the perpetuated, multigenerational trauma inflicted upon Black birthing people cannot be understated. The stench of that trauma lingers. Green, Killings, and Clare (2021) discuss the broad array of factors impacting infant feeding decisions today. These include not only forced wet nursing and enslavement but also the dubious past of the medical establishment as it relates to Black bodies, leading to disdain, distrust, and the resulting hesitance to adhere to medical recommendations. Black birthing people make personal health decisions within the context of not only their lived experiences but also well-known historical tragedies such as Dr. J. Marion Sims's cruel experimentation, the Tuskegee experiment, Fannie Lou Hamer's hysterectomy and other Mississippi appendectomies without consent, and forced sterilizations.

Current factors compounding the challenge include inadequate infant feeding counseling and problematic marketing by formula companies. Lack of workplace support for nursing parents, lack of access to informed and respectful care, racism in the birthing space equating to medical neglect, and forced parent-baby separations when seeking care are all pressing issues. Yet, Black birthing people persist in their pursuit of healthy infant feeding options. The overwhelming majority (74%) of Black infants receive some human milk (Chiang et al. 2019), and that number continues to increase steadily. This is extraordinary given the many historical and current factors at play to thwart breastfeeding and chestfeeding success. A great deal of the credit for recent gains in Black breastfeeding and chestfeeding rates is owed to local and national services and programs that have raised awareness and provided direct support to families and communities.

THE ANSWERS LIE WITHIN THE COMMUNITY: SERVICES AND SOCIAL AND ECONOMIC RESOURCES

The persistence of inequities in Black breastfeeding is rooted in structural and systemic racism. Services and social and economic resources must focus on addressing racism, poor access to resources and support for Black pregnant and birthing persons, and inadequate diversity in the lactation workforce. Black birthing persons face barriers in the perinatal period, limiting their ability to achieve their feeding goals. Explicit and implicit biases by health care professionals/workers (HCWs), especially in hospital settings, negatively affect Black breastfeeding and chestfeeding. Interpersonal, sociocultural, and institutional barriers for Black birthing persons include lack of paid leave from work, lack of access to electric pumps, social pressures to initiate formula supplementation, fears that breastfeeding renders infants overly dependent on parental care, and a lack of breastfeeding role models and/or support networks to normalize longer-term breastfeeding (Deubel et al. 2019). Lack of HCW knowledge of the historical, cultural, and social context of feeding in the Black community, specifically wet nursing, may lead to poor maternity care practices (Green, Killings, and Clare 2021).

There are also higher rates of formula feeding among Black infants—that is, nine times the rate of white infants—and disparate care of Black infants in the neonatal intensive care unit setting (Asiodu, Bugg, and Palmquist 2021).

Since Black communities are not a monolith, it is important to further distinguish Black subgroups and the impact on feeding practices for those groups. Significant differences in breastfeeding initiation were noted between Black immigrants and African Americans enrolled in a District of Columbia Supplemental Nutrition Program for *Women, Infants, and Children* (WIC) program. By combining African American and Black immigrant subgroups, significant differences are masked, and rates of breastfeeding (chestfeeding was not distinguished in this study) are overestimated among African Americans. This, in turn, overestimates the impact of interventions among African Americans, leading to missed opportunities for targeted interventions and policies to improve breastfeeding.

Furthermore, within the WIC program, there has been an underreporting of breastfeeding behavior to obtain formula vouchers or overreporting to receive additional maternal food package issuances, both important financial challenges to feeding goals. Pertinent information should be gathered with care. For example, when relying on primary language spoken at home as an identifier, Black subgroups in the District of Columbia may be underestimated in data collection, especially among immigrant groups from English-speaking countries (Roess et al. 2022).

Older data from the 2007-2008 Louisiana Pregnancy Risk Assessment Monitoring System described Black birthing persons as less likely to receive breastfeeding instruction and support from health care professionals. They are also less likely to receive phone numbers for support and to participate in rooming-in practices, and less likely to have breastfed at all or exclusively while in the hospital (Gee, Zerbib, and Luckett 2012).

Despite the common narrative of poor rates among Black birthing individuals, they *are* breastfeeding and chestfeeding their infants. Some culturally appropriate services that have been offered to support these individuals include the Baby Friendly Hospital Initiative (BFHI), which supports hospital- and community-based resources for breastfeeding and chestfeeding. Hospitals that are serving mostly Black populations may not be appropriately following the Ten Steps to Successful Breastfeeding of the BFHI or may not have that designation. Community, local, state, and national initiatives that are Black-led can increase the rates of Black infant feeding, including Reaching Our Sisters Everywhere, the Black Mothers' Breastfeeding Association, the Center for Social Inclusion, HealthConnect One, and Black Mamas Matter Alliance, among others. The creation of Black Breastfeeding Week, online support groups, and community-centered peer-to-peer breastfeeding trainings have also been successful (Asiodu, Bugg, and Palmquist 2021).

The 2011 Call to Action to Support Breastfeeding by the Surgeon General outlined several strategies for communities and community-based organizations (HHS 2011), such as the following:

1. increasing peer-to-peer support;
2. ensuring continuity of care;
3. increasing maternity care practices that are supportive of breastfeeding;
4. funding nonprofit organizations that support breastfeeding, especially in Black, Brown, and Indigenous communities;
5. ensuring that all public health programs include breastfeeding education and support;
6. developing community and national campaigns to promote breastfeeding; and
7. ensuring the application of the World Health Organization International Code of Marketing of Breast-Milk Substitutes (WHO Code; 1981).

Public health policies call for an investment of additional resources and investment with community partners (Asiodu, Bugg, and Palmquist 2021).

National and local efforts to increase feeding support in the United States from 2009 to 2015 included policies that protect the right to breast- and chestfeed in public, time and space to express milk at work, the expansion of training for physicians and other health care professionals, and access to professional lactation support. Nevertheless, Black birthing people may experience relatively poor access to breastfeeding programs and supports, further widening inequities in breastfeeding and chestfeeding between Black and white parents (Li et al. 2019).

The COVID-19 pandemic further amplified the need for creative approaches to address the feeding goals of Black birthing people. Notable challenges included restrictive hospital visitation policies at the onset of the initial surge in 2020; the elimination of birth and breastfeeding and chestfeeding education; reductions and shortages of staff, especially the lactation workforce; program elimination or closure; service transitions to online, virtual, and telehealth platforms; and parental separation based on severe acute respiratory syndrome coronavirus 2 (SARS-CoV-2)-positive or under-investigation status, affecting bonding, skin-to-skin opportunities, and the initiation of breastfeeding and chestfeeding (Asiodu, Bugg, and Palmquist 2021).

Asiodu, Bugg, and Palmquist (2021) describe decolonializing breastfeeding and chestfeeding research centered on Eurocentrism and white supremacy. Clinical practices, including Black, Brown, and Indigenous people of the global majority, and expanding lactation support persons (e.g., international board-certified lactation consultants, certified lactation counselors and specialists, certified lactation educators, breastfeeding peer counselors), are critical to breastfeeding and chestfeeding services for patients. Collaboration among Black birth workers such as obstetrician-gynecologists, midwives, doulas, nurses, and dietitians is needed, alongside lactation workers. Resilient rather than deficit-focused models of research with the inclusion of diverse researchers and research teams maintain this pro-Blackness approach. In addition, including more Black, Brown, and Indigenous researchers allows them to examine more pertinent inquiries about the lived experiences of Black pregnant and birthing persons, evidence-based interventions, data collection and analysis, and recommendation dissemination (Asiodu, Bugg, and Palmquist 2021).

Tele-lactation services support disenfranchised and marginalized communities who potentially have limited access to professional lactation support by International Board-certified lactation consultants, particularly those racially and ethnically concordant to birthing persons. The first randomized-controlled clinical trial to examine the impact of tele-lactation on breastfeeding duration and exclusivity, and acceptability of and experiences among Black and Latino/a/e/x parents, began in 2022 (Uscher-Pines et al. 2022). This ongoing work will provide a context for Black birthing persons beyond the COVID-19 pandemic and the utility of tele-lactation in a variety of situations.

Insurance coverage is an important access point, especially for Black, Brown, and Indigenous people of the global majority. Kapinos, Bullinger, and Gurley-Calvez (2017) noted that the Affordable Care Act-mandated coverage of lactation services increased breastfeeding initiation among privately insured individuals relative to those covered by Medicaid. This translated into about 47,000 more infants for whom breastfeeding was initiated in 2014. Larger effects were demonstrated among Black, less educated, and unmarried parents. However, the long-term effects at 6- and 12-months postpartum for breastfeeding and chestfeeding rates are yet to be determined (Kapinos, Bullinger, and Gurley-Calvez 2017).

Additional support for Black birthing persons considers maximizing breastfeeding and chestfeeding goals based on type of work. For example, white, nonworking persons breastfed the longest, while those in the service and labor workforce breastfed for the shortest duration. Among Black individuals, those in professional and managerial work breastfed for longer than those in the other two occupational categories. In addition, Black individuals may experience less flexibility in job functions or face racially discriminatory practices by supervisors and employers. Inequities in hiring, firing, and layoff practices between Black and white workers are other structural barriers. Needed workplace services involve the Business Case for Breastfeeding (a comprehensive program designed to educate employers about the value of supporting breastfeeding employees in the workplace; US Department of Health and Human Services, Office of Women's Health n.d.), lactation programs for employees, and corporate initiatives to reduce work-family conflict and increase the control of employee schedules with broad implementation and tailoring to the needs of Black workers (Whitley, Ro, and Palma 2021).

In a study of self-reported reasons for breastfeeding and chestfeeding cessation during the first year postpartum in those participating in the WIC program, Gallo, Kogan, and Kitsantas (2019) reported that food security, parity, country of birth, education, and marital status may lead to cessation of desired infant feeding. Black primiparous patients were more likely to discontinue feeding due to problems with suckling and latch, further illustrating the importance of in-hospital support services for this population by culturally sensitive HCWs. In addition, Black birthing persons with very low food security stopped breastfeeding or chestfeeding due to wanting or needing someone else to feed their baby (Gallo, Kogan, and Kitsantas 2019).

A successful program called the Bosom Buddy Program, sponsored by grant funding by the Indiana Black Breastfeeding Coalition in 2012, offered breastfeeding support groups with trained peer mentors (Friesen, Hormuth, and Curtis 2015). Specific challenges between breastfeeding intention and duration have been described in Black and Hispanic women, including experiences during the birth hospitalization, access to or receipt of professional lactation services, family and community-level support for breastfeeding, affordable childcare, and experiences within workplace environments. The use of WIC peer counselors or participation in a WIC peer breastfeeding support group have addressed such barriers (Hamner et al. 2021).

Home visiting services support families seeking and accessing care. For example, six programs located in Chicago, Illinois, are funded by state and federal governments: Chicago Family Case Management, Early Intervention, Family Focus, Healthy Start, Healthy Families Illinois, and Family Connects Chicago. Family Connects Chicago is a universal postpartum nurse home visiting service for families, providing one to three visits starting about three-weeks postpartum. The benefits of a universal service include the reduction of stigma, assessment of population risks, and the connection of those with specialized needs to resources. Nurses in these programs have lactation training and can refer participants to community-based lactation care providers and/or WIC services (Butler et al. 2021).

Funding needs for Black, Brown, and Indigenous people of the global majority to support breast- and chest-feeding have been addressed by community-based organizations and federally qualified health centers. Sufficient funding from institutions and funding agencies must include lactation services to address breastfeeding barriers within socioeconomically marginalized communities and to expand the multilevel lactation care workforce. Community-led approaches for Black birthing persons are especially important to combat inconsistencies between breast- and chestfeeding information provided by lactation providers and that of the hospital-based delivery team. Selective investment in certain communities leads to increased vulnerability in settings of hospital closures in poorly resourced neighborhoods. A mismatch in priorities occurs between lactation care workers and hospital staff, who may often interrupt or delay early breast- and chest-feeding efforts due to limited or lack of knowledge about breast- and chestfeeding best practices (Butler et al. 2021). Therefore, additional education is needed for HCWs or physicians.

The National Medical Association Breastfeeding Alliance was created from a grant by the W.K. Kellogg Foundation in 2014 to educate Black physicians and the patients that they serve about the benefits of breastfeeding. This was an attempt to decrease inequities in breast- and chestfeeding rates among Black birthing persons. Through educational conferences, didactic lectures, community outreach, presentations, and the identification of physician champions, the Alliance impacted the training of the physician workforce on feeding practices (National Medical Association n.d.).

The Project Dads in Nutrition Education interventional program in Georgia highlights the need for multilevel support for a Black birthing person's ability to maintain nutrition and breastfeeding knowledge, attitudes, and self-efficacy by including the role of nongestational parents, specifically fathers, as part of a Healthy Start program. Father involvement is an interpersonal factor impacting maternal health. Parental involvement in sustaining breast- and chestfeeding education and addressing gestational and nongestational parents is pivotal. This intervention is one of a few discussing father involvement for breastfeeding support and healthy eating lifestyles (Rollins et al. 2022).

The role of the partner cannot be understated in the discussion of support for the nursing parent. Just as with other types of support systems, coparents and life partners play an integral role in reinforcing efficacy and affirming the intentions to reach breast- and chestfeeding goals.

According to Mitchell-Box et al. (2013), partner attitudes toward breast- and chestfeeding directly correlate to the nursing parent's attitudes toward and intentions regarding infant feeding. When partners are supportive and advocate for long-term nursing, the outcomes are often even better than the nursing parent intended (Rempel, Rempel, and Moore 2017).

Indeed, opening support groups to partners increases the likelihood that the nursing parent will attend, as bringing a trusted companion into an unfamiliar space provides comfort and confidence. At the forefront of empowering fathers as breast- and chest-feeding advocates is the organization Reaching Our Sisters Everywhere with their extension organization, Reaching Our Brothers Everywhere (ROBE). This latter independent organization, whose mission is to "educate, equip, and empower men to impact an increase in breastfeeding rates and a decrease in infant mortality rates within the African-American communities," hosts informative sessions and support groups for Black fathers of nurslings (ROBE 2019).

Fathers and nongestational parents play a key role in supporting Black pregnant, birthing, and lactating persons in their breast- and chestfeeding goals not only in the intention to breast- and chestfeed but also to reduce risk of problems, to improve rates of exclusive breast- and chestfeeding, and to improve the knowledge and attitudes toward breast- and chestfeeding of the gestational parent. In addition, paternal emotional support, responsiveness to needs and decisions, assistance with household and childcare tasks, and help with breast- and chestfeeding difficulties may improve outcomes (Backman 2021).

Social media platforms have been piloted for interventions supporting the feeding goals of Black birthing persons. A pilot study of a local WIC program demonstrated that using electronic, smartphone apps with social media, such as #BlackBreastsMatter, benefits recruitment and health education intervention studies. Such messaging and resources reinforce and educate parents about breast- and chestfeeding and provide lactation support. Authors have suggested the use of metrics for data analysis, such as "Group Insight," to capture prenatal and postnatal educational interventions, live lactation opportunities, especially for racially concordant services, and web-based systems to support WIC and peer counselors. Culturally sensitive interventions that address socioeconomic and structural barriers, parental perceptions of breastfeeding benefits and difficulties, and improvements in postnatal lactation and doula support may foster a more inclusive culture of breastfeeding and chestfeeding (Dauphin et al. 2020).

CONCLUSION

Reclaiming Black power in infant feeding for Black pregnant and birthing persons must center the sociocultural and historical context in which breastfeeding and chestfeeding is practiced. Removal of the interpersonal, structural, and institutional racism; bias; and discriminatory practices and barriers in birthing systems and among the lactation workforce is key to liberate Black birthing persons and their lived experiences in a reproductive justice framework. Bolstering programs and services that are culturally congruent, locally targeted to community needs, and national in reach and impact are vital components to a balanced and effective set of solutions that will give way to continued increases in Black breastfeeding and chestfeeding rates in the United States.

REFERENCES

Asiodu IV, Bugg K, Palmquist AEL. Achieving breastfeeding equity and justice in Black communities: past, present, and future. *Breastfeed Med*. 2021;16(6):447–451. https://doi.org/10.1089/bfm.2020.0314

Backman D. The importance of family engagement in breastfeeding programs. Association of State and Territorial Health Officials. August 27, 2021. Available at: https://www.astho.org/communications/blog/importance-of-family-engagement-in-breastfeeding-programs

Brown WW. *Narrative of William W. Brown, a fugitive slave*. Boston, MA: The Anti-slavery Office; 1847. Available at: https://www.loc.gov/item/14004708

Brown WW, Cashin JE. *Clotel, or the President's Daughter*. New York, NY: Routledge; 2016. https://doi.org/10.4324/9781315285139

Butler M, Allen JA, Hoskins-Wroten J, et al. Structural racism and barriers to breastfeeding on Chicagoland's South Side. *Breastfeed Med*. 2021;16(2):112–115. https://doi.org/10.1089/bfm.2020.0311

Chiang KV, Li R, Anstey EH, Perrine CG. Racial and ethnic disparities in breastfeeding initiation—United States, 2019. *MMWR Morb Mortal Wkly Rep*. 2021;70(21):769–774. http://dx.doi.org/10.15585/mmwr.mm7021a1

Dauphin C, Clark N, Cadzow R, et al. #BlackBreastsMatter: process evaluation of recruitment and engagement of pregnant African American women for a social media intervention study to increase breastfeeding. *J Med Internet Res*. 2020;22(8):e16239. https://doi.org/10.2196/16239

Deubel TF, Miller EM, Hernandez I, Boyer M, Louis-Jacques A. Perceptions and practices of infant feeding among African American women. *Ecol Food Nutr*. 2019;58(4):301–316. https://doi.org/10.1080/03670244.2019.1598977

Friesen CA, Hormuth LJ, Curtis TJ. The Bosom Buddy Project: a breastfeeding support group sponsored by the Indiana Black Breastfeeding Coalition for Black and minority women in Indiana. *J Hum Lact*. 2015;31(4):587–591. https://doi.org/10.1177/0890334415581617

Gallo S, Kogan K, Kitsantas P. Racial and ethnic differences in reasons for breastfeeding cessation among women participating in the Special Supplemental Nutrition Program for Women, Infants, and Children. *J Midwifery Womens Health*. 2019;64(6):725–733. https://doi.org/10.1111/jmwh.13031

Gee RE, Zerbib LD, Luckett BG. Breastfeeding support for African American women in Louisiana hospitals. *Breastfeed Med*. 2012;7(6):431–435. https://doi.org/10.1089/bfm.2011.0150

Green VL, Killings NL, Clare CA. The historical, psychosocial, and cultural context of breastfeeding in the African American community. *Breastfeed Med*. 2021;16(2):116–120. https://doi.org/10.1089/bfm.2020.0316

Hacker JD. From "20. and odd" to 10 million: the growth of the slave population in the United States. *Slavery Abol*. 2020;41(4):840–855. https://doi.org/10.1080/0144039x.2020.1755502

Hamner HC, Beauregard JL, Li R, Nelson JM, Perrine CG. Meeting breastfeeding intentions differ by race/ethnicity, Infant and Toddler Feeding Practices Study-2. *Matern Child Nutr*. 2021;17(2):e13093. https://doi.org/10.1111/mcn.13093

Heuman GJ, Walvin J, eds. *The Slavery Reader*. Vol. 1. New York, NY: Psychology Press; 2003.

Kapinos KA, Bullinger L, Gurley-Calvez T. Lactation support services and breastfeeding initiation: evidence from the Affordable Care Act. *Health Serv Res*. 2017;52(6):2175–2196. https://doi.org/10.1111/1475-6773.12598.

Li R, Perrine CG, Anstey EH, Chen J, MacGowan CA, Elam-Evans LD. Breastfeeding trends by race/ethnicity among US children born from 2009 to 2015. *JAMA Pediatr*. 2019;173(12):e193319. https://doi.org/10.1001/jamapediatrics.2019.3319

Mitchell-Box K, Braun KL, Hurwitz EL, Hayes DK. Breastfeeding attitudes: association between maternal and male partner attitudes and breastfeeding intent. *Breastfeed Med*. 2013;8(4):368–373. https://doi.org/10.1089/bfm.2012.0135

National Medical Association. Breastfeeding. Available at: https://www.nmanet.org/page/Breastfeeding?&hhsearchterms=%22breastfeeding+and+alliance%22

Owens DC, Fett SM. Black maternal and infant health: historical legacies of slavery. *Am J Public Health.* 2019;109(10):1342–1345. https://doi.org/10.2105/AJPH.2019.305243

Reaching Our Brothers Everywhere. Our mission statement. 2019. Available at: https://breastfeedingrobe.org

Rempel LA, Rempel JK, Moore KCJ. Relationships between types of father breastfeeding support and breastfeeding outcomes. *Matern Child Nutr.* 2017;13(3):e12337. https://doi.org/10.1111/mcn.12337

Roess AA, Robert RC, Kuehn D, et al. Disparities in breastfeeding initiation among African American and Black immigrant WIC recipients in the District of Columbia, 2007–2019. *Am J Public Health.* 2022;112:671–674. https://doi.org/10.2105/AJPH.2021.306652

Rollins L, Giddings T, Henes S, et al. Design and implementation of a nutrition and breastfeeding education program for Black expecting mothers and fathers. *J Nutr Educ Behav.* 2022;54(8):794–803. https://doi.org/10.1016/j.jneb.2022.03.011

Steckel R. A dreadful childhood: the excess mortality of American slaves. *Soc Sci Hist.* 1986;10(4):427–466.

Tannenbaum RJ. *Health and Wellness in Colonial America.* Santa Barbara, CA: Greenwood; 2012.

US Department of Health and Human Services. Office of Women's Health. Business Case for Breastfeeding. Available at: https://www.womenshealth.gov/breastfeeding/breastfeeding-home-work-and-public/breastfeeding-and-going-back-work/business-case

US Department of Health and Human Services. The Surgeon General's call to action to support breastfeeding. Washington, DC: Office of the Surgeon General; 2011.

Uscher-Pines L, Demirci J, Waymouth M, et al. Impact of telelactation services on breastfeeding outcomes among Black and Latinx parents: protocol for the Tele-MILC randomized controlled trial. *Trials.* 2022;23(1):5. https://doi.org/10.1186/s13063-021-05846-w

Whitley MD, Ro A, Palma A. Work, race and breastfeeding outcomes for mothers in the United States. *PLoS One.* 2021;16(5):e0251125. https://doi.org/10.1371/journal.pone.0251125

World Health Organization. WHO International Code of Marketing Breastmilk Substitutes. January 27, 1981. Available at: https://www.who.int/publications/i/item/9241541601

18

Fertility, Infertility, and Family-Building Considerations Among Black Women

Jerrine R. Morris, MD, MPH, Tia Jackson-Bey, MD, MPH, and Torie Comeaux Plowden, MD, MPH

Infertility, defined as the inability to conceive after 12 months of unprotected intercourse, impacts one in eight American couples (Centers for Disease Control and Prevention [CDC] 2023). American women have poor knowledge of reproductive physiology, which may be magnified amongst Black women. This knowledge gap coupled with a lack of fertility awareness presents significant challenges for Black women when trying to build their families. Due to a host of social, economic, and historical factors, infertility is commonly regarded as an issue that only impacts wealthy white women. By contrast, population survey data indicate that infertility may be more prevalent in historically excluded communities (Chandra, Copen, and Stephen 2013). Whether due to intrinsic false beliefs, social stigma of infertility, or reticence from providers to call attention to fertility-related issues in communities of color, Black women are particularly vulnerable to infertility and often suffer in silence.

This chapter covers several important topics including the origins of misconceptions surrounding fertility in Black women and age-related fertility decline and gynecologic conditions that may affect fertility or contribute to infertility, particularly those that disproportionately impact Black women. We examine the impact of bias and racism in medicine and its consequences on fertility and infertility in Black women. We also discuss family-building considerations for Black members of the lesbian, gay, bisexual, transgender, queer, and questioning plus (LGBTQ+) community and third-party reproduction, including utilization of donation and surrogacy among Black women.

DISPARITIES IN FERTILITY TREATMENT AND OUTCOMES

The desire to procreate is a basic human right. Black women often have difficulty navigating their reproductive journeys secondary to myriad biological, social, cultural, and political factors. Although the use of fertility treatment has increased in the last decade, a recent study found that Black and Hispanic women had a 70% lower likelihood of receiving treatment for infertility when compared with non-Hispanic white women (Dongarwar et al. 2022). Even when Black women do utilize fertility treatment, they have a lower likelihood of pregnancy and a higher likelihood of miscarriage when compared to white women (Seifer et al. 2020). Disparities in outcomes have persisted for the past 20 years despite overall advances in the field of reproductive medicine. These are the result of disparities in sexually transmitted infections (STIs), tubal sterilization, and fertility preservation, which have downstream consequences, particularly contributing to the increased prevalence of infertility seen in Black women.

Acquisition of Sexually Transmitted Infections

Both the incidence and prevalence of STIs have increased in the United States across all racial and ethnic populations. Human papillomavirus (HPV) continues to be the most prevalent with more than three million individuals diagnosed with HPV and close to 5.4 million living with this infection (Kreisel et al. 2018). In a study using data from the 2006-2010 National Survey of Family Growth exploring HPV vaccination initiation, Black women were 51% less likely to have initiated vaccination even after adjusting for sociodemographic characteristics including age, household income, and health care access (Gelman et al. 2013). In a retrospective cohort comprising the same population but data from 2002 to 2015, Black women were more likely to undergo HIV testing, but less likely to report any contraception use, effective contraception use, and HPV vaccination (Horwitz, Pace, and Ross-Degnan 2018). Rates of HPV unfortunately have been shown to be greater among Black women (Lin et al. 2015). Despite access to a health care provider and previous STI testing, Black women had lower odds of having heard about HPV and the vaccine (Amboree et al. 2021). Gaps in knowledge of the infection and differences in vaccine initiation hampers stage 1 prevention of cervical cancer and exacerbates disparities in HPV prevalence among Black women.

Ascending infections, which begin in the vagina and spread from the endocervix into the endometrium and fallopian tubes (CDC 1991), are responsible for more than 50% of tubal disease (Practice Committee of the American Society for Reproductive Medicine 2021). Chlamydia and gonorrhea are the most common, most curable, and extremely preventable. The vast majority of new diagnoses of chlamydia and gonorrhea occur in Black females between the ages of 15 and 24 years. Black women are more than eight and 20 times more likely to contract chlamydia and gonorrhea, respectively, when compared to white women. Sexual practices including inconsistent condom use, multiple partners, and early age of sexual debut have all been shown to be more commonly identified among Black women when compared to white women (Pflieger et al. 2013). Decreasing the prevalence of STIs among Black women, particularly adolescents and young adults who may not have considered childbearing, is essential given the risks for tubal infertility that may result from a diagnosis.

Tubal Sterilization

Tubal ligation, a procedure to remove part or the entire connection between the fallopian tube and the uterus through cutting or banding, remains the most common method for contraception among reproductive-aged women 15 to 44 years, with postpartum sterilization the reason for greater than 50% of procedures (American College of Obstetricians and Gynecologists [ACOG] 2019). While incredibly effective, with failure rates around 1% with surgical removal of one or both fallopian tubes, compared to other methods, the risk of regret is not insignificant. In fact, close to 20% of women younger than than age 30 at the time of sterilization expressed regret after undergoing the procedure. This figure was doubled to 40% among women aged 18 to 24 years (ACOG 2019). Both Black race and use of public insurance have been shown to be significant predictors of postpartum tubal sterilization (Garcia et al. 2015). In a survey of women who had undergone tubal sterilization, Black women were more likely to think sterilization was easily reversible or would resolve with time as compared with white women. They were also less likely to have heard of the intrauterine device (IUD), a known effective and reversible contraceptive option (Borrero 2011).

In the United States, there has been a long-standing tradition of ignoring reproductive autonomy and policing female bodies, particularly among women of color, and sterilization is no exception to this. Health inequities have perpetuated both coercive sterilization practices after inadequate or absent counseling as well as restrictive practices limiting access to sterilization when highly desired. Employing a shared decision-making model when counseling Black women—particularly those aged younger than 30 years, who are at greater risk for regret—on contraceptive options, while avoiding racial as well as other biases, may decrease disparities in sterilization (ACOG Committee on Ethics 2017).

Unequal Utilization of Fertility Preservation for Both Oncologic and Non-Oncologic Indications

The American Society of Clinical Oncology, American Society for Reproductive Medicine, American Academy of Pediatrics, and World Professional Association for Transgender Health are a few of the national professional organizations and societies recommending all patients at risk for subfertility due to medication or radiation that causes direct damage to the ovary (gonadotoxic treatment), surgery on one or both ovaries including partial or complete removal (gonadal surgery), or prolonged hormone therapy receive fertility counseling and be offered fertility preservation (Coleman et al. 2012; Practice Committee of the American Society for Reproductive Medicine 2019; Neblett and Hipp 2019; Oktay et al. 2018). However, studies have shown disparities in fertility preservation counseling and utilization among Black women.

In a retrospective cohort of women diagnosed with breast, gynecologic, hematologic, or gastrointestinal cancer at an academic medical center from 2008 through 2010, non-white women eligible for a fertility preservation consultation were less likely to complete it (Goodman, Kim, and Mersereau 2012). In 2010, Letourneau et al. surveyed women identified through the California Cancer Registry on whether they pursued fertility preservation. Of the 2,532 women contacted, 1,041 (41%) completed this survey, and 4% of them endorsed undergoing fertility preservation. Of the 31 African American women who completed the questionnaire, none of them underwent fertility preservation despite similarities in parity and reported access to fertility preservation counseling (Letourneau et al. 2012). By contrast, in an oncofertility program in Denver, Colorado, around a similar time (2012), adolescents newly diagnosed with cancer who underwent a fertility preservation consultation were included. Among those who opted for fertility preservation, they were 3.3 times more likely to be white compared to another race or ethnicity (Flink, Sheeder, and Kondapalli 2017).

Finally, when modeling the observed versus expected number of fertility preservation services by race and ethnicity among women with cancer in New York City, Black women were significantly less likely to be represented (Voigt et al. 2020). While the sample sizes in these studies are small with often aggregated results for historically excluded populations, there is some suggestion that Black women with cancer have been less likely to undergo fertility preservation when compared to white women. Limitations in current studies to assess this as well as absent data assessing racial and ethnic disparities in fertility preservation among transmasculine individuals should be a target of future studies.

DISPARITIES IN CAUSES OF SUBFERTILITY AND INFERTILITY AMONG BLACK WOMEN PRESENTING FOR EVALUATION

There are causes of subfertility (e.g., unwanted delay in conception, such as the result of tubal disease) and infertility (e.g., absolute inability to conceive) that are more prevalent in Black women compared to women from other racial and ethnic backgrounds. Some are a function of age at seeking care and its contribution to the diagnosis; others are a direct result of systemic inequities in access to full-spectrum care and the impact provider bias may have on disease perpetuation. This section reflects on the differential impact certain conditions exert on Black women in terms of future fertility and pregnancy outcomes.

Age at Presentation and Diminished Ovarian Reserve

Egg (oocyte) age has well-known effects on the likelihood of chromosomal normality, with older age more associated with an abnormal number of chromosomes. Yet, studies have consistently shown that Black women suffer with infertility longer than white women before undergoing an evaluation, leading them to have a greater age at presentation for care and treatment. In a population of women who presented for care at an academic center in Boston, Massachusetts, Black women waited one year longer than white women (4.3 years vs 3.3 years; Jain 2006). These findings were consistent in another cross-sectional study performed in Chicago, Illinois, a state that similarly has comprehensive fertility treatment coverage. Missmer, Seifer, and Jain (2011) found that Black and Hispanic women attempted to conceive for 20 months longer than white women before seeking care.

Obtaining an appointment and finding a doctor that they were comfortable with were two of the most common barriers cited among Black women when compared to white women or those from other racial and ethnic groups (Missmer, Seifer, and Jain 2011). At the macro level, when examining national trends from 2014 to 2016, the age distribution of Black versus white women revealed a similar trend, with white women more represented among the groups aged younger than 35 years and 35 to 37 years, while Black women were more represented in the group aged 38 to 40 years and roughly 15% more represented in the group aged 41 years and older. An increase in diagnoses of diminished ovarian reserve among Black women when compared to white women (27.4% vs 21.5%) is unsurprising given their greater age when proceeding with treatment for infertility through assisted reproductive technology (ART; Seifer et al. 2020).

Finally, Black women are among the fastest growing group of professionals in the United States. Delayed childbearing is a well-recognized cause of infertility, and in a study of female physicians, nearly 25% of respondents were diagnosed with infertility, which is greater than the national average. Interestingly, close to 30% of respondents would have attempted conception earlier, 17% would have gone into a different specialty, and those who were pregnant during training perceived less workplace support than when in practice (Stentz 2016). In a survey specifically of Black obstetrician-gynecologists, 66% of respondents felt the need to postpone childbearing due to medical training, and 70% felt all women planning medical training should consider planned oocyte cryopreservation (Wiltshire et al. 2022).

Uterine Fibroids

Uterine myomas, or fibroids, are common tumors of the uterine myometrium that affect up to 70% of women of reproductive age and are known to increase during one's reproductive lifespan. Black women have been shown to have larger, more numerous fibroids, and an earlier age of fibroid onset as compared with white women. For example, in a population of young women aged 18 to 30 years without symptoms and a known history of fibroids who underwent a transvaginal ultrasound, Black women were more than four times more likely to be diagnosed with a fibroid than white women (25.6% vs 6.9%; Marsh 2013). Racial differences in infertility diagnosis and treatment outcomes using data from the Society for Assisted Reproductive Technology Clinic Outcome Reporting System (SART CORS) were assessed from 2014 through 2016. These findings were similarly compared to those previously reported and, as such, Seifer et al. (2020) found that Black women were three times more likely to have a uterine factor contributing to infertility when compared to white women.

Due to differences in characteristics across current studies, there are insufficient data to conclude that fibroids reduce the likelihood of achieving pregnancy for those trying to conceive both spontaneously and with ART (Practice Committee of the American Society for Reproductive Medicine 2017). However, previous systematic reviews as well as several retrospective cohort studies support resection of fibroids that bulge into the uterus to improve clinical pregnancy rates. As mentioned, there are limitations of the data and the ability to assess the impact of multiple fibroids and degree of cavity distortion on the probability of conception, impact on reproductive outcomes of fibroids that grow within the muscle tissues of the uterus, and the value of surgical removal on ART outcomes in particular (Practice Committee of the American Society for Reproductive Medicine 2017). Given the higher independent risk for uterine fibroids that Black women face, exploring its contribution to subfertility is paramount.

Tubal Factor Infertility

Ectopic pregnancy is when a pregnancy implants outside of the uterus with implantation sites often including the fallopian tube, ovary, or abdomen. Risk factors for an ectopic pregnancy include a previous ectopic pregnancy, history of pelvic infection or endometriosis, and cesarean delivery, to name a few (ACOG 2018a). Black women enrolled in Medicaid from 2004 to 2008 were more likely to experience an ectopic pregnancy than white women from a similar demographic population (Stulberg 2016).

In a retrospective cohort study of women aged 15 to 60 years with a previous ectopic pregnancy treated from 2006 through 2015, factors associated with medical versus surgical management of ectopic pregnancy were assessed. There was no statistically significant difference in medical therapy when comparing Black to white women, though there was a trend toward lower use. On the other hand, Black women were less likely to undergo tubal conserving surgery through salpingostomy (removal of the ectopic pregnancy in which the fallopian tube remains in place) compared to white women (Hsu et al. 2017).

Salpingostomy is similarly as effective as salpingectomy (removal of part or the entire fallopian tube with the ectopic pregnancy) with mixed data associated with increased risk for recurrence rendering it as a viable option for the management of an ectopic pregnancy (ACOG 2018a). Even though one study showed an increased risk for repeat ectopic with salpingostomy, the absolute difference increased from 4% to 10%. This implies a 90% chance that another ectopic would not occur. With the risk for tubal pathology already greater in Black women, serious consideration should be given regarding discussion of tubal conserving options for the management of ectopic pregnancy (ACOG 2018a).

Endometriosis

Endometriosis is a common gynecologic condition affecting up to 10% of reproductive-aged women, leading to pain and infertility. Endometriotic implants in the pelvis can proliferate, leading to lesions that penetrate surrounding organs. Particularly in more advanced cases, this persistent inflammatory state can lead to the formation of ovarian cysts and adhesions, which may affect the patency or function of fallopian tubes (ACOG 2010; Ziegler 2010).

Infertility conveys about a 30% chance of underlying endometriosis; this figure rises to 50% if infertility is in the presence of moderate to severe pain with menses (Ziegler 2010). However, Black women are much less likely to receive a diagnosis of endometriosis. In a meta-analysis including 16 studies, the likelihood of receiving a diagnosis of endometriosis was compared between white and Black women. Black women were 51% less likely to receive this diagnosis. This meta-analysis did not find that this difference persisted among infertile women, but only two studies were included in that assessment (Bougie et al. 2019).

Endometriosis, particularly as it advances to stage 3 or 4, can have clear impacts on fertility. However, whether due to attributing pain to other causes including pelvic inflammatory disease and fibroids, less awareness of endometriosis as a cause for one's painful menstrual periods, or even implicit biases that lead physicians to be less sensitive to Black women's pain, endometriosis is less commonly diagnosed in Black women and can have profound impacts on one's future fertility. A recent study utilized a national database to investigate outcomes in more than 11,000 women undergoing surgery for endometriosis. The authors found that Black women were more likely to undergo surgical removal of the ovary at an earlier age, were less likely to have a hysterectomy performed via a minimally invasive procedure, and had higher complication rates (Orlando 2022).

In the 1930s, an American gynecologist, Joseph Meigs, linked endometriosis with delayed childbearing as he more frequently diagnosed endometriosis in his private patients (Bougie et al. 2019). During that time frame in America, "private" patients were white and wealthy women, whereas "ward" patients were Black and/or of a lower socio-economic status (Bougie et al. 2019). Several studies in the 1950s and 1960s demonstrated that the incidence of endometriosis was similar in Black and white patients (Lloyd 1964; Cavanagh 1951). Ultimately, the idea that endometriosis was a disease exclusive to wealthy white women became firmly entrenched in the medical community (Bougie et al. 2019).

Dr. Donald Chatman, a Black gynecologist, published about the detrimental impact this assumption had on patients (Chatman 1976). He found that 20% of his private Black patients had laparoscopy-confirmed evidence of endometriosis. Yet, almost 40% of those endometriosis cases had been previously misdiagnosed with pelvic inflammatory disease, noting that the myth about Black women being immune to endometriosis along with the erroneous stereotype about their promiscuity contributed to delayed diagnosis and inappropriate treatment (Chatman 1976).

Polycystic Ovary Syndrome

Polycystic ovary syndrome (PCOS) is a complex multisystem disorder characterized by ovulatory dysfunction (<8 cycles per year), excess levels of androgen hormones (both clinical and biochemical), and/or polycystic ovaries (ACOG 2018b). PCOS affects 6% to 12% of women, with the prevalence often dependent on the population studied and diagnostic criteria used, but it is still regarded as the most common endocrinological disorder affecting reproductive-aged women. Given the systemic effects, women diagnosed with PCOS may suffer from irregular or absent periods resulting in infertility; have a higher prevalence of diabetes, preeclampsia, and preterm birth during pregnancy; and have increased risks for metabolic syndrome and cardiovascular disease later in life (Legro et al. 2013).

While differences in PCOS prevalence based on race and ethnicity are fairly mixed, multiple studies have suggested increased prevalence of metabolic syndrome in Black women. In a longitudinal cohort study of 247 adult women with elevated androgens and PCOS, the incidence of metabolic syndrome was higher in Black women when compared to white women, even among women who were specifically aged younger than 30 years. Furthermore, Black women aged younger than 30 years with PCOS who did not have metabolic syndrome at their initial visit were more likely to develop this when compared to similarly aged white women (28.7% vs 11.6%; $P<.01$; Lee et al. 2022). Metabolic syndrome is associated with infertility and pregnancy complications, particularly in women with PCOS (Arya et al. 2021; Grieger 2018). The impact of infertility, particularly in Black women with PCOS, has been shown to impact one's quality of life (Alur-Gupta et al. 2021). Even with similar prevalence of PCOS, Black women are at greater risk for metabolic syndrome, which is associated with infertility, decreased quality of life, pregnancy complications, and greater long-term morbidity and mortality due to cardiovascular disease.

FAMILY-BUILDING CONSIDERATIONS

In communities of color, particularly Black communities, infertility treatment, including third-party reproduction, is less often utilized. Furthermore, when used, outcomes are substandard.

Stigma Associated With Infertility and Fertility Treatment

Black women often report a lack of communication regarding sex and reproductive health in their communities (Crooks et al. 2019). Several studies have noted that Black women tend to have less knowledge related to fertility (Alexander et al. 2019). This lack of accurate knowledge may fuel some of the fertility misconceptions Black women report. Infertility stigma is an issue. In one study, 49% of Black women were disturbed about infertility stigma (Missmer, Seifer, and Jain 2011). Previous studies have demonstrated that Black women are less likely to perceive themselves as infertile or are more averse to being labeled infertile (Missmer, Seifer, and Jain 2011; White and Greil 2006). A qualitative study of Black women with infertility found that infertility had a negative impact on one's self-worth (Ceballo, Graham, and Hart 2015). A significant number of women (32%) associated motherhood with womanhood and reported that an inability to conceive made them feel a sense of failure. Women in this study often did not share their infertility diagnosis with close friends and family, leading to feelings of isolation (Ceballo, Graham, and Hart 2015).

Another study examining Black women who sought evaluation for infertility reported delaying disclosure of infertility to their peers (Cebert-Gaitors 2022). Taken together, these studies all indicate that Black women with infertility have less social support. Infertility care itself has also been associated with stigma and can be a reason why women of color do not seek care (Jackson-Bey 2021; Kirubarajan 2021). Indeed, the social and cultural context surrounding the pursuit of fertility among Black women is complex (Greil, Stauson-Blevins, and McQuillan 2010).

Part of the stigma associated with infertility among Black women is directly correlated with the presumption of hyperfertility and sexuality in this community. Race-based sexual stereotypes are very prevalent in the media and are utilized to portray negative images of Black women (Bond et al. 2021; Wilson 2009). Black women themselves are likely to have internalized the media images that portray them as hyperfertile (Roberts 1997). As a result, many Black women believe that infertility is uncommon in their community (Ceballo 1999). This misperception may play a role in delaying treatment in this population.

Access to Social Support

Undoubtedly, stress is also of particular importance when considering infertility issues, as the physiological processes associated with stress directly affect hormonal regulation, which can, in turn, affect the chances of conception (Galst 2018). Low levels of disclosure impact ability to use normal social support resources. However, access to supportive social interactions provide the opportunity for lowering stress and increasing self-esteem, mood, general trust, confidence, and a feeling of safety during infertility treatment (Malina, Głogiewicz, and Piotrowski 2019). Partner support is also an important element of coping with infertility. Partner support significantly lowers negative emotions, pressure, and worries (Koss, Rudnik, and Bidzan 2014).

Implicit and Explicit Biases in the Medical System

Reproductive health disparities are not limited to obstetrics. Black women also experience inequities in gynecological care, including care related to infertility access and treatment. Even in the setting of cancer, Black women are less likely to be referred to an infertility specialist for fertility preservation counseling (Goodman, Kim, and Mersereau 2012; Lawson et al. 2017). Black women are vulnerable to inequitable care and may not receive appropriate infertility referrals in a timely fashion because of provider bias or racist practices in institutions (Cebert-Gaitors et al. 2022). In addition, Black women have reported negative interactions when seeking infertility care, encountering health care providers who made assumptions about their ability to afford care and about their sexual promiscuity (Ceballo, Graham, and Hart 2015). Furthermore, unmarried Black women may be less likely to be referred for care because they identify as single (White and Greil 2006). Historically, refusal to treat unmarried women was a practice that was very common among infertility physicians. The American Society for Reproductive Medicine has recently stated that it is unethical to refuse to treat infertile patients because of marital status (Ethics Committee of the American Society for Reproductive Medicine 2021). Some physicians and health care providers involved in basic gynecologic care do not have adequate knowledge about risk factors of infertility, particularly in Black women (Ceballo, Abbey, and Schooler 2010). Inexperience may also be a component in inappropriate referral patterns. Whatever the cause, lack of referral for infertility treatment plays a role in hindering access of Black women to appropriate infertility care.

Insurance Coverage for Fertility Treatment in Black Women

In 1986, Dr. Shellee Colen coined "stratified reproduction" to describe the phenomenon of prioritizing the reproduction of privileged groups over the reproduction of under privileged groups (i.e., women of color; Colen 1986). Conversations around stratified reproduction often center contraception and sterilization practices (Greil et al. 2011). However, infertility diagnosis and access to treatment must also be included. In the United States, where many infertility treatments are not covered by insurance, women of color and women of lower socioeconomic status are often left without the ability to receive the necessary treatment to expand their families. This conveys a message that the reproductive hopes and goals of historically excluded women are not prioritized. Indeed, this is the latest form of stratified reproduction.

In an equal-access-to-care population, utilization of ART services increased among Black women relative to the US ART population (Feinberg et al. 2006). These findings contrasted in Massachusetts, a state with mandated and comprehensive insurance coverage of fertility treatment, where authors found disparities in access persisted; in vitro fertilization (IVF) services were most accessed by highly educated, wealthy, white women (Jain and Hornstein 2005). Bitler and Schmidt (2006) also examined this question and did not find evidence that insurance mandates improved racial, ethnic, or socioeconomic disparities in access to care. Black women at an academic center were twice as likely to report income as a barrier to obtaining fertility treatment when compared to white women (Galic et al. 2021).

Thus, the intersection between race and socioeconomic status often exponentially increases the barriers faced in accessing fertility treatment among Black women. While data are mixed, certainly women residing in states without insurance coverage, those with governmental insurance, and those who are uninsured have limited access to comprehensive fertility treatment, which often places the burden of infertility on the shoulders of women, namely Black women.

Comfort With Provider

Currently, only 5% of physicians are Black (Association of American Medical Colleges 2019). There is a significant and persistent pipeline problem that has limited the increase of Black physicians, including in the field of reproductive endocrinology and infertility (Richard-Davis 2021). Black women have reported difficulty finding a physician with whom they felt connected (Missmer, Seifer, and Jain 2011). A recent large survey study of more than 1,400 women undergoing infertility treatment revealed that 42.3% of Black women surveyed perceived that their physician did not understand their cultural background (Galic et al. 2021). Another study investigating Black women who sought infertility treatment noted the importance in receiving culturally competent care (Cebert-Gaitors et al. 2022). Of note, in that study no Black physicians were employed by the infertility clinic; thus, Black women relied on reports that the physicians had good relationships with other Black women patients (Cebert-Gaitors et al. 2022). Available evidence suggests that when there is racial concordance between patients and physicians, the patients have a more positive experience of care (Martinez et al. 2016). The ongoing lack of Black reproductive health specialists further compounds the difficulty Black women face in assessing empathetic, culturally competent care.

Fertility Considerations in LGBTQ+ Communities

Members of the LGBTQ+ community often need assistance to build their families and have considerations and concerns that are different from those of heterosexual couples (Raja and Moravek 2022). Indeed, more lesbian couples are utilizing ART and are choosing to expand their families in a variety of ways that may involve one or both partners conceiving and carrying a pregnancy (Carpinello, Nulsen, and Benadiva 2016). In a Canadian qualitative study, lesbian patients noted a lack of support from their health care team. They wanted greater assistance "in navigating a complex and costly medical journey through a system largely designed for the needs of heterosexual patients" (Gregory, Mielke, and Neiterman 2022).

LGBTQ+ individuals have reported that health providers may not possess an understanding of their reproductive health priorities (Wingo and Roberts 2018). Until recently, it was assumed that most transgender individuals did not desire parenthood; however, many transgender people are parents (Raja and Moravek 2022). More transgender patients are now being counseled about fertility preservation options than in the past (Cooper, Long, and Aye 2022). Black women who are also members of the sexual minority community have an additional set of barriers and biases when navigating health care. Studies have indicated that Black sexual minority women experience worse health care–related quality of life than white heterosexual women (Yette 2018). These people experience compounded oppression, including racism, sexism, and homophobia, which further hinders access to ART (Tam 2021).

Disparities in Treatment Outcomes

Access to fertility treatment is undoubtedly a barrier among Black women; however, when Black women are able to navigate these barriers, outcomes remain suboptimal. In a secondary analysis of a retrospective cohort study of women who underwent IVF at an academic practice between 2001 and 2010 and were followed through 2014, individuals whose first fresh IVF cycle was unsuccessful were queried to explore patterns of treatment discontinuation and time to return for a second IVF cycle (Bedrick et al. 2019). Black women were significantly more likely to discontinue treatment when compared to other patients. Among patients who returned for a second cycle, Black women also had a longer time to return to treatment as compared to other women. Both of these findings were adjusted for income, distance from clinic, insurance coverage, and age (Bedrick et al. 2019).

Black women who continue with fertility treatment, particularly IVF, are also less likely to achieve a clinical pregnancy and, when they do, are more likely to experience a miscarriage. In a large private practice in Illinois, Black women who underwent their first cycle from 2010 through 2012 were shown to have fewer mature oocytes, fewer fertilized oocytes, lower blastocyst development, higher cancellation rates, and higher rates of miscarriage when compared to white women (McQueen et al. 2015). Similarly, in an analysis of national SART CORS data from 2014 to 2016, Black women had a lower live birth rates irrespective of age, body mass index, infertility diagnosis, and parity (Seifer et al. 2020). These findings unfortunately did not differ from previous analyses of SART CORS data from the same group, reflecting essentially stable disparities since 1999 (Seifer, Zackula, and Grainger 2010).

Finally, as the field of infertility continues to take advantage of new technologies to improve treatment outcomes, the potential for widening disparities between Black and white populations is evident. In addition to undergoing IVF, patients can undergo screening of embryos for chromosomal abnormalities or preimplantation genetic testing for ploidy, to prevent transmission of single gene defects or translocations (ACOG 2020). Patients treated at an academic practice from 2018 through 2019 were sent a questionnaire on perspectives surrounding genetic testing. Black respondents were significantly less likely to report undergoing genetic carrier screening when compared to white respondents. Interestingly, in this same study, Black respondents were more likely to agree with sex selection compared to white respondents (McQueen et al. 2021). This suggests the low number of carrier screenings may not be due to dismissal of the technology but other patient versus systems-based factors. Furthermore, as these new technologies emerge, they are often validated among those of European ancestry with limitations in generalizability among populations without shared ancestry (Forzano et al. 2022). Genetic testing in the field of reproductive medicine is one of many examples of how differences in validation and utilization of new technologies can only exacerbate disparities seen among Black women.

Utilization of Third-Party Reproduction

Third-party reproduction (TPR) including the use of donor eggs, donor embryos, or a gestational surrogate is a way many individuals in the United States can build their families. Using data from SART CORS from 2004 through 2013, the prevalence of TPR use was examined by race and ethnicity. In this analysis, Black women were significantly less likely to utilize TPR than non-Hispanic white women. Furthermore, among the TPR utilized, Black women were most likely to use sperm donation and least to utilize surrogacy even in the setting of increased uterine-factor infertility diagnoses (Shapiro et al. 2017).

Whether decreased rates of utilization are a function of cost, awareness, or culture is up for debate, but when Black women do utilize TPR, success rates are lower. In a retrospective analysis of close to 1,000 egg recipients who underwent a fresh embryo transfer at an academic center between 2009 and 2015, Black women had a lower clinical pregnancy rate (and live birth rate) when compared to white recipients after adjustment for age, body mass index, and primary infertility diagnosis (Zhou 2020). In a similar retrospective study conducted using data from a national oocyte bank through a private center from 2008 to 2015, live birth rates of oocyte recipients by race and ethnicity were explored. Liu et al. (2020) found embryo transfer cycles to Black recipients had a lower probability of live birth than those to white recipients. Current data suggest lower rates of utilization of TPR among Black women as well as worse outcomes among users. Further data are necessary to explore the barriers to use and factors associated with worse outcomes that potentiate these disparities seen among Black women, particularly as TPR utilization becomes more widespread.

CONCLUSION

Despite pervasive stereotypical images of Black hyperfertility, the stark reality is that Black women are often impacted by infertility. Social and cultural factors significantly influence if Black women decide to build a family, how they go about doing so, if they encounter difficulty conceiving, and their decision to access care and treatment. Public health initiatives must work to explicitly dispel the myth that Black women can get pregnant at any time—both in Black communities as well as in medical communities. Reproductive justice states that women should have the right to conceive (depending on their individual desires) and the right to parent their children in safe and sustainable communities (SisterSong Women of Color Reproductive Justice Collective n.d.). For Black women hoping to start or expand their families, stratified reproduction must be eliminated. Family building is not just an issue that impacts only wealthy white women. We must prioritize systems and policies that ensure all women can access needed fertility care.

REFERENCES

Alexander KA, Perrin N, Jennings JM, Ellen J, Trent M. Childbearing motivations and desires, fertility beliefs, and contraceptive use among urban African-American adolescents and young adults with STI histories. *J Urban Health*. 2019;96(2):171–180. https://doi.org/10.1007/s11524-018-0282-2

Alur-Gupta S, Lee I, Chemerinski A, et al. Racial differences in anxiety, depression, and quality of life in women with polycystic ovary syndrome. *F S Rep*. 2021;2(2):230–237. https://doi.org/10.1016/j.xfre.2021.03.003

Amboree T, Sonawane K, Deshmukh AA, Montealegre JR. Regular healthcare provider status does not moderate racial/ethnic differences in human papillomavirus (HPV) and HPV vaccine knowledge. *Vaccines (Basel)*. 2021;9(7):802. https://doi.org/10.3390/vaccines9070802

American College of Obstetricians and Gynecologists. ACOG Practice Bulletin No. 191: Tubal ectopic pregnancy. *Obstet Gynecol*. 2018a;131(2):e65–e77. https://doi.org/10.1097/AOG.0000000000002464

American College of Obstetricians and Gynecologists. ACOG Practice Bulletin No. 194: Polycystic ovary syndrome. *Obstet Gynecol*. 2018b;131(6):e157–e171. https://doi.org/10.1097/AOG.0000000000002656

American College of Obstetricians and Gynecologists. Management of endometriosis. *Obstet Gynecol*. 2010;116(1):223–236. https://doi.org/10.1097/AOG.0b013e3181e8b073

American College of Obstetricians and Gynecologists Committee. Preimplantation genetic testing: ACOG Committee Opinion, Number 799. *Obstet Gynecol.* 2020;135(3):e133–e137. https://doi.org/10.1097/AOG.0000000000003714

American College of Obstetricians and Gynecologists Committee on Ethics. Committee Opinion No. 695: Sterilization of women: ethical issues and considerations. *Obstet Gynecol.* 2017;129(4):e109–e116. https://doi.org/10.1097/AOG.0000000000002023

Arya S, Hansen KR, Peck JD, Wild RA, National Institute of Child Health and Human Development Reproductive Medicine Network. Metabolic syndrome in obesity: treatment success and adverse pregnancy outcomes with ovulation induction in polycystic ovary syndrome. *Am J Obstet Gynecol.* 2021;225(3):280.e281–280.e211. https://doi.org/10.1016/j.ajog.2021.03.048

Association of American Medical Colleges. Diversity in medicine: facts and figures 2019. 2019. Available at: https://www.aamc.org/data-reports/workforce/interactive-data/figure-18-percentage-all-active-physicians-race/ethnicity-2018

Bedrick B, Anderson K, Broughton D, Hamilton B, Jungheim E. Factors associated with early in vitro fertilization treatment discontinuation. *Fertil Steril.* 2019;112(1):105–111. https://doi.org/10.1016/j.fertnstert.2019.03.007

Bitler M, Schmidt L. Health disparities and infertility: impacts of state-level insurance mandates. *Fertil Steril.* 2006;85(4):858–865. https://doi.org/10.1016/j.fertnstert.2005.11.038

Bond KT, Leblanc NM, Williams P, Gabriel CA, Amutah-Onukagha NN. Race-based sexual stereotypes, gendered racism, and sexual decision making among young Black cisgender women. *Health Educ Behav.* 2021;48(3):295–305. https://doi.org/10.1177/10901981211010086

Borrero S, Abebe K, Dehlendorf C, Schwarz EB, Creinin MD, Nikoljaski C, Ibrahim SA. Racial variation in tubal sterilization rates: the role of patient-level factors. *Fertil Steril.* 2011;95(1):17–22. https://doi.org/10.1016/j.fertnstert.2010.05.031

Bougie O, Healey J, Singh SS. Behind the times: revisiting endometriosis and race. *Am J Obstet Gynecol.* 2019;221(1):35.e31–35.e35. https://doi.org/10.1016/j.ajog.2019.01.238

Bougie O, Yap MI, Sikora L, Flaxman T, Singh S. Influence of race/ethnicity on prevalence and presentation of endometriosis: a systematic review and meta-analysis. *BJOG.* 2019;126:1104–1115. https://doi.org/10.1111/1471-0528.15692

Carpinello OJ, Jacob MC, Nulsen J, Benadiva C. Utilization of fertility treatment and reproductive choices by lesbian couples. *Fertil Steril.* 2016;106(7):1709–1713.e1704. https://doi.org/10.1016/j.fertnstert.2016.08.050

Cavanagh WV. Fertility in the etiology of endometriosis. *Am J Obstet Gynecol.* 1951;61(3):539–547. https://doi.org/10.1016/0002-9378(51)91399-3

Ceballo R. "The only Black woman walking the face of the earth who cannot have a baby": two women's stories. In: Romero M, Stewart AJ, eds. *Women's Untold Stories: Breaking Silence, Talking Back and Voicing Complexity.* New York, NY: Taylor & Frances/Routledge; 1999: 3–19.

Ceballo R, Abbey A, Schooler D. Perceptions of women's infertility: what do physicians see? *Fertil Steril.* 2010;93(4):1066–1073. https://doi.org/10.1016/j.fertnstert.2008.11.019

Ceballo R, Graham ET, Hart J. Silent and infertile: an intersectional analysis of the experiences of socioeconomically diverse African American women with infertility. *Psychol Women Q.* 2015;39(4):497–511. https://doi.org/10.1177/0361684315581169

Cebert-Gaitors M, Shannon-Baker PA, Silva SG, et al. Psychobiological, clinical and sociocultural factors that influence Black women seeking treatment for infertility: a mixed-methods study. *F S Rep.* 2022;3(2):29-39. https://doi.org/10.1016/j.xfre.2022.02.004

Centers for Disease Control and Prevention. Infertility FAQs. 2023. Available at: https://www.cdc.gov/reproductivehealth/infertility/index.htm

Centers for Disease Control and Prevention. Pelvic inflammatory disease: guidelines for prevention and management. *MMWR Recomm Rep.* 1991;40(RR-5):1-25.

Chandra A, Copen CE, Stephen EH. Infertility and impaired fecundity in the United States, 1982-2010: data from the National Survey of Family Growth. *Natl Health Stat Rep.* 2013;(67):1-18.

Chatman DL. Endometriosis in the Black woman. *Am J Obst Gynecol.* 1976;125(7):987-989. https://doi.org/10.1016/0002-9378(76)90502-0

Coleman E, Bockting W, Botzer M, et al. Standards of care for the health of transsexual, transgender, and gender-nonconforming people, version 7. *Int J Transgend.* 2012;13(4):165-232. https://doi.org/10.1080/15532739.2011.700873

Colen S. "With respect and feelings": voices of West Indian child care workers in New York City. In: Cole JB, ed. *All American Women: Lines That Divide, Ties That Bind.* New York, NY: Free Press; 1986:46-70.

Cooper HC, Long J, Aye T. Fertility preservation in transgender and non-binary adolescents and young adults. *PloS One.* 2022;17(3):e0265043. https://doi.org/10.1371/journal.pone.0265043

Crooks N, King B, Tluczek A, Sales JM. The process of becoming a sexual Black woman: a grounded theory study. *Perspect Sex Reprod Health.* 2019;51(1):17-25. https://doi.org/10.1363/psrh.12085

Dongarwar D, Mercado-Evans V, Adu-Gyamfi S, Laracuente ML, Salihu HM. Racial/ethnic disparities in infertility treatment utilization in the US, 2011-2019. *Syst Biol Reprod Med.* 2022;68(3):180-189. https://doi.org/10.1080/19396368.2022.2038718

Ethics Committee of the American Society for Reproductive Medicine. Access to fertility treatment irrespective of marital status, sexual orientation, or gender identity: an Ethics Committee opinion. *Fertil Steril.* 2021;116(2):326-330. https://doi.org/10.1016/j.fertnstert.2021.03.034

Feinberg E, Larsen F, Catherino W, Zhang J, Armstrong A. Comparison of assisted reproductive technology utilization and outcomes between Caucasian and African American patients in an equal-access-to-care setting. *Fertil Steril.* 2006;85(4):888-894. https://doi.org/10.1016/j.fertnstert.2005.10.028

Flink D, Sheeder J, Kondapalli LA. A review of the oncology patient's challenges for utilizing fertility preservation services. *J Adolesc Young Adult Oncol.* 2017;6(1):31-44. https://doi.org/10.1089/jayao.2015.0065

Forzano F, Antonova O, Clarke A, et al. The use of polygenic risk scores in pre-implantation genetic testing: an unproven, unethical practice. *Eur J Hum Genet.* 2022;30(5):493-495. https://doi.org/10.1038/s41431-021-01000-x

Galic I, Swanson A, Warren C, et al. Infertility in the Midwest: perceptions and attitudes of current treatment. *Am J Obstet Gynecol.* 2021;225(1):61.e1-61.e11. https://doi.org/10.1016/j.ajog.2021.02.015

Galst JP. The elusive connection between stress and infertility: a research review with clinical implications. *J Psychother Integr.* 2018;28(1):1-13.

Garcia G, Richardson DM, Gonzales KL, Cuevas AG. Trends and disparities in postpartum sterilization after cesarean section, 2000 through 2008. *Womens Health Issues.* 2015;25(6):1-7. http://dx.doi.org/10.1016/j.whi.2015.07.006

Gelman A, Miller E, Schwarz EB, Akers AK, Jeong K, Borrero S. Racial disparities in human papillomavirus vaccination: does access matter? *J Adolesc Health.* 2013;53(6):756-762. https://doi.org/10.1016/j.jadohealth.2013.07.002

Goodman LR, Balthazar U, Kim J, Mersereau JE. Trends of socioeconomic disparities in referral patterns for fertility preservation consultation. *Hum Reprod.* 2012;27(7):2076-2081. https://doi.org/10.1093/humrep/des133

Gregory KB, Mielke JG, Neiterman E. Building families through healthcare: experiences of lesbians using reproductive services. *J Patient Exp.* 2022;9:23743735221089459. https://doi.org/10.1177/23743735221089459

Greil AL, McQuillan J, Shreffler KM, Johnson KM, Slauson-Blevins KS. Race-ethnicity and medical services for infertility: stratified reproduction in a population-based sample of US women. *J Health Soc Behav.* 2011;52(4):49-509. https://doi.org/10.1177/0022146511418236

Greil AL, Slauson-Blevins K, McQuillan J. The experience of infertility: a review of recent literature. *Soc Health Illn.* 2010;32(1):140-162. https://doi.org/10.1111/j.1467-9566.2009.01213.x

Grieger J, Bianco-Miotto T, Grzeskowiak LE, et al. Metabolic syndrome in pregnancy and risk for adverse pregnancy outcomes: a prospective cohort of nulliparous women. *PloS Med.* 2018;15(12):e1002710. https://doi.org/10.1371/journal.pmed.1002710

Horwitz ME, Pace LE, Ross-Degnan D. Trends and disparities in sexual and reproductive health behaviors and service use among young adult women (aged 18-25 years) in the United States, 2002-2015. *Am J Public Health.* 2018;108(suppl 4):S336-S343. https://doi.org/10.2105/AJPH.2018.304556

Hsu JY, Chen L, Gumer AR, et al. Disparities in the management of ectopic pregnancy. *Am J Obstet Gynecol.* 2017;217(1):49.e1-49.e10. https://doi.org/10.1016/j.ajog.2017.03.001

Jackson-Bey T, Morris J, Jasper E, et al. Systematic review of racial and ethnic disparities in reproductive endocrinology and infertility: where do we stand today? *Fertil Steril Rev.* 2021;2(3):169-188. https://doi.org/10.1016/j.xfnr.2021.05.001

Jain T. Socioeconomic and racial disparities among infertility patients seeking care. *Fertil Steril.* 2006;85(5):876-881. https://doi.org/10.1016/j.fertnstert.2005.07.1338

Jain T, Hornstein MD. Disparities in access to infertility services in a state with mandated insurance coverage. *Fertil Steril.* 2005;84(1):221-223. https://doi.org/10.1016/j.fertnstert.2005.01.118

Kirubarajan A, Patel P, Leung S, Prethipan T, Sierra S. Barriers to fertility care for racial/ethnic minority groups: a qualitative systematic review. *Fertil Steril Rev.* 2021;2(2):150-159. https://doi.org/10.1016/j.xfnr.2021.01.001

Koss J, Rudnik A, Bidzan M. Experiencing stress and the obtained social support among women with high-risk pregnancies. Preliminary report. *Fam Forum.* 2014;4:183-201.

Kreisel K, Spicknall IH, Gargano J, et al. Sexually transmitted infections among US women and men: prevalence and incidence estimates, 2018. *Sex Transm Dis.* 2018;48(4):208-214. https://doi.org/10.1097/OLQ.0000000000001355

Lawson AK, McGuire JM, Noncent E, Olivieri JF Jr, Smith KN, Marsh EE. Disparities in counseling female cancer patients for fertility preservation. *J Womens Health (Larchmt)*. 2017;26(8):886-891. https://doi.org/10.1089/jwh.2016.5997

Lee I, Vresilovic J, Irfan M, Gallop R, Dokras A. Higher incidence of metabolic syndrome in Black women with polycystic ovary syndrome: a longitudinal study. *J Clin Endocrinol Metab*. 2022;107(4):e1558-e1567. https://doi.org/10.1210/clinem/dgab840

Legro R, Arslanian SA, Ehrmann DA, et al.; Endocrine Society. Diagnosis and treatment of polycystic ovary syndrome: an Endocrine Society clinical practice guideline. *J Clin Endocrinol Metab*. 2013;98(12):4565-4592. https://doi.org/10.1210/jc.2013-2350

Letourneau JM, Smith JF, Ebbel EE, et al. Racial, socioeconomic, and demographic disparities in access to fertility preservation in young women diagnosed with cancer. *Cancer*. 2012;118(18):4579-4588. https://doi.org/10.1002/cncr.26649

Lin L, Benard VB, Greek A, Hawkins NA, Roland KB, Saraiya M. Racial and ethnic differences in human papillomavirus positivity and risk factors among low-income women in federally qualified health centers in the United States. *Prev Med*. 2015;81:258-261. https://doi.org/10.1016/j.ypmed.2015.08.027

Liu Y, Hipp H, Nagy ZP, Capelouto SM, Shapiro DB, Spencer JB, Gaskins AJ. The effect of donor and recipient race on outcomes of assisted reproduction. *Am J Obstet Gynecol*. 2020;224(4):374. e1-374.e12. https://doi.org/10.1016/j.ajog.2020.09.013

Lloyd FP. Endometriosis in the Negro woman: a five-year study. *Am J Obstet Gynecol*. 1964;89:468-469. https://doi.org/10.1016/0002-9378(64)90549-6

Malina A, Głogiewicz M, Piotrowski J. Supportive social interactions in infertility treatment decrease cortisol levels: experimental study report. *Front Psychol*. 2019;10:2779. https://doi.org/10.3389/fpsyg.2019.02779

Marsh EE, Ekpo GE, Cardozo ER, Brocks M, Dune T, Cohen LS. Racial differences in fibroid prevalence and ultrasound findings in asymptomatic young women (18-30 years old): a pilot study. *Fertil Steril*. 2013;99(7):1951-1957. https://doi.org/10.1016/j.fertnstert.2013.02.017

Martinez KA, Resnicow K, Williams GC, et al. Does physician communication style impact patient report of decision quality for breast cancer treatment? *Patient Educ Couns*. 2016;99(12):1947-1954. https://doi.org/10.1016/j.pec.2016.06.025

McQueen D, Schufreider A, Lee SM, Feinberg E, Uhler M. Racial disparities in in vitro fertilization outcomes. *Fertil Steril*. 2015;104(2):398-402.e1. http://dx.doi.org/10.1016/j.fertnstert.2015.05.012

McQueen D, Warren CM, Xiao AH, Shulmamn LP, Jain T. Disparities among infertility patients regarding genetic carrier screening, sex selection, and gene editing. *J Assist Reprod Genet*. 2021;38(9):2319-2325. https://doi.org/10.1007/s10815-021-02261-7

Missmer SA, Seifer DB, Jain T. Cultural factors contributing to health care disparities among patients with infertility in Midwestern United States. *Fertil Steril*. 2011;95(6):1943-1949. https://doi.org/10.1016/j.fertnstert.2011.02.039

Neblett M, Hipp H. Fertility considerations in transgender persons. *Endocrinol Metab Clin North Am*. 2019;48(2):391-402. https://doi.org/10.1016/j.ecl.2019.02.003

Oktay K, Harvey B, Partridge A, et al. Fertility preservation in patients with cancer: ASCO clinical practice guideline update. *American Society of Clinical Oncology*. 2018;36(19). https://doi.org/10.1200/JCO.2018.78.1914

Orlando MS, Luna Russo MA, Richards EG, et al. Racial and ethnic disparities in surgical care for endometriosis across the United States. *Am J Obstet Gynecol*. 2022;226(6):824.e1–824.e11. https://doi.org/10.1016/j.ajog.2022.01.021

Pflieger J, Cook E, Niccolai LM, Connell CM. Racial/ethnic differences in patterns of sexual risk behavior and rates of sexually transmitted infections among female young adults. *Am J Public Health*. 2013;103(5):903–909. https://doi.org/10.2105/AJPH.2012.301005

Practice Committee of the American Society for Reproductive Medicine. Fertility preservation in patients undergoing gonadotoxic therapy or gonadectomy: a committee opinion. *Fertil Steril*. 2019;112(6):1022–1033. https://doi.org/10.1016/j.fertnstert.2019.09.013

Practice Committee of the American Society for Reproductive Medicine. Removal of myomas in asymptomatic patients to improve fertility and/or reduce miscarriage rate: a guideline. *Fertil Steril*. 2017;108(3):416–425. https://doi.org/10.1016/j.fertnstert.2017.06.034

Practice Committee of the American Society for Reproductive Medicine. Role of tubal surgery in the era of assisted reproductive technology: a committee opinion. *Fertil Steril*. 2021;115(5):1143–1150. https://doi.org/10.1016/j.fertnstert.2021.01.051

Raja NS, Russell CB, Moravek MB. Assisted reproductive technology: considerations for the nonheterosexual population and single parents. *Fertil Steril*. 2022;118(1):47–53. https://doi.org/10.1016/j.fertnstert.2022.04.012

Richard-Davis G. The pipeline problem: barriers to access of Black patients and providers in reproductive medicine. *Fertil Steril*. 2021;116(2):292–295. https://doi.org/10.1016/j.fertnstert.2021.06.044

Roberts D. *Killing the Black Body: Race, Reproduction, and the Meaning of Liberty*. New York, NY: Penguin Random House; 1997.

Seifer D, Simsek B, Wantman E, Kotlyar AM. Status of racial disparities between Black and white women undergoing assisted reproductive technology in the US. *Reprod Biol Endocrinol*. 2020;18(1):113. https://doi.org/10.1186/s12958-020-00662-4

Seifer DB, Zackula R, Grainger DA. Trends of racial disparities in assisted reproductive technology outcomes in Black women compared with white women: Society for Assisted Reproductive Technology 1999 and 2000 vs. 2004-2006. *Fertil Steril*. 2010;93(2):626–635. https://doi.org/10.1016/j.fertnstert.2009.02.084

Shapiro AJ, Darmon SK, Barad DH, Albertini DF, Gleicher N, Kushnir VA. Effect of race and ethnicity on utilization and outcomes of assisted reproductive technology in the USA. *Reprod Biol Endocrinol*. 2017;15(1):44. https://doi.org/10.1186/s12958-017-0262-5

SisterSong Women of Color Reproductive Justice Collective. Reproductive justice. Available at: https://www.sistersong.net/reproductive-justice

Stentz NC, Griffith K, Perkins E, DeCastro Jones R, Jagsi R. Fertility and childbearing among American female physicians. *J Womens Health (Larchmt)*. 2016;25(10):1059–1065. http://doi.org/10.1089/jwh.2015.5638

Stulberg D, Cain L, Dahlquist I, Lauderdale D. Ectopic pregnancy morbidity and mortality in low-income women, 2004–2008. *Hum Reprod.* 2016;31(3):666–671. https://doi.org/10.1093/humrep/dev332

Tam MW. Queering reproductive access: reproductive justice in assisted reproductive technologies. *Reprod Health.* 2021;18(1):164. https://doi.org/10.1186/s12978-021-01214-8

Voigt P, Blakemore JK, McCulloh D, Fino E. Equal opportunity for all? An analysis of race and ethnicity in fertility preservation in New York City. *J Assist Reprod Genet.* 2020;37(12):3095–3102. https://doi.org/10.1007/s10815-020-01980-7

White L, McQuillan J, Greil AL. Explaining disparities in treatment seeking: the case of infertility. *Fertil Steril.* 2006;85(4):853–857. https://doi.org/10.1016/j.fertnstert.2005.11.039

Wilson PA, Valera P, Ventuneac A, Balan I, Rowe, M, Carballo-Dieguez A. Race-based sexual stereotyping and sexual partnering among men who use the internet to identify other men for bareback sex. *J Sex Res.* 2009;46(5):399–413. https://doi.org/10.1080/00224490902846479

Wiltshire A, Ghidei L, Lantigua-Martinez M, et al. Planned oocyte cryopreservation and the Black obstetrician gynecologist: utilization and perspectives. *Reprod Sci.* 2022;29(7):2060–2066. https://doi.org/10.1007/s43032-022-00914-1

Wingo E, Ingraham N, Roberts SCM. Reproductive health care priorities and barriers to effective care for LGBTQ people assigned female at birth: a qualitative study. *Womens Health Issues.* 2018;28(4):350–357. https://doi.org/10.1016/j.whi.2018.03.002

Yette EM, Ahern J. Health-related quality of life among Black sexual minority women. *Am J Prev Med.* 2018;55(3):281–289. https://doi.org/10.1016/j.amepre.2018.04.037

Zhou X, McQueen DB, Schufreider A, Lee SM, Uhler M, Feinberg EC. Black recipients of oocyte donation experience lower live birth rates compared with white recipients. *Reprod BioMed Online.* 2020;40(5):668–673. https://doi.org/10.1016/j.rbmo.2020.01.008

Ziegler D, Borghese B, Chapron C. Endometriosis and infertility: pathophysiology and management. *Lancet.* 2010:376(9742):730–738. https://doi.org/10.1016/S0140-6736(10)60490-4

19

Changing Our Perception of the Change: The Impact of Chronic Stress on Menopausal Black Women

Lesley L. Green-Rennis, EdD, MPH, Lisa Grace-Leitch, EdD, MPH, MA, and Gloria Shine McNamara, PhD, MS

This chapter discusses perimenopause and menopause among Black women and their public health significance. Specifically, we examine the role chronic stress plays in the experience of menopause among Black women and provide a framework for lifestyle programs to address the menopause transition holistically.

WHAT REALLY HAPPENS DURING "THE CHANGE"

Menopause, the slow reduction of estrogen and progesterone hormones that leads to the end of menstruation, can be thought of as puberty in reverse. Studies suggest that Black women may begin menopause earlier, experience more intense effects, and have a longer transition period (Li et al. 2013; Santoro et al. 2021; Harlow et al. 2022). In the United States, Black women reach menopause at a median age of 49 years, two years earlier than the national median age, making it more likely that they will experience longer menopausal transitions and symptoms (Bromberger et al. 1997; Harlow et al. 2022; El Khoudary et al. 2019). Age of onset and length of menopause transition are markers of aging and health status that have been linked to risk for heart disease, stroke, osteoporosis, bone fracture, and overall life expectancy (Cooper and Sandler 1998). Studies also show that Black women are more likely to experience menopausal symptoms. These symptoms include depression and mood disturbances, hot flashes, dizziness, difficulty concentrating, poor coordination and/or clumsiness, urine leakage, and vaginal dryness. Though common for all menopausal women, these symptoms, particularly hot flashes, increase with age in Black women.

Though often discussed as a single event, menopause occurs over an extended period of time. The menopause transition begins with perimenopause, or "around menopause," and is characterized by changes in hormones, energy balance, and body composition. Women of all races and ethnicities enter perimenopause 8 to 10 years ahead of the final stage of menopause. The gradual cessation of menses and the accompanying hormonal changes can last anywhere from a few months to 10 years; the average length of perimenopause is about four years. The best predictor of when a woman will enter menopause is the age at which her mother began menopause.

The first sign of perimenopause is typically a change in the menstrual cycle. Changes may include a much earlier or later monthly cycle, experiencing heavier-than-normal periods, and/or skipping months entirely. Some women report no symptoms at all. Significant changes occur during perimenopause. The body decreases the amount of hormones it makes, particularly estrogen. In those assigned female at birth, estrogen is responsible for developing and maintaining their reproductive system and for secondary sex characteristics such as breast development and female-patterned hair growth. It is secreted by the ovaries during the reproductive age and regulates the menstrual cycle. As women age, ovarian function declines, and estrogen levels decrease. The decline and eventual cessation of estrogen production has been shown to cause most of the symptoms experienced by women during menopause. Research shows that estrogen levels impact almost every organ system (Sherwin 2003).

The body makes three main estrogens: (1) estrone (E1), the main type of estrogen present in the body after menopause, made primarily in adipose tissues; (2) estradiol (E2), the strongest estrogen made by the ovaries and present in the body before menopause; and (3) estriol (E3), the weakest estrogen, present in the body primarily during pregnancy. The body has two main receptors to which estrogen binds: alpha receptors that promote cell growth and beta receptors that inhibit cell growth. Each type of estrogen binds with varying affinity to these receptors, resulting in either cell proliferation or cell inhibition. Besides the direct effects of estrogen in the body, its metabolites are also important (Kolan 2020).

Estrogen is broken down into 2-hydroxyestrone or 16-hydroxyestrone, each of which has distinct functions in the body. Two-hydroxyestrone has multiple health benefits including blocking cell proliferation and subsequent cancer growth. Conversely, 16-hydroxyestrone increases cell proliferation and is associated with inflammation, excess levels of omega-6 fatty acids, obesity, and hypothyroidism. A small amount of estrogen is metabolized into 4-hydroxyestrone, which is thought to promote cancer by damaging DNA. Healthy estrogen production favoring more of 2-hydroxyestrone is important for women's health during and after menopause and is key to healthy aging for women. Unbalanced hormones during the menopause transition trigger symptoms such as weight gain, hot flashes, sleep disturbances, and vaginal dryness. Estrogen dominance, the condition of increased estrogen levels relative to progesterone levels, may be the result of changes in estrogen metabolism, or an imbalance in the estrogen to progesterone ratio, and has been associated with chronic health diseases such as breast cancer (Kolan 2020).

Weight Gain

Weight gain and difficulty losing weight during menopause are major concerns for women and important public health concerns. The prevalence of overweight and obesity combined, which is closely associated with cardiovascular risk, increases significantly in American women after they reach age 40; the prevalence reaches 65% between ages 40 and 59 years and 73.8% in women aged older than 60 years (Flegal 2010). The reasons for weight gain in menopausal women are not fully understood. However, there is accumulating evidence that the absence of estrogen promotes metabolic dysfunction, leading to weight gain and obesity. Estrogen and estrogen receptors regulate various aspects of glucose and lipid metabolism. Studies show that estrogens regulate body weight and energy metabolism like that of leptin, the hormone that regulates energy metabolism in the brain (Gao et al. 2007). Disturbances of metabolic signals lead to the development of metabolic syndrome, characterized by increased blood pressure, high blood glucose levels, lipid profile variations, and predominant abdominal fat accumulation. Lower levels of estrogen are also associated with reductions in the amount of energy the body uses to perform essential physical functions and increases in energy intake. More energy intake results in a positive energy balance leading to further weight gain and increased fat deposits in the abdominal region.

A recent large-scale national study found Black women were 50% more likely to gain weight during the menopause transition than white women (Ford et al. 2021). According to researchers, the higher risk of weight gain is not due to differences in initial weight alone but to biological, social, cultural, and economic differences. Other studies show that Black women are particularly concerned about menopausal weight gain (Kracht et al. 2022).

Heart Health

Black women are particularly at risk of cardiovascular disease (CVD), including coronary heart disease, which is largely responsible for heart attacks and strokes and kills nearly 50,000 Black women annually (American Heart Association [AHA] 2022). Only 36% of African American women know that heart disease is their greatest health risk. More than 40% of Black Americans have high blood pressure, often developing it earlier in life than other races (AHA 2022).

The absence of estrogen during menopause is a contributing factor to the onset of CVD, a major public health threat to women. The various metabolic changes linked to menopause increase the risk of cardiometabolic diseases. About 1 in 2.7 women will eventually die of CVD compared to 1 in 4.6 women dying of cancer (Zhang 2010). About one in three women (34.9%) in the United States has some form of CVD. In both men and women, risk factors such as hypertension, high blood cholesterol level, smoking, lack of physical activity, and obesity increase the probability of developing CVD. Black women have a disproportionately higher rate of developing CVD than any other group. The 2020 Heart Disease and Stroke Statistics Update showed that 57.1% of Black women have CVD compared to 43.4% of white, 42.6% of Hispanic, and 37.2% of Asian women (Virani et al. 2020). Menopause, oral contraceptive use, and the removal of both ovaries in premenopausal women also increase the risk of CVD in women. CVD is the greatest killer of African American females in the United States.

Estrogen is an anti-inflammatory agent, and research shows that inflammation can increase during menopause because of declining estrogen levels. Clinical research reports that estrogen reduces atherosclerosis by reducing low-density lipoproteins (LDL) and inflammatory processes in the vasculature (Ruediger et al. 2021). Studies point to estrogen's role in regulating vascular function, acting directly on the vascular endothelium through the production of nitric oxide, as the mechanism by which it serves as a vasodilator and hypotensive agent. The decline in estrogen production throughout menopause is associated with chronic elevations in blood pressure as well as progressive declines in peripheral conduit arterial endothelial function across the stages of menopause (Ruediger et al. 2021). As a consequence, decreasing estrogen leads to higher levels of LDL and lower levels of high-density lipoproteins (HDL), contributing to the buildup of fat and cholesterol in the arteries.

Brain Health

Both the brain and ovaries are a part of the neuroendocrine system. There is a constant back-and-forth communication between the two. Women's brains age differently than men's, and menopause plays a key role in the difference. The brain's interaction with the reproductive system impacts how the brain ages in women. Brain–reproductive system interactions are mediated by hormones. Unlike testosterone, which ceases to be produced slowly over time until late in life, estrogen levels start to decrease earlier and have more dramatic effects on the body. Symptoms like hot flashes, night sweats, memory loss, depression, and anxiety are neurological symptoms that start in the brain. Estrogen hormones are key for energy production in the brain. Estrogen regulates the glucose delivery to brain cells. As estrogen levels decline, neurons slow down and age faster, making it more difficult to deliver glucose to the brain.

In addition, midlife women's brains are more sensitive to hormonal aging. Studies show a significant reduction in brain glucose uptake during perimenopause (Wang, Mishra, and Brinton 2020). This interference with glucose delivery can lead to the formation of amyloid plaques, a risk factor for Alzheimer's disease (Scheyer et al. 2018). Furthermore, the imbalance of estrogen in the region of the amygdala, the emotional center of the brain, impacts memory and mood, triggering depression and anxiety. Hot flashes occur when estrogen fails to activate the hypothalamus, the gland responsible for regulating body temperature. When estrogen does not activate the brain stem correctly, women demonstrate trouble sleeping.

Research suggests Black Americans are more likely than white Americans to suffer from age-related brain disorders and less likely to focus on their brain health (Alzheimer's Association 2018). Matthews et al. (2019) found that Black American women had the highest prevalence (15.1%) of Alzheimer's disease and related dementias among the nearly five million people (aged ≥65 years) diagnosed in 2014. Participants in a study of older African American adults believed that their life circumstances required a greater focus on day-to-day survival than preventive brain health (Bardach et al. 2019). Other studies highlight the significant correlation between vascular risk factors (e.g., diabetes, high blood pressure, excess abdominal fat, high blood pressure, high cholesterol) and declines in cognitive processing among African Americans. Studies also connect experiences of systemic racism to higher rates of depression, which can lead to dementia in later life (Paradies et al. 2015).

Sexual Health

Low estrogen levels can interfere with sexual function. Genitourinary syndrome of menopause (GSM) is the term adopted to accurately describe the multiple changes that occur to a woman's external genitalia, pelvic floor tissues, bladder, and urethra, and the sexual sequelae that follow, specifically loss of sexual function and libido, during menopause. The term is more expansive than the vulvovaginal symptoms, a term commonly used to describe changes in the vagina during the menopause transition (vaginal dryness, dyspareunia, vaginal irritation, itching sensation, vaginal tenderness, vaginal bleeding or spotting during intercourse). GSM includes not only genital and sexual symptoms but also lower urinary tract symptoms, such as dysuria, urgency, frequency, nocturia, urinary incontinence, and recurrent urinary tract infections (Kim et al. 2015).

GSM is caused by reduced estrogen levels during the menopause transition and postmenopausal period. The loss of estrogen causes anatomical and functional changes, leading to physical symptoms in genitourinary tissues. The tissues lose collagen and elastin, have altered smooth muscle cell function, and have a reduced number of blood vessels accompanied by an increase in connective tissue—all leading to thinning of the epithelium, diminished blood flow, and reduced elasticity. These changes result in a loss of labial and vulvar fullness, vaginal shortening and narrowing, pelvic floor weakening, vaginal dryness, alkaline pH changes leading to vaginal microbiome changes, loss of clitoral stimulation, and changes in the discharge and odor of the vagina. Symptoms increase with age and range from mild to moderately debilitating. Studies have found that 50% of women aged 50 to 60 years report symptoms, increasing to 72% in women aged older than 70 years (Nappi and Kokot-Kierpea 2012).

Few studies of older women's sexuality focus on older Black women. Because Black women are likely to enter the menopausal transition earlier and remain there longer, they are at increased risk for adverse outcomes related to aging and sexuality. Black women are also more likely to experience chronic illnesses that lead to decreased sexual desire. Hartmann et al. (2004) identified the following factors as influencing sexual desire: ethnicity, culture, religion, social background, age, and sexual performance expectations. A qualitative study of Black women aged 57 to 82 years identified four major themes of older Black women's sexuality: having (often unfulfilled) sexual desire, engaging in less sexual activity with advancing age, facing sexuality changes stemming from absence of a spouse, and having control over one's sexual life in older age. The authors concluded that older Black women were reluctant to disclose information about their sexuality (White and Laganá 2013; Ford et al. 2021).

HEALTH DISPARITIES IN BLACK MENOPAUSAL WOMEN

The ongoing physical and emotional changes that happen throughout menopause can be stressful for all women. However, for Black women, who already face multiple chronic stressors linked to poor health, the risk for negative menopausal symptoms and outcomes is greater. Despite overall gains in active life expectancy and efforts to reduce health disparities in the United States, Black–white and socioeconomic inequalities in life expectancy and the prevalence of chronic disease persist (Flegal 2002; Geronimus et al. 1996; Levine et al. 2001; Mokdad et al. 2001; Wong et al. 2002). This is true for menopause as well. Compared to white women, Black women have a higher prevalence and longer duration of bothersome vasomotor symptoms (i.e., hot flashes and night sweats), have shorter sleep duration and less-efficient sleep, and have lower energy expenditure and physical activity (Kracht et al. 2022). Black women are also more likely to experience increases in depressive symptoms and declines in sexual function over the menopause transition compared to white women (Kracht et al. 2022). In addition, Black women may face systemic barriers to obtaining sufficient guidance from medical professionals compared to white women.

The Study of Women's Health Across the Nation (SWAN), a multisite, multiracial/ethnic longitudinal cohort study of the menopause transition, focuses on the biological and psychosocial antecedents and sequelae of menopause in an ethnically and racially diverse sample of midlife women (El Khoudary et al. 2019). SWAN findings reveal that Black women experience poor outcomes across multiple health indicators for midlife women. The study is the longest ongoing multiracial study of menopause. SWAN's robust design and the breadth of information collected over approximately two decades enabled the investigators to unravel the contribution of the menopause transition versus chronological aging in several physiological systems and health domains. The study posits that unmeasured socioeconomic, cultural, and nontraditional biological factors likely play a role in racial/ethnic menopause transition differences.

The Black Women's Health Study (BWHS), a prospective bi-annual follow up study of 59,000 African American women from across the United States, began in 1995 and assesses risk factors for cancers and other major illnesses in Black women. The BWHS found that natural menopause before the age of 40 years was associated with a higher rate of all-cause and cause-specific mortality for Black women. These findings support the theory that natural menopause before age 40 may be a marker of accelerated somatic aging among Black women (Li et al. 2013). The most pronounced differences in health between US Black and white women are seen in middle age, suggesting, at least metaphorically, an accelerated aging process (Geronimus 2001). Geronimus hypothesized that this age pattern of US Black health disadvantage reflects a process of biological weathering (Geronimus 1992, 2001). That is, US Blacks may be biologically older than whites of the same chronological age due to the cumulative impact of repeated exposure to and high-effort coping with stressors. These studies propose that some of the disparities that exist between white women and women of color in perimenopause and menopause are likely attributable to structural racism in the United States.

STRESS AND MENOPAUSE

Though menopause itself can be stressful, the combined effects of fluctuating hormones and life's stressors often result in women feeling completely overwhelmed. Career and familial responsibilities peak around the time of menopause. Issues such as the demands of adolescent children, children leaving home, aging parents, midlife spouses, and career changes converge on women during these years, exacerbating symptoms associated with menopause and increasing their overall stress level.

Like menopause, the body's stress response is governed primarily by hormones. The body is designed to respond to stressors through the cooperative work of the sympathetic nervous system (SNS) and hypothalamic–pituitary–adrenal (HPA) axis. An efficient response to an acute stressor involves activation of the SNS to direct resources for the "fight-or-flight" response. Increases in the hormones cortisol and adrenaline provide energy, focus, and increased alertness to fight back physically or emotionally. However, exposure to chronic stress and repeated activation of the stress response results in an allostatic load on the body's systems (McEwen 1998).

During menopause, the adrenal glands (i.e., the stress glands) take over some of the work of the diminishing ovaries by producing small amounts of progesterone and estrogen. However, when stressed, overtaxed adrenal glands cannot produce healthy levels of these hormones; the body chooses survival over fertility, producing more cortisol and adrenaline instead of estrogen and progesterone. Subsequently, chronically high levels of cortisol lead to adrenal fatigue and burnout, and menopausal symptoms increase. Women experiencing higher levels of depression, food cravings, weight gain, exhaustion, insomnia, and foggy thinking often compensate with unhealthy behaviors (i.e., consumption of

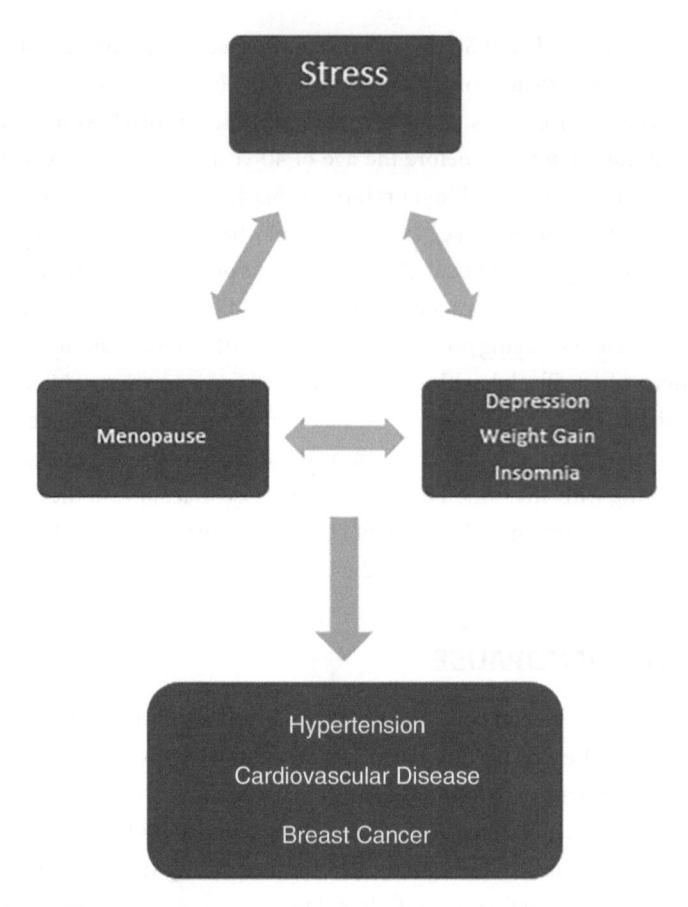

Figure 19-1. Stress–Menopause Cycle

processed sugary foods, forgoing exercise, and poor stress management). They feel stuck in a cycle of stress, menopause, and physical and emotional symptoms, often resulting in long-term chronic health conditions (Figure 19-1).

For Black women, the stress of midlife is complicated by discrimination, sexism, and navigating ongoing financial and health care challenges propagated by systemic racism and social inequities. Diverse literature from sociology, economics, anthropology, and public health documents that US Blacks are more likely to experience stressful situations, such as material hardship (Charles and Guryan 2008; Mayer and Jencks 1989), interpersonal discrimination (Barnes et al. 2004; Taylor and Turner 2002), structural discrimination in housing and employment (Charles and Hurst 2002; Darity and Mason 1998; Holzer, Offner, and Sorensen 2005; Ondrich Ross and Yinger 2003; Yinger 1998), and multiple caregiving roles (Dilworth-Anderson, Williams, and Gibson 2002; Lum 2005) than whites. By age 30, Black women exhibit a greater risk of having high allostatic load scores than Black men or than white men or women. This risk gap increases through midlife and is most severe among Black women who are poor and who often bear central responsibility for the social and economic survival of their families and communities (Burton and Whitfield 2003; Geronimus et al. 2006; Jarrett and Burton 1999; Lancaster 1989; Mullings and Wali 2001; Stack and Burton 1993; Warren-Findlow 2006). Ultimately, this gap leads to greater wear and tear on the body over time, overtaxing various hormonal and biological factors, and resulting in worse outcomes related to menopause.

MENOPAUSAL BLACK WOMEN—SUPPORT OF HEALTH CARE PROVIDERS

In developed countries, where life spans have been extended, women will spend more than half of their lives in a state of estrogen deficiency (Lizcano and Guzmán 2014). Despite our current understanding of the symptoms and sequalae of menopause, many Black women are unprepared for the transition and how it impacts their lives. The lack of knowledge, misinformation, and silence around menopause has created a sense of helplessness.

Hormonal imbalances and related chronic conditions are complicated. Thus, the need for health care providers who specialize in the health of women of color is crucial to their well-being. Finding a supportive provider whom Black women can trust, establish a close relationship with, and fully disclose their medical record to is the first step in the process. A complete review of symptoms and medical history will enable the provider to recommend a personalized treatment protocol to address hormone balance to the extent possible. Open provider-patient communication will facilitate effective interventions. Black women need access to culturally sensitive providers who are willing to discuss the range of options available and assist with their transition into menopause.

Providers who care for Black women must go beyond the physiology of menopause and understand the role of impalpable stressors, such as systemic racism and its long-term consequences. The allostatic load that comes from the accumulation of stress and triggers the inflammatory response leads to greater risk of lowered resilience (Velez 2021). Specialists need to help Black women recognize signs of lowered resilience. They should be taught to recognize exhaustion, fatigue, and detachment as signs of the weathering effect and seek the help of others, be it a circle of friends or support groups.

SUPPORT BEYOND HEALTH CARE PROVIDERS

Black women want help managing their menopausal symptoms (Kracht et al. 2022). They want to learn more about menopause alongside other women and receive social support, accountability for healthy living, and motivation from other Black women. It is important that this support be inclusive and equity focused, welcoming lesbian, bisexual, gay, transgender, and queer individuals and acknowledging experiences outside of the cisgendered, heteronormative experience. Public health programs should establish support groups for Black women experiencing menopause so their perspectives can be acknowledged.

Lifestyle Programs

According to Omisade Burney-Scott (2022), host of the *Black Girl's Guide to Surviving Menopause* podcast, Black women should see the menopause transition as a time to recalibrate their bodies and figure out how to achieve good health, stress-free living, rest, and pleasure. Public health programs targeting Black women in midlife should address factors most likely to disrupt the stress–menopause cycle. Specifically, such lifestyle programs should address the following areas:

1. Prioritize healthy diets and food choices.
   a. There are many components to a diet that, when enacted, have the capacity to counter the adverse effects of menopause. Studies have shown postmenopausal women who lost 10% of their body weight over a year were more likely to eliminate hot flashes and night sweats (Brown 2022). Thus, a small reduction in daily caloric intake over time can lead to gradual weight loss and help alleviate menopausal symptoms.
   b. In choosing carbohydrate sources, menopausal women should focus on those high in fiber, such as fruits and vegetables, as they tend to have lower glycemic indices. Avoidance of refined, processed carbohydrates is advised as they tend to have higher glycemic indices leading to a quick spike in blood glucose levels following digestion (Brown 2017).
   c. When considering the mineral content of healthful diets for menopausal women, it should also be adequate in calcium (1,000–1,200 mg daily) for proper bone density and strength (Brown 2017). Hormonal changes during menopause can cause bones to weaken and may lead to osteoporosis.
   d. It is important to include anti-inflammatory agents and antioxidants in the diet of menopausal women. Vitamin D can serve as an anti-inflammatory agent once absorbed by the body (Brown 2022). Vitamins C and E, and beta-carotene, the precursor for vitamin A, act as antioxidants when metabolized and effectively combat oxidative damage (Brown 2017).
   e. Phytoestrogens are naturally occurring plant substances that mimic the effect of estrogen in the body. When consumed they may help lower the risk of menopausal symptoms (Desmawati and Sulastri 2019).
   f. Menopausal women should consume adequate protein throughout the day to help prevent the loss of lean muscle mass that occurs with aging (Brown 2022).
2. Make physical activity a priority.
   a. Exercise during and after menopause offers many benefits, including mood elevation; reducing the risk of CVD, cancer, and other chronic diseases; and

prevention of weight gain. Exercise also slows down the age-related processes of sarcopenia (muscle loss), osteopenia (loss of bone mineral density), and osteoporosis (weak and brittle bones). Strength training is particularly beneficial for women during the menopause transition.
3. Help Black women adopt effective, convenient, and varied strategies for managing stress.
   a. Public health interventions should address the unique social and psychological issues that arise during midlife for Black women and assist in navigating these challenges. Black women should be encouraged to engage regularly in stress management techniques, such as prayer, meditation, and deep breathing, and seek assistance in balancing work and familial responsibilities. For some, this may include therapy.
   b. Prioritize getting enough rest. Getting more rest can decrease cortisol levels and restore balance to the body's systems.
4. Help Black women investigate food-grade supplements and/or hormone-replacement therapy or other medical interventions.
   a. Dietary supplements are under consideration for the treatment of menopausal symptoms. It is a relatively new area of research and, as such, is limited in its findings. More research is needed with larger study samples of menopausal women representing diverse racial and ethnic groups before recommendations can be generalized to this population.
   b. Current scientific evidence suggests that among symptomatic menopausal women younger than age 60 or within 10 years of menopause, the benefits of menopausal hormone therapy (HT) may outweigh the risks (Mehta, Kling, and Manson 2021). Such benefits include a potential reduction in mortality from osteoporotic fractures and coronary heart disease (Nicholoson et al. 1999). With the higher underlying coronary heart disease mortality rate among Black women, hormone replacement therapy may be an important preventive therapy on multiple levels. While there are advantages to HT, the risks must also be considered; these include a possible increase in breast and endometrial cancer (Nicholson et al. 1999). HT prescribing practices have evolved over the last few decades guided by the improved understanding of the effects of HT. Black women should ask their provider for a detailed explanation of types, formulations, routes of administration, risks, and benefits of HT.

REFERENCES

Agarwal A, Doshi, S. The role of oxidative stress in menopause. *J Midlife Health*. 2013;4(3):140. https://doi.org/10.4103/0976-7800.118990

Alzheimer's Association. 2018 Alzheimer's disease facts and figures. *Alzheimers Dement*. 2018;14(3):367–429. https://doi.org/10.1016/j.jalz.2018.02.001

American Heart Association. Heart disease in African American women. June 2022. Available at: https://www.goredforwomen.org/en/about-heart-disease-in-women/facts/heart-disease-in-african-american-women

Bardach SH, Benton B, Walker C, et al. Perspectives of African American older adults on brain health. *Alzheimer Dis Assoc Disord.* 2019;33(4):354–358. https://doi.org/10.1097/wad.0000000000000335

Barnes LL, de Leon CFM, Wilson RS, Bienias JL, Bennett DA, Evans DA. Racial differences in perceived discrimination in a community population of older Blacks and whites. *J Aging Health.* 2004;16(3):315–337. https://doi.org/10.1177/0898264304264202

Bromberger JT, Matthews KA, Kullerr LH, et al. Prospective study of the determinants of age at menopause. *Am J Epidemiol.* 1997;145:124–133. https://doi.org/10.1093/oxfordjournals.aje.a009083

Brown MJ. Eleven natural remedies for menopause relief. *Healthline.* 2022. Available at: https://www.healthline.com/nutrition/11-natural-menopause-tips

Brown J. *Nutrition Now.* Boston, MA: Cengage Learning; 2017.

Burney-Scott O. All you gotta do is say "Yes"! [audio podcast]. March 16, 2022. Available at: https://blackgirlsguidetosurvivingmenopause.com

Burton LM, Whitfield KE. "Weathering" towards poorer health in later life: co-morbidity in urban low-income families. *Public Policy Aging Rep.* 2003;13(3):13–18. https://doi.org/10.1093/ppar/13.3.13

Charles K, Guryan J. Prejudice and wages: an empirical assessment of Becker's *The Economics of Discrimination. J Polit Econ.* 2008;116(5):773–809. https://doi.org/10.1086/593073

Charles KK, Hurst E. The transition to home ownership and the Black–white wealth gap. *Rev Econ Stat.* 2002;84(2):281–297. https://doi.org/10.1162/003465302317411532

Cooper GS, Sandler DP. Age at natural menopause and mortality. *Ann Epidemiol.* 1998;8(4):229–235. https://doi.org/10.1016/S1047-2797(97)00207-X

Darity WA, Mason PL. Evidence on discrimination in employment: codes of color, codes of gender. *J Econ Perspect.* 1998;12(2):63–90. https://doi.org/10.1257/jep.12.2.63

Desmawati D, Sulastri D. Phytoestrogens and their health effect. *Open Access Maced J Med Sci.* 2019;7(3):495–499. https://doi.org/10.3889/oamjms.2019.044

Dilworth-Anderson P, Williams IC, Gibson BE. Issues of race, ethnicity, and culture in caregiving research: a 20-year review (1980–2000). *Gerontologist.* 2002;42(2):237–272. https://doi.org/10.1093/geront/42.2.237

El Khoudary SR, Greendale G, Crawford SL, et al. The menopause transition and women's health at midlife: a progress report from the Study of Women's Health Across the Nation (SWAN). *Menopause.* 2019;26(10):1213–1227. https://doi.org/10.1097/gme.0000000000001424

Flegal KM. Prevalence and trends in obesity among US adults, 1999–2000. *JAMA.* 2002;288(14):1723. https://doi.org/10.1001/jama.288.14.1723

Flegal KM. Prevalence and trends in obesity among US adults, 1999–2008. *JAMA.* 2010;303(3):235. https://doi.org/10.1001/jama.2009.2014

Ford CN, Chang S, Wood AC, et al. On the joint role of non-Hispanic Black race/ethnicity and weight status in predicting postmenopausal weight gain. *PLoS One.* 2021;16(3):e0247821. https://doi.org/10.1371/journal.pone.0247821

Gao Q, Mezei G, Nie Y, et al. Anorectic estrogen mimics leptin's effect on the rewiring of melanocortin cells and Stat3 signaling in obese animals. *Nat Med.* 2007;13(1):89-94. https://doi.org/10.1038/nm1525

Geronimus AT. The weathering hypothesis and the health of African-American women and infants: evidence and speculations. *Ethn Dis.* 1992;2(3):207-221.

Geronimus AT, Bound J, Waidmann TA, Colen CG, Steffick D. Inequality in life expectancy, functional status, and active life expectancy across selected Black and white populations in the United States. *Demography.* 2001;38(2):227-251. https://doi.org/10.1353/dem.2001.0015

Geronimus AT, Bound J, Waidmann TA, Hillemeier MM, Burns PB. Excess mortality among Blacks and whites in the United States. *N Engl J Med.* 1996;335(21):1552-1558. https://doi.org/10.1056/nejm199611213352102

Geronimus AT, Hicken M, Keene D, Bound J. "Weathering" and age patterns of allostatic load scores among Blacks and whites in the United States. *Am J Public Health.* 2006;96(5):826-833. https://doi.org/10.2105/ajph.2004.060749

Geronimus AT, Hicken MT, Pearson JA, Seashols SJ, Brown KL, Cruz TD. Do US Black women experience stress-related accelerated biological aging? *Hum Nat.* 2010;21(1):19-38. https://doi.org/10.1007/s12110-010-9078-0

Harlow SD, Burnett-Bowie SAM, Greendale GA, et al. Disparities in reproductive aging and midlife health between Black and white women: the Study of Women's Health Across the Nation (SWAN). *Womens Midlife Health.* 2022;8(1):3. https://doi.org/10.1186/s40695-022-00073-y

Hartmann U, Philippsohn S, Heiser K, Rüffer-Hesse C. Low sexual desire in midlife and older women: personality factors, psychosocial development, present sexuality. *Menopause.* 2004;11(6):726-740. https://doi.org/10.1097/01.gme.0000143705.42486.33

Holzer HJ, Offner P, Sorensen E. Declining employment among young Black less-educated men: the role of incarceration and child support. *J Policy Analysis Manag.* 2005;24(2):329-350. https://doi.org/10.1002/pam.20092

Jarrett RL, Burton LM. Dynamic dimensions of family structure in low-income African American families: emergent themes in qualitative research. *J Compar Fam Stud.* 1999;30(2):177-187. https://doi.org/10.3138/jcfs.30.2.177

Kim HK, Kang SY, Chung YJ, Kim JH, Kim MR. The recent review of the genitourinary syndrome of menopause. *J Menopausal Med.* 2015;21(2):65-71. https://doi.org/10.6118/jmm.2015.21.2.65

Kolan A. *Estrogen Dominance.* Whole Health Library. Washington, DC: US Department of Veterans Affairs; 2020.

Kracht CL, Romain JS, Hardee JC, Santoro N, Redman LM, Marlatt KL. "It just seems like people are talking about menopause, but nobody has a solution": a qualitative exploration of menopause experiences and preferences for weight management among Black women. *Maturitas.* 2022;157:16-26. https://doi.org/10.1016/j.maturitas.2021.11.005

Lancaster JB. Evolutionary and cross-cultural perspectives on single parenthood. In: Bell RW, Bell NJ, eds. *Interfaces in Psychology, Sociobiology, and the Social Sciences.* Lubbock, TX: Texas Tech University Press; 1989: 63-72.

Levine RS, Foster JE, Fullilove RE, et al. Black-white inequalities in mortality and life expectancy, 1933-1999: implications for Healthy People 2010. *Public Health Rep.* 2001;116(5):474-483. https://doi.org/10.1016/s0033-3549(04)50075-4

Li S, Rosenberg L, Wise LA, Boggs DA, LaValley M, Palmer JR. Age at natural menopause in relation to all-cause and cause-specific mortality in a follow-up study of US Black women. *Maturitas.* 2013;75(3):246-252. https://doi.org/10.1016/j.maturitas.2013.04.003

Lizcano F, Guzmán G. Estrogen deficiency and the origin of obesity during menopause. *Biomed Res Int.* 2014:1-11. https://doi.org/10.1155/2014/757461

Lum TY. Understanding the racial and ethnic differences in caregiving arrangements. *J Gerontol Soc Work.* 2005;45(4):3-21. https://doi.org/10.1300/j083v45n04_02

Matthews KA, Xu W, Gaglioti AH, et al. Racial and ethnic estimates of Alzheimer's disease and related dementias in the United States (2015-2060) in adults aged ≥65 years. *Alzheimers Dement.* 2019;15(1):17-24. https://doi.org/10.1016/j.jalz.2018.06.3063

Mayer SE, Jencks C. Poverty and the distribution of material hardship. *J Hum Resources.* 1989;24(1):88-114. https://doi.org/10.2307/145934

McEwen BS. Protective and damaging effects of stress mediators. *N Engl J Med.* 1998;338(3):171-179. https://doi.org/10.1056/nejm199801153380307

Mehta J, Kling JM, Manson JE. Risks, benefits, and treatment modalities of menopausal hormone therapy: current concepts. *Front Endocrinol (Lausanne).* 2021;12:564781. https://doi.org/10.3389/fendo.2021.564781

Mokdad AH, Ford ES, Bowman BA, et al. The continuing increase of diabetes in the US. *Diabetes Care.* 2001;24(2):412. https://doi.org/10.2337/diacare.24.2.412

Mullings L, Wali A. *Stress and Resilience: The Social Context of Reproduction in Central Harlem.* New York, NY: Springer Science & Business Media; 2001.

Nappi RE, Kokot-Kierepa M. Vaginal health: insights, views & attitudes (VIVA)—results from an international survey. *Climacteric.* 2011;15(1):36-44. https://doi.org/10.3109/13697137.2011.647840

Nicholson WK, Brown AF, Gathe J, Grumbach K, Washington AE Pérez-Stable EJ. Hormone replacement therapy for African American women: missed opportunities for effective treatment. *Menopause.* 1999;6(2):147-155.

Ondrich J, Ross S, Yinger J. Now you see it, now you don't: why do real estate agents withhold available houses from Black customers? *Rev Econ Stat.* 2003;85(4):854-873. https://doi.org/10.1162/003465303772815772

Paradies Y, Ben J, Denson N, et al. Racism as a determinant of health: a systematic review and meta-analysis. *PLoS One.* 2015;10(9):e013851. https://doi.org/10.1371/journal.pone.0138511

Ruediger SL, Koep JL, Keating SE, Pizzey FK, Coombes JS, Bailey TG. Effect of menopause on cerebral artery blood flow velocity and cerebrovascular reactivity: systematic review and meta-analysis. *Maturitas.* 2021;148:24-32. https://doi.org/10.1016/j.maturitas.2021.04.004

Santoro N, Roeca C, Peters BA, Neal-Perry G. The menopause transition: signs, symptoms, and management options. *J Clin Endocrinol Metab.* 2021;106(1):1-15. https://doi.org/10.1210/clinem/dgaa764

Scheyer O, Rahman A, Hristov H, et al. Female sex and Alzheimer's risk: the menopause connection. *J Prev Alzheimers Dis.* 2018;5(4), 225-230. https://doi.org/10.14283/jpad.2018.34

Sherwin BB. Estrogen and cognitive functioning in women. *Endocrine Rev.* 2003;24(2):133-151. https://doi.org/10.1210/er.2001-0016

Stack C. *All Our Kin: Strategies for Survival in a Black Community.* New York, NY: Harper and Row; 1974.

Stack CB, Burton LM. Kinscripts. *J Compar Fam Stud.* 1993;24(2):157-170. https://doi.org/10.3138/jcfs.24.2.157

Taylor J, Turner RJ. Perceived discrimination, social stress, and depression in the transition to adulthood: racial contrasts. *Soc Psychol Q.* 2002;65(3):213. https://doi.org/10.2307/3090120

Velez A. Menopause is different for women of color. EndocrineWeb. March 10, 2021. Available at: https://www.endocrineweb.com/menopause-different-women-color

Virani S, Alonso A, Benjamin EJ, et al. Heart disease and stroke statistics—2020 update: a report from the American Heart Association. *Circulation.* 2020;141(9):e139–e596. https://doi.org/10.1161/CIR.0000000000000757

Wang Y, Mishra A, Brinton RD. Transitions in metabolic and immune systems from pre-menopause to post-menopause: implications for age-associated neurodegenerative diseases. *F1000Res.* 2020; 9:F1000 Faculty Rev-68. https://doi.org/10.12688/f1000research.21599.1

Warren-Findlow, J. Weathering: stress and heart disease in African American women living in Chicago. *Qual Health Res.* 2006;16(2):221-237. https://doi.org/10.1177/1049732305278651

White T, Laganá L. Factors influencing older Black women's sexual functioning and their disclosure of sexual concerns. *OA Women's Health.* 2013;1(1):10. https://doi.org/10.13172/2053-0501-1-1-788

Wong MD, Shapiro MF, Boscardin WJ, Ettner SL. Contribution of major diseases to disparities in mortality. *N Engl J Med.* 2002;347(20):1585-1592. https://doi.org/10.1056/NEJMsa012979

Yinger J. Evidence on discrimination in consumer markets. *J Econ Perspect.* 1998;12(2):23-40. https://doi.org/10.1257/jep.12.2.23

Zhang Y. Cardiovascular diseases in American women. *Nutr Metab Cardiovasc Dis.* 2010;20(6): 386-393. https://doi.org/10.1016/j.numecd.2010.02.001

20

Sexual Agency, Behaviors, and Decision-Making Throughout the Life Span

Torie Comeaux Plowden, MD, MPH, and Camille A. Clare, MD, MPH

Sexual well-being is a significant, but often overlooked, contributor of overall quality of life and satisfaction. In fact, overall well-being is positively correlated with sexual satisfaction and sexual pleasure. For Black women, feeling empowered sexually can often be a goal that is out of reach. Constant messaging and images that negatively impact self-esteem, media portrayals of hypersexualized Black women, changing cultural norms (e.g., "hookup" culture), and the gender ratio disparities can make attaining sexual wellness difficult for Black women of any age. Endorsing hegemonic beauty ideals can lead to sexual guilt and shame as well as decrease sexual agency. This chapter will focus on research related to sexual agency, behaviors, and decision-making among women in various stages of reproductive life—adolescents, college-aged and young women, women in their 30 and 40s, and peri- and postmenopausal women—with a specific focus on the public health impact of sexual mores in Black women relative to reproductive justice.

SEXUAL WELL-BEING, SEXUAL SATISFACTION, AND SEXUAL AGENCY

Sexual well-being is an important factor of wellness and quality of life. Overall well-being is positively associated with sexual satisfaction, sexual well-being, and sexual pleasure (Anderson 2013). Black women face many barriers that may inhibit them from fully achieving sexual satisfaction and sexual agency.

Existing literature in sex research involving Black women is very limited. Indeed, a content analysis of sexualities research on Black women conducted from 1972 to 2018 discovered that one-third of publications focused on risky sexual behaviors and sexually transmitted infections (STIs; Hargons et al. 2021). In 46 years of sexual health research, only 6.5% of the articles used a "sex-positive discourse" (Hargons et al. 2021, p. 1287). In 2009, McGruder noted that because sexuality studies in Black women are often problem-focused, the stigma that Black sexuality is nonnormative continues (McGruder 2009).

Sociocultural Context

Sexual Mores and Taboos

Historically, the worth of Black women in America has been tied to their ability to procreate. From 1619 until the mid-1800s, enslaved African women and their descendants did not have any agency over their own bodies; nor did they have the freedom to choose when or with whom to conceive. Through sexual manipulation and reproductive coercion, Black enslaved women were forced to have as many children as possible without any consideration of their own desires. As a means of justifying the rape and sexual exploitation of enslaved women, the Jezebel stereotype was born, portraying Black women as sexually promiscuous and as having an insatiable sexual appetite (Collins 2004).

Research has indicated that Black women's awareness of the Jezebel stereotype can inform their sexual agency. This stereotype leads Black women to subscribe to sexual scripts that objectify them, champion sexual passivity, and decrease regard for their own sexual desires (Leath et al. 2022; Crooks et al. 2019; French 2013; Stephens and Phillips 2003). Indeed, Black women with a stronger awareness of the Jezebel stereotype demonstrated more emotional avoidance behaviors, tended to participate in sexual distancing, displayed significant feelings of sexual objectification, and had poorer sexual outcomes (Leath et al. 2022). Conversely, when Black women rejected the Jezebel stereotype and embraced positive feelings about their identity as a Black woman, they experienced more sexual satisfaction (Leath et al. 2022; Crooks et al. 2019).

Race-based sexual stereotypes (RBSS) have been defined as the implicit expectations and inferred beliefs of sexual encounters or experiences based on the partner's race (Wilson et al. 2009). A recent qualitative study sought to understand how race-based sexual stereotyping could impact sexual decisions that Black women make. Participants revealed that RBSS may cause Black women to become resistant to learning about safer sexual practices. In addition, RBSS made Black women feel less empowered in sexually intimate encounters and relationships (Bond et al. 2021).

Another study sought to explore the role of endorsement of femininity scripts and how the strong Black women (SBW) ideal influenced sexual assertiveness and self-silencing behaviors in Black women (Avery et al. 2022). Femininity scripts are common in American culture, and endorsement of that script is associated with sexual passivity, submission, and self-silencing behaviors, which can ultimately stifle sexual agency and sexual expression (Lentz and Zaikman 2021; Eaton and Matamala 2014). Many Black women are socialized to embrace the SBW standard, which also prioritizes the needs of others over one's own needs and champions self-silencing behaviors (Avery et al. 2022). The authors found that self-silencing behaviors were negatively associated with all measures of sexual assertiveness (communication assertiveness, refusal assertiveness, and pleasure-focused assertiveness). Furthermore, the strong endorsement of the SBW schema led to decreased pleasure-focused sexual assertiveness (Avery et al. 2022). The authors concluded that gendered sexual norms in Black women are complicated; self-silencing behaviors in this group diminish sexual agency and may make it difficult for these women to advocate for their sexual safety and wellness (Avery et al. 2022).

Beauty Ideals and Self-Esteem

In America, Eurocentric standards of beauty are highly valued, while Afrocentric aesthetics are often considered less desirable and less feminine (Avery et al. 2021; Awad et al. 2015). Internalization and endorsement of these hegemonic feminine beauty ideals has been shown to decrease self-esteem and is associated with poorer body image (Avery et al. 2021). A study of more than 600 Black college women was conducted to investigate if endorsement of hegemonic beauty ideals was associated with measures of sexual well-being. The investigators found that women who endorsed hegemonic beauty ideals experienced greater sexual guilt, shame, sexual self-consciousness, and emotional distancing, while also experiencing less sexual assertiveness and satisfaction (Avery et al. 2021).

Emerging Sexuality in Black Women

Guided by principles from grounded theory, an in-depth qualitative study elucidated information to better understand the phases Black women go through as they become sexual Black women (Crooks et al. 2019). The three phases identified were girl, grown, and woman. The girl phase was characterized by early sexual development and minimal sexual knowledge. The grown phase was a time in which participants were transitioning from childhood to adulthood and was marked by beginning to engage in sexual activity. It is critical to note that in this phase women expressed that they were heavily influenced by peers and often engaged in high-risk sexual behaviors, such as promiscuity and unprotected sex. The woman phase was described as time in which participants gained a strong sense of themselves and the ability to better define their own image of what it means to be a Black woman. At this phase, women often rejected stereotypes of Black women and began to embrace their sexuality more fully.

One theme that emerged from this study was the importance of protecting young girls as they traveled through this process (Crooks, King, and Tluczek 2020; Crooks et al. 2019). Many participants expressed that their own sexual development was a bit surprising and faster compared to their peers'. As such, they were often sexually objectified by older men and made to feel quite self-conscious as adolescents. These women discussed the "culture of silence" that often exists in Black communities surrounding sexuality (Crooks et al. 2019). Protecting Black female sexuality ultimately means developing safe spaces for Black adolescents, sharing personal stories, and providing accurate knowledge about topics related to sexual health and reproduction (Crooks et al. 2019).

Mothers are often the primary sex educators, and previous research indicates that mothers who explore open communication with their daughters can more effectively guide them to successfully navigate future sexual relationships (Grigsby 2018; Aronowitz and Agbeshie 2012). Early sexual discussion between mothers and daughters can positively impact health behaviors (e.g., remaining abstinent longer, having fewer sexual partners) and ultimately improve the health outcomes of adolescent girls (Grigsby 2018; Aronowitz and Eche 2013). A qualitative study noted that Black women draw from their own experiences, their faith, and their values when discussing sexual topics with their daughters (Grigsby 2018).

Influence of the Black Church and Religion

Several studies have indicated that higher levels of religiosity in adolescent females is protective against high-risk sexual behaviors (Rew and Wong 2006; McCree et al. 2003; Miller and Gur 2002). And, yet, many young Black women voiced that when religious beliefs enforced the idea that sex was sinful, feelings of guilt and shame led them to feel silenced (Crooks, King, and Tluczek 2020). One study examined the relationship of religiosity, spirituality, and sexual risk-taking behaviors in 100 Black female college students attending a Historically Black College or University (HBCU) in the South. The authors found that although religion and spirituality is an important part of the HBCU experience, it was not protective in limiting sexual risk-taking behavior (Thomas and Freeman 2011).

Sexual Health, Behaviors, and Decision-Making

Black women are disproportionately impacted by adverse reproductive and sexual health outcomes potentially related to their sexual behaviors and decision-making. Race itself does not purport greater reproductive and sexual risk; instead, behaviors, access to appropriate medical care, education (or lack thereof), and other social contexts associated with particular behaviors confer risk (Centers for Disease Control and Prevention [CDC] 2022; McCord 2014; McGruder 2009). Racism on all levels—institutionalized, personally mediated, and internalized—negatively impacts the health outcomes of Black people in America (Jones 2000). Public health interventions focusing only on behaviors will not be successful unless structural racism is also addressed (Bailey et al. 2017).

College-Age and Adult Women

Young adult women (aged 18-25) who engage in sexual activity may be particularly vulnerable due to risky sexual behaviors (Murray Horrowitz, Pace, and Ross-Degnan 2018). "Hookups"—defined as casual sexual encounters without being involved in a romantic relationship—have become very common on college campuses and are considered a normal part of sexual experimentation among many college-age students (Jenkins Hall and Tanner 2016). This phenomenon has been understudied in Black women.

Hookup scenarios underscore power imbalances that Black women experience in relationships (Jenkins Hall and Tanner 2016). Research indicates that, despite a desire for committed monogamous relationship, many Black college women engaged in casual nonmonogamous hookups because campus men were not interested in a more committed partnership (Hall, Lee, and Witherspoon 2014). As such, Black men wielded considerable power in their relationships. Black women on predominately white college campuses may navigate hookup culture differently. In that setting, racism and sexism limit this group's options for suitable partners and may cause them to seek out romantic and sexual relationships outside of their university (Anakaraonye et al. 2019).

Previous studies have demonstrated that gender ratio imbalance (more women than men) on college campuses was a contributor to high-risk sexual practices. Specifically, female students may be less likely to enforce strict condom usage (Ferguson et al. 2006). In addition, this may influence female students to choose male partners who take part in high-risk behaviors, such as having multiple sexual partners, using substances, or having sex with other men (Jenkins Hall and Tanner 2016; Ferguson et al. 2006).

The male-to-female sex ratio and lack of committed partnerships issue extends beyond college campuses. Communities with higher male incarceration rates and resulting low sex ratio have been shown to also have higher risk behaviors. A qualitative study of reproductive age (18–39 years), heterosexual, unmarried Black women who had been sexually active in the past 90 days examined partner availability. All women interviewed were from one of two US neighborhoods: one with a high male incarceration rate and an imbalanced sex ratio and one with a low male incarceration rate and an equitable sex ratio (Dauria et al. 2015). In the first neighborhood, Black heterosexual women reported that because of lower numbers of higher-quality partners (e.g., financially stable, monogamous, more understanding), relationships were often shorter and were more focused on sexual activity, often with higher-risk sexual partners. Women living in the second neighborhood reported that marriage rates were the cause of low numbers of desirable partners. Regardless of the cause of imbalanced sex ratio, its presence can heavily influence sexual risk behaviors.

Hypermasculine behaviors may play a role in Black relationships, particularly in the context of unintended pregnancy and STI risk. Risky sexual behaviors have been linked to hypermasculinity and include a tendency for Black men to have multiple sexual partners and a strong dislike of condom usage (Wolfe 2003). A qualitative study of Black men seeking care at a public STI clinic explored beliefs that these men held about sexual partner concurrency (Carey et al. 2010). From this discussion, multiple themes arose, including that having more than one sexual partner was normative and acceptable for men but not necessarily acceptable for women (Carey et al. 2010). Navigation of this potential sexual double standard represents yet another hurdle for young Black women as they negotiate their sexual agency and warrants further research (Fasula, Carry, and Miller 2014).

In addition, socioeconomic status has been found to be a contributor to sexual behavior and decision-making among Black women. A study of 524 Black women aged 18 to 49 years (mean age, 23.3 years) sheds light on this issue. Almost 80% of women had completed high school, and 7% were college graduates. Most women in the study (67.9%) reported a history of participating in unwanted sex, often due to fear. The authors concluded that socio-behavioral moderators—including fear of violence (verbal or physical abuse), fear of loss of relationship, and fear of loss of shelter—played an important role in high-risk sexual behavior. These women had low levels of sexual assertiveness and control in their sexual relationships (Whyte 2006).

Reproductive Coercion

Reproductive coercion is a phenomenon in which a partner interferes with a woman's contraception (sabotage of birth control efforts), pressures a female partner to become pregnant against her will, or pressures a female partner to continue or terminate a pregnancy (control of pregnancy outcomes; Nikolajski et al. 2015). Previous research indicates that reproductive coercion may be more commonly experienced by Black women (Basile et al. 2021; Holliday et al. 2017; Grace and Anderson 2018; Nikolajski et al. 2015).

To better understand if reproductive coercion could impact Black women's disparate risk of unintended pregnancy, Nikolajski et al. conducted a qualitative study of 66 women (36 Black women and 30 white women). More Black women reported becoming pregnant as a direct result of reproductive coercion, suggesting that Black participants in this study also offered insight as to why men might coerce women into a pregnancy, noting that lack of social support, barriers to stable housing and employment, and incarceration may be motivating factors. These findings highlight how social instability in low-income Black communities, as well as high incarceration rates, may contribute to sexual risk behavior (Nikolajski et al. 2015).

A qualitative study involving young Black men (n = 25; aged 18-25 years) living in an urban community (Baltimore, Maryland) explored childbearing motivations in the context of reproductive coercion. Twenty-six percent of participants reported exhibiting reproductive coercion behaviors toward a sexual partner. Men in this study perceived that the childbearing motivations behind reproductive coercion were reflective of displays of masculinity and personal dreams for fatherhood (Alexander et al. 2021). Interestingly, this cohort of men perceived that the motivation for female partner-led reproductive coercion was entrapment.

Women of Later Reproductive Age

There has been an emphasis on understanding the sexual risk behavior in younger women. However, recent information in New York City notes that 25% of its new HIV cases have occurred in women in their late 30s (Pahl et al. 2019). A recent study surveyed 343 Black and Puerto Rican women aged 30 to 39 years to elucidate information on sexual practices of these women and their sexual partners. Many of the women in the study (n = 233) categorized their sexual relationship as exclusive. Two-thirds of the women in exclusive sexual relationships (ESR) reported engaging in unprotected vaginal intercourse, even though 33.5% had partners with a history of concurrent relationships and 66.1% of their partners were at risk for HIV and STI transmission. Of the women in ESRs, 7.3% reported not being monogamous and 18.9% reported that their partner was not monogamous. This study demonstrates that women in their late 30s may still be at significant risk for STIs even when reporting being in an ESR (Pahl et al. 2019).

Postmenopausal Women

Recently, there has been more interest in understanding sexual and dating behaviors in older Black women. This group of older Black women may have historically been less likely to discuss their sexual experiences for myriad reasons (Salisu and Dacus 2021; Laganá et al. 2021). Within the context of slavery and the value placed on Black women's fertility, women who were past childbearing age were "stripped of any sexuality, considered worthless, and faced with an increased risk of psychological and physical abuse" (Salisu and Dacus 2021, p. 307). To truly understand the lived experiences of older Black women in relation to their sexual and reproductive well-being, this historical context must be considered. Yet, motivations behind sexual decision-making in older Black women continue to be understudied.

Older sexually active adults have specific issues and concerns that may be significantly different than those of reproductive-age adults. For instance, a systematic review of HIV sexual risk in older Black women noted that this group often views condoms mainly as a contraceptive tool. Subsequently, postmenopausal women who are no longer worried about the possibility of pregnancy may be more likely to engage in risky sexual behaviors and are not considering the benefit of condom usage for prevention of STIs (Smith and Larson 2015). Another study of Black women aged 45 to 60 years noted that having sex without condoms may be done because that is what these women have become used to. Some women in this qualitative study noted that after re-entering the dating pool as a new divorcée or widow, a person might not use condoms because she has been accustomed to having unprotected sex for many years (McCord 2014).

One study examined sexual health behavior and mental health among Black women aged 50 to 80 years. Interestingly, more than 65% of the respondents reported that physicians told them that addressing sexual health practices was unnecessary given their age. Many women in this study did not feel comfortable discussing sexual health with their physicians and cited a lack of rapport as a major reason to avoid the conversation; indeed, many women also did not feel comfortable discussing sexual health with their partners or their friends. Women who engaged in high-risk sexual behaviors noted that feelings of depression, self-esteem issues, and loneliness influenced those behaviors (Thames et al. 2018).

A systematic review from 2015 also noted that psychosocial factors, such as depression, stress, and history of trauma, played a role in sexual decision-making in older Black women (Smith and Larson 2015). This review also found that women of a lower socioeconomic status, those who utilized drugs and/or alcohol, and those with less education were also at higher risk of contracting HIV (Smith and Larson 2015). Of note, a qualitative study of older Black women who were mostly well-educated and middle-class also made poor decisions related to sexual risk behaviors (McCord 2014). Despite being well-educated and having access to resources, women in this study still demonstrated a knowledge gap related to the prevalence of STIs (including HIV) and accurately assessing their personal risk of contracting an STI (McCord 2014).

Several recent qualitative studies have been conducted regarding older Black women and dating behaviors. One such study noted major themes that influenced these women's decisions to date, including valuing independence versus pursuing intimacy, unavailability of Black men in their age range, and perceptions of lack of approval of their family members (Salisu 2022). Qualitative work has attempted to examine how older single and widowed Black women (aged 60-75 years) reconciled their familial responsibilities and how they viewed their sexuality, especially considering the centralized roles that these women play in their families (Salisu and Dacus 2021). These nuanced conversations are necessary to better understand the sexual health decisions older Black women may face.

Black Sexual Minoritized Women

Black sexual minoritized women exist at the intersection of their race, gender identity, and sexuality. This combination of minoritized race, gender identity, and sexual minoritized status has been called "triple jeopardy" (Greene 1996). Black women who engage in sex with both women who have sex with women (WSW) and women who have sex with women and men (WSWM) have been found to have higher rates of STIs than Black women who exclusively have sex with WSW (Muzny et al. 2011). Another study found that WSWM appreciate their risks of STIs, particularly regarding their male partners, but not necessarily with their female partners. Some women in the study employed perceived risk-reducing behaviors with their female partners, such as proper hygiene (e.g., washing before and after sex, sanitizing sex toys) and sharing STI testing results (Muzny et al. 2013a). Other studies in this population document that Black WSW perceive few options for safer sex between women including the use of barriers (e.g., condoms on sex toys, use of dental dams; Muzny et al. 2013a; Muzny et al. 2013b).

CONCLUSION

Sexual and reproductive well-being are an integral part of the overall enhanced quality of life for all women. Black women have long been excluded from sexuality research that does not present their sexuality as "other." Future public health interventions will not be successful without a deeper and more nuanced understanding of the historical and sociocultural context in which Black women live their lives and navigate the world. Research indicates that positive rapport can make Black women more willing to pursue a discussion surrounding sexual health with their health care providers (Thames et al. 2018). Physicians, health care providers, public health practitioners, and researchers must be cognizant of Black women's experiences and the inequities they face. Seeing Black women as fully human and fully sexual beings throughout their lifespan is an integral part of achieving sexual well-being.

REFERENCES

Alexander KA, Arrington Sanders R, Grace KT, Thorpe RJ, Doro E, Bowleg L. "Having a child meant I had a real life": reproductive coercion and childbearing motivations among young Black men living in Baltimore. *J Interpers Violence.* 2021;36(17–18):NP9197–NP9225. https://doi.org/10.1177/0886260519853400

Anakaraonye AR, Mann ES, Annang Ingram L, Henderson AK. Black US college women's strategies of sexual self-protection. *Cult Health Sex.* 2019;21(2):160–174. https://doi.org/10.1080/13691058.2018.1459844

Anderson RM. Positive sexuality and its impact on overall well-being. *Bundesgesundheitsblatt Gesundheitsforschung Gesundheitsschutz.* 2013;56(2):208–214. https://doi.org/10.1007/s00103-012-1607-z

Aronowitz T, Agbeshie E. Nature of communication: voices of 11-14 year old African-American girls and their mothers in regard to talking about sex. *Issues Compr Pediatr Nurs.* 2012;35(2):75–89. https://doi.org/10.3109/01460862.2012.678260

Aronowitz T, Eche I. Parenting strategies African American mothers employ to decrease sexual risk behaviors in their early adolescent daughters. *Public Health Nurs.* 2013;30(4):279–287. https://doi.org/10.1111/phn.12027

Avery LR, Stanton AG, Ward LM, Cole ER, Trinh SL, Jerald MC. "Pretty hurts": acceptance of hegemonic feminine beauty ideals and reduced sexual well-being among Black women. *Body Image.* 2021;38:181–190. https://doi.org/10.1016/j.bodyim.2021.04.004

Avery LR, Stanton AG, Ward LM, Trinh SL, Cole ER, Jerald MC. The strong, silent (gender) type: the strong Black woman ideal, self-silencing, and sexual assertiveness in Black college women. *Arch Sex Behav.* 2022;51(3):1509–1520. https://doi.org/10.1007/s10508-021-02179-2

Awad GH, Norwood C, Taylor DS, et al. Beauty and body image concerns among African American college women. *J Black Psychol.* 2015;41(6):540–564. https://doi.org/10.1177/0095798414550864

Bailey ZD, Krieger N, Agénor M, Graves J, Linos N, Bassett MT. Structural racism and health inequities in the USA: evidence and interventions. *Lancet.* 2017;389(10077):1453–1463. https://doi.org/10.1016/S0140-6736(17)30569-X

Basile KC, Smith SG, Liu Y, Miller E, Kresnow MJ. Prevalence of intimate partner reproductive coercion in the United States: racial and ethnic differences. *J Interpers Violence.* 2021;36(21–22):NP12324–NP12341. https://doi.org/10.1177/0886260519888205

Bond KT, Leblanc NM, Williams P, Gabriel CA, Amutah-Onukagha NN. Race-based sexual stereotypes, gendered racism, and sexual decision making among young Black cisgender women. *Health Educ Behav.* 2021;48(3):295–305. https://doi.org/10.1177/10901981211010086

Carey MP, Senn TE, Seward DX, Vanable PA. Urban African-American men speak out on sexual partner concurrency: findings from a qualitative study. *AIDS Behav.* 2010;14(1):38–47. https://doi.org/10.1007/s10461-008-9406-0

Centers for Disease Control and Prevention. HIV and Black/African American people in the US. 2022. Available at: https://www.cdc.gov/nchhstp/newsroom/fact-sheets/hiv/black-african-american-factsheet.html

Collins PH. *Black Sexual Politics: African Americans, Gender, and the New Racism.* New York, NY: Routledge; 2004.

Crooks N, King B, Tluczek A. Protecting young Black female sexuality. *Cult Health Sex.* 2020;22(8):871–886. https://doi.org/10.1080/13691058.2019.1632488

Crooks N, King B, Tluczek A, Sales JM. The process of becoming a sexual Black woman: a grounded theory study. *Perspect Sex Reprod Health.* 2019;51(1):17–25. https://doi.org/10.1363/psrh.12085

Dauria EF, Oakley L, Arriola KJ, Elifson K, Wingood G, Cooper HL. Collateral consequences: implications of male incarceration rates, imbalanced sex ratios and partner availability for heterosexual Black women. *Cult Health Sex.* 2015;17(10):1190–1206. https://doi.org/10.1080/13691058.2015.1045035

Eaton AA, Matamala A. The relationship between heteronormative beliefs and verbal sexual coercion in college students. *Arch Sex Behav.* 2014;43(7):1443–1457. https://doi.org/10.1007/s10508-014-0284-4

Fasula AM, Carry M, Miller KS. A multidimensional framework for the meanings of the sexual double standard and its application for the sexual health of young Black women in the US. *J Sex Res.* 2014;51(2):170–183. https://doi.org/10.1080/00224499.2012.716874

Ferguson YO, Quinn SC, Eng E, Sandelowski M. The gender ratio imbalance and its relationship to risk of HIV/AIDS among African American women at Historically Black Colleges and Universities. *AIDS Care.* 2006;18(4):323–331. https://doi.org/10.1080/09540120500162122

Finer LB, Zolna MR. Declines in unintended pregnancy in the United States, 2008–2011. *N Engl J Med.* 2016;374(9):843–852. https://doi.org/10.1056/NEJMsa1506575

French B. More than Jezebels and freaks: exploring how Black girls navigate sexual coercion and sexual scripts. *J Afr Am Stud.* 2013;17(1):35–50. https://doi.org/10.1007/s12111-012-9218-1

Grace KT, Anderson JC. Reproductive coercion: a systematic review. *Trauma Violence Abuse.* 2018;19(4):371–390. https://doi.org/10.1177/1524838016663935

Greene B. Lesbian women of color: triple jeopardy. *J Lesbian Stud.* 1996;1(1):109–147. https://doi.org/10.1300/J155v01n01_09

Grigsby SR. Giving our daughters what we never received: African American mothers discussing sexual health with their preadolescent daughters. *J Sch Nurs.* 2018;34(2):128-138. https://doi.org/10.1177/1059840517707241

Hall NM, Lee AK, Witherspoon DD. Factors influencing dating experiences among African American emerging adults. *Emerg Adulthood.* 2014;2(3):184-194. https://doi.org/10.1177/2167696813520154

Hargons CN, Dogan J, Malone N, Thorpe S, Mosley DV, Stevens-Watkins D. Balancing the sexology scales: a content analysis of Black women's sexuality research. *Cult Health Sex.* 2021;23(9):1287-1301. https://doi.org/10.1080/13691058.2020.1776399

Holliday CN, McCauley HL, Silverman JG, et al. Racial/ethnic differences in women's experiences of reproductive coercion, intimate partner violence, and unintended pregnancy. *J Womens Health (Larchmt).* 2017;26(8):828-835. https://doi.org/10.1089/jwh.2016.5996

Jenkins Hall W, Tanner AE. US Black college women's sexual health in hookup culture: intersections of race and gender. *Cult Health Sex.* 2016;18(11):1265-1278. https://doi.org/10.1080/13691058.2016.1183046

Jones CP. Levels of racism: a theoretic framework and a gardener's tale. *Am J Public Health.* 2000;90(8):1212-1215. https://doi.org/10.2105/ajph.90.8.1212

Laganá L, Balian OA, Nakhla MZ, Zizumbo J, Greenberg S. A preliminary model of health regarding sexual and ethnic minority older adults. *Cult Health Sex.* 2021;23(3):333-348. https://doi.org/10.1080/13691058.2019.1710566

Leath S, Jones M, Jerald MC, Perkins TR. An investigation of Jezebel stereotype awareness, gendered racial identity and sexual beliefs and behaviours among Black adult women. *Cult Health Sex.* 2022;24(4):517-532. https://doi.org/10.1080/13691058.2020.1863471

Lentz AM, Zaikman Y. The big "O": sociocultural influences on orgasm frequency and sexual satisfaction in women. *Sex Cult.* 2021;25:1096-1123. https://doi.org/10.1007/s12119-020-09811-8.

McCord LR. Attention HIV: older African American women define sexual risk. *Cult Health Sex.* 2014;16(1):90-100. https://doi.org/10.1080/13691058.2013.821714

McCree DH, Wingood GM, DiClemente R, Davies S, Harrington KF. Religiosity and risky sexual behavior in African-American adolescent females. *J Adolesc Health.* 2003;33(1):2-8. https://doi.org/10.1016/s1054-139x(02)00460-3

McGruder K. Black sexuality in the US: presentations as non-normative. *J Afr Am Stud.* 2009;13(3):251-262. http://www.jstor.org/stable/41819211

Miller L, Gur M. Religiousness and sexual responsibility in adolescent girls. *J Adolesc Health.* 2002;31(5):401-406. https://doi.org/10.1016/s1054-139x(02)00403-2

Murray Horwitz ME, Pace LE, Ross-Degnan D. Trends and disparities in sexual and reproductive health behaviors and service use among young adult women (aged 18-25 years) in the United States, 2002-2015. *Am J Public Health.* 2018;108(suppl 4):S336-S343. https://doi.org/10.2105/AJPH.2018.304556

Muzny CA, Harbison HS, Pembleton ES, Austin EL. Sexual behaviors, perception of sexually transmitted infection risk, and practice of safe sex among southern African American women who have sex with women. *Sex Transm Dis.* 2013a;40(5):395-400. https://doi.org/10.1097/OLQ.0b013e31828caf34

Muzny CA, Harbison HS, Pembleton ES, Hook EW, Austin EL. Misperceptions regarding protective barrier method use for safer sex among African-American women who have sex with women. *Sex Health.* 2013b;10(2):138-141. https://doi.org/10.1071/SH12106

Muzny CA, Sunesara IR, Martin DH, Mena LA. Sexually transmitted infections and risk behaviors among African American women who have sex with women: does sex with men make a difference? *Sex Transm Dis.* 2011;38(12):1118-1125. https://doi.org/10.1097/OLQ.0b013e31822e6179

Nikolajski C, Miller E, McCauley HL, et al. Race and reproductive coercion: a qualitative assessment. *Womens Health Issues.* 2015;25(3):216-223. https://doi.org/10.1016/j.whi.2014.12.004

Pahl K, Lee JY, Capasso A, Lekas HM, Brook JS, Winters J. Sexual risk behaviors among Black and Puerto Rican women in their late thirties: a brief report. *J Immigr Minor Health.* 2019;21(6):1432-1435. https://doi.org/10.1007/s10903-019-00877-7

Rew L, Wong YJ. A systematic review of associations among religiosity/spirituality and adolescent health attitudes and behaviors. *J Adolesc Health.* 2006;38(4):433-442. https://doi.org/10.1016/j.jadohealth.2005.02.004

Salisu MA. Dating behaviors of older Black women. *J Gerontol Soc Work.* 2022;65(3):337-357. https://doi.org/10.1080/01634372.2021.1967547

Salisu MA, Dacus JD. Living in a paradox: how older single and widowed Black women understand their sexuality. *J Gerontol Soc Work.* 2021;64(3):303-333. https://doi.org/10.1080/01634372.2020.1870603

Smith TK, Larson EL. HIV sexual risk behavior in older Black women: a systematic review. *Womens Health Issues.* 2015;25(1):63-72. https://doi.org/10.1016/j.whi.2014.09.002

Stephens DP, Phillips LD. Freaks, gold diggers, divas, and dykes: the sociohistorical development of adolescent African American women's sexual script. *Sex Cult.* 2003;7(1):3-49. https://doi.org/10.1007/BF03159848

Thames AD, Hammond A, Nunez RA, et al. Sexual health behavior and mental health among older African American women: the Sistahs, Sexuality, and Mental Health Well-Being Project. *J Womens Health (Larchmt).* 2018;27(9):1177-1185. https://doi.org/10.1089/jwh.2017.6777

Thomas TL, Freeman A. Project genesis: self-reported religiosity and spirituality and sexual risk-taking in young African-American women attending a historically African-American college. *J Natl Black Nurses Assoc.* 2011;22(1):27-35.

Wilson PA, Valera P, Ventuneac A, Balan I, Rowe M, Carballo-Dieguez A. Race-based sexual stereotyping and sexual partnering among men who use the internet to identify other men for bareback sex. *J Sex Res.* 2009;46(5):399-413. https://doi.org/10.1080/00224490902846479

Whyte IV J. Sexual assertiveness in low-income African American women: unwanted sex, survival, and HIV risk. *J Community Health Nurs.* 2006;23(4):235-244. https://doi.org/10.1207/s15327655jchn2304_4

Wolfe WA. Overlooked role of African-American males' hypermasculinity in the epidemic of unintended pregnancies and HIV/AIDS cases with young African-American women. *J Natl Med Assoc.* 2003;95(9):846-852.

21

Creating Hope and Ending Stigma: A Holistic Approach to HIV/AIDS

Ashleigh LoVette, PhD, MA, Brenice Duroseau, MSN, Angela Wangari Walter, PhD, MPH, MSW, and Kamila A. Alexander, PhD, MPH, RN

Using socio-structural perspectives from multiple disciplines, this chapter outlines multilevel protective and risk factors contributing to optimal HIV prevention, treatment, and care among Black women. We emphasize how holistic approaches to primary and secondary HIV prevention incorporating concepts of pleasure, safety, and reproductive justice are critical for effective and culturally relevant sexual health promotion efforts among Black women in the United States (Wyatt 2009). We also highlight the importance of implementing tailored HIV prevention and care services and discuss how the process of aging shapes health care access and usage among Black women living with HIV (BWLH). To close the chapter, we apply a strengths-based lens to explore future directions that emphasize the utility of using research and practices that create hope through actions of resilience and healing.

BLACK WOMEN AND HIV

In 2020, Black people represented 13% of the US population, but 40% of the people living with HIV, with Black women being the largest percentage (57%) of all women living with HIV in the United States (Centers for Disease Control and Prevention [CDC] 2022a). Black women in the United States also experienced the highest rate of new HIV diagnoses when compared to women of other races (CDC 2022b). While the rates of new HIV diagnoses among Black women in the United States have declined in recent years, racial and gendered disparities in HIV persist, with a reported HIV prevalence of 62% among Black transgender women (Adimora et al. 2021; CDC 2022b).

Efforts to address this disproportionate burden of HIV among Black women include initiatives such as Black Women First (https://targethiv.org/BlackWomen), which supports the development, implementation, and evaluation of bundled interventions addressing the needs of this community while also leveraging partnerships between the US government, scientists, and community organizations. To prevent HIV and promote sexual health among Black women in the United States, we must continue to support culturally relevant efforts that consider how the lived experiences of Black women, as well as the contexts in which these experiences occur, contribute to observed disparities in sexual health.

CDC cites several barriers that Black women might encounter while trying to prevent acquisition of HIV, including racism and other social issues, as well as longstanding systemic inequities, such as economic and relationship power differentials (2022b). In addition, lack of knowledge about HIV status and biomedical HIV prevention tools, lack of awareness of sex partners' risk factors, intimate partner violence (IPV), and biological vulnerabilities due to receptive sexual activity can affect Black women's sexual health (CDC 2022b). However, exclusive use of risk paradigms focused on individual sexual behaviors may reflect stereotypes that frequently underpin scientific and programmatic assumptions (Crooks, King, and Tluczek 2020). Links to individual, or partner-based, desires and social identities often go unexplored, and the decentralization of US public health and health care systems reiterates that fears should be centered on prevention of one potential sexual health problem at a time.

This decentralization, along with historical and structural disadvantage, leads to varied experiences around HIV prevention and care for Black women throughout the United States. Black women living in poverty, along with those living in the southern United States, have some of the highest HIV incidence rates (Adimora et al. 2021). The structural and social drivers of HIV incidence also contribute to disparities in access to HIV care for those living with HIV, reflecting inequitable distributions of medical and public health resources. The experiences of racial, HIV-related, and gendered discrimination faced by BWLH is associated with higher barriers to care (Dale et al. 2019). Research also shows medical mistrust is correlated with lower engagement in health care among Black women who have sex with women, and, while studies focused on Black transgender women living with HIV are limited, one study identified gender stigma as well as peer and institutional distrust as barriers to HIV care (Brenick et al. 2017; Wilson, Arayasirikul, and Johnson 2013).

When we refer to Black women throughout this chapter, we are referring to both Black cisgender and transgender women unless specified otherwise. Transgender women experience similar and distinct disparities in HIV risk when compared to cisgender women, due to discrimination and exclusion based on gender identity and its intersections (Poteat, Reisner, and Radix 2014). The inclusion of Black transgender women in HIV prevention and care efforts is critical not only to promote health equity but also to better understand how experiences of Black women across gender identities influence sexual health and well-being. We also note that despite exclusion and structural disadvantage, Black women holding multiple identities have worked to improve HIV prevention and treatment efforts through the development and implementation of research and policy as well as advocacy efforts. Thus, social determinants of health impacted by systems of disadvantage are also influenced by resilience and healing practices of Black women working to create hope and reduce stigma across the United States and globally.

HIV/AIDS AND STIGMA

Despite advances in HIV prevention and treatment, HIV-related stigma persists. Stigma refers to "an attribute that is deeply discrediting" and often aligned with membership in marginalized social groups, including those living with HIV (Goffman 1963, p. 3). HIV-related stigma across multiple sociocultural levels can negatively impact health-seeking behaviors and outcomes (Earnshaw and Chaudoir 2009). HIV-related stigma can also result in suboptimal access to and quality of care (Reif, Wilson, and McAllaster 2018; Turan et al. 2017). In addition, internalized manifestations of stigma (i.e., the acceptance and adoption of negative societal beliefs and attitudes about one's HIV diagnosis) can lead to poor mental and emotional wellness and less perceived social support and mental health severity (Whetten et al. 2008).

HIV-related stigma is layered and multidimensional, and understanding these aspects is critical for addressing stigma among BWLH in a way that centers equity. Black women living with HIV experience stigma at individual, interpersonal, and systemic levels, and face higher risks for lower engagement in HIV care due to intersecting stigmas related to their gender, race, and socioeconomic status (Geter, Sutton, and Hubbard McCree 2018). Throughout this chapter, we will apply this sociocultural and multidimensional lens to the concept of stigma and highlight the need for holistic approaches for HIV prevention, as well as care, for Black women living in the context of HIV/AIDS.

HOLISTIC APPROACHES TO ADDRESS HIV/AIDS AMONG BLACK WOMEN

Strengths-Based Approaches

Strengths-based approaches, as opposed to deficit-based approaches, are a more holistic way to address HIV/AIDS among Black women and create space for an asset-based counternarrative of Black women who are frequently stigmatized and problematized in HIV prevention and sexual health promotion efforts. A deficit-based approach focuses on unhealthy behaviors and what Black women are doing wrong, while a strengths-based approach focuses on what Black women are doing well, despite individual, community, and structural barriers.

Recent work has emphasized the importance of using holistic and strengths-based approaches in HIV programming and policies for Black women living with and without HIV. In addition, organizations promoting the sexual health of Black women have incorporated strengths-based concepts, like resilience and healing, in their work. We will highlight research, programs, and organizations using these approaches to address health disparities and promote sexual health among Black women. To address stigma and effectively prevent and treat HIV/AIDS among Black women, we must move beyond individual and deficit-focused approaches and take cues from Black women throughout the United States who have been creating hope by tackling stigma in the community.

Life Course Approach

Applying a life course perspective to HIV/AIDS among Black women complements strengths-based approaches through its emphasis on understanding how time and context shape health. A life course approach considers how cumulative experiences throughout an individual's life, and across generations, influences health outcomes (Kuh et al. 2003). According to the life course perspective, early life experiences, such as childhood trauma and social support, can shape the health of an individual as they age. For example, research using a life course perspective has highlighted unique considerations for addressing HIV risk among Black women across various stages of development and aging, including adolescence, emerging adulthood, and older adulthood (Smith and Larson 2015; Taggart et al. 2020). We discuss how both younger and older Black women face unique barriers and leverage distinct resources based on not only developmental stage but also how they experience aging as Black women in the context of the United States.

INTEGRATED CONCEPTS AND FRAMEWORKS FOR HIV PREVENTION AND CARE
Integrated Concepts for Primary and Secondary Prevention

Despite what we know about the health disparities faced by Black women, HIV prevention messaging continues to focus on changing individual-level behavior and often disregards system-level changes that support healthy sexual practices and outcomes. Studies have long debunked the notion that Black women are "more promiscuous" than other races of women as an explanation for the disproportionate impact of HIV/AIDS and other sexually transmitted infections (STIs). Therefore, primary and secondary prevention efforts should focus on safety, reproductive justice, and pleasure to create systems change while also making comprehensive HIV prevention a shared value.

Safety

HIV/AIDS and associated epidemics, such as substance use and violence, shift sexual health prevention paradigms to ones associated with risk, danger, and pathology (Sharps, Njie-Carr, and Alexander 2021; Nydegger and Claborn 2020). As definitions of safety are created through personal and sociocultural experiences, Black women bear disproportionate consequences from behaviors connected to historical and contemporary structural injustices and interpersonal power imbalances (Davis, Montaque, and

Jackson 2022). Thus, sexual health messaging used in primary and secondary prevention initiatives often shapes communication about sex as well as sexual decision-making (Chmielewski, Bowman, and Tolman 2020) and should reflect contextual realities of Black women's lives. Furthermore, exclusive risk paradigms might not attend to the personalized processes of resilience each woman brings to their sexual experiences (Catabay et al. 2019).

IPV and other forms of gender-based violence are well-documented predictors of negative sexual and reproductive health outcomes, including HIV transmission, heightening safety risks among Black women compared to women of other racial and ethnic groups (Holliday et al. 2017). Experiences of IPV impact the ability of Black women of all ages to engage in various aspects of HIV prevention and care. Black women experiencing several types of IPV (i.e., psychological, physical, and sexual) are less likely to access HIV health care (Lilly and Graham-Bermann 2009; Stockman, Hayashi, and Campbell 2015) and might also be experiencing unprotected sex, simultaneously raising risks for HIV transmission and unintended pregnancy.

To date, HIV prevention efforts for Black women have focused primarily on evidence-based behavioral interventions that rely on successful use of the male condom. Pre-exposure prophylaxis (PrEP), a women-controlled option for HIV prevention, is underutilized among Black women (Ojikutu et al. 2018). Researchers have found that multilevel factors influence acceptability and uptake of women-controlled methods, and emerging research highlights factors affecting awareness and potential adoption of PrEP among Black women (Pyra et al. 2022). However, like many interventions, there remain challenges to navigate mistrust of health care providers (Sharpless et al. 2022) and medically inaccurate myths about the efficacy of the drug (Ojikutu et al. 2020), as well as potential interference from partners (O'Malley et al. 2020) that must be considered in broader HIV prevention efforts.

Interventions that focus solely on individual-level HIV/STI prevention may not address the full scope of Black women's lived experiences. There are calls to build on community and institutional-level ties to strengthen the sustainability of comprehensive interventions that are tailored for Black women (Ware, Thorpe, and Tanner 2019). Therefore, safety as a concept has broader implications for Black women's health. Integrated approaches for intervention are moving beyond "safe sex" to promoting safe environments more deeply connected to Black women's lives, thereby reducing HIV-related stigma and addressing entrenched sexual health inequities.

Reproductive Justice

A singular approach to preventing HIV among Black women ignores broader implications for their sexual health. This approach also ignores desires around pregnancy, parenting, and autonomy that are reflected in the concept of reproductive justice. A human rights-focused concept, reproductive justice is deeply connected to notions of safety and pleasure. An integrated approach to HIV/AIDS highlights the connections between these three concepts and offers a holistic lens to promote HIV prevention and treatment among Black women that moves beyond disciplinary boundaries. Reproductive justice is rooted in the right to maintain bodily autonomy, the right to have or not have children, the right to parent children in a safe and sustainable community, and the right to access quality health care (Ross and Solinger 2017). Importantly, collectives like SisterSong and reproductive justice organizers have long advocated for access to reproductive health care in addition to advocating for issues linked to prevention of HIV, such as violence, sex education, and STI prevention and care, that continue to disproportionately impact Black women.

Research has also highlighted how a reproductive justice framework, with its focus on systems and power, can draw attention to the structural factors driving sexual health disparities and increased HIV risk among Black women (Jolly 2021; Thompson et al. 2022). A reproductive justice lens can also attend to issues such as reproductive coercion. Reproductive coercion, a form of abuse, is defined as a group of controlling behaviors that compromise a woman's reproductive autonomy (Alexander et al. 2021). A reproductive justice framework has the potential to address issues such as reproductive coercion in a culturally relevant way that considers the sexual health needs and desires of Black women holistically. Thus, reproductive justice efforts are intertwined with HIV prevention and sexual health promotion among Black women, and achieving reproductive justice can result in a more equitable place for Black women affected by HIV/AIDS while also emphasizing autonomy, safety, and pleasure.

Pleasure

Another growing area of HIV and sexual health research has highlighted the need for a sex-positive approach to promoting sexual health among Black women (Townes et al. 2021). This shift in focus acknowledges that framing sexual activity as physiologically hazardous discounts the concept of pleasure, as well as aspects of emotionality like love, feelings, and empowerment. Promoting sex-positive approaches that support healthy views of sexual development and exploration as universal experiences can aid in overall well-being (Cruz, Greenwald, and Sandil 2017). Although the World Health Organization (2017) includes pleasure as a key component in its definition of sexual health, its inclusion in research and policy has been limited, especially within work focused on Black women's sexual health (Hargons et al. 2021).

Research among Black cisgender women living in the southern United States identified three key dimensions of sexual pleasure that incorporated mental, physical, and emotional aspects of sex while also offering a more nuanced understanding of pleasure (Thorpe et al. 2022). Ensuring pleasurable and safe sexual experiences for all who want them is important and relevant for both primary and secondary HIV prevention efforts. In fact, pleasure as a strategy in HIV and other STI interventions can motivate increased and more effective condom use as well as facilitate knowledge and attitudes about sexual safety (Ojikutu et al. 2018). A recent public health HIV prevention campaign, PrEP4Love, used a health equity and sex-positive approach to reach more than one million individuals, including Black women at risk for HIV, in Chicago, Illinois (Dehlin et al. 2019). Additional research has also identified ways to integrate pleasure and sex-positivity into trauma-informed approaches that acknowledge experiences across an individual's life course (Fava and Fortenberry 2021).

Programming and advocacy in this area also create opportunities for community-engaged approaches to HIV prevention and treatment. Community-engaged approaches are needed to identify the priorities and needs from the perspective of Black women, including those rooted in sex positivity and pleasure. To successfully elicit and incorporate community feedback throughout HIV prevention programming and policy initiatives, we need to recognize the nuanced social contexts in which Black women make sexual health decisions as well as Black women's desires, reproductive needs, and safety. These tailored efforts are also important to consider throughout the life course as sexual needs and desires, along with HIV care for those living with HIV, may change as women age.

Integrated Concepts for Comprehensive HIV Care

The Role of Aging in HIV Care

Medical advances with antiretroviral therapy (ART) have significantly increased the life expectancy of people living with HIV (PLWH; Ball 2014). However, older populations living with HIV have been referred to as a "silent generation" because of age-related comorbid conditions that impact their health and quality of life and the lack of tailored and equitable approaches for HIV treatment among this population as they move along the HIV care continuum (Inelman et al. 2014). The HIV care continuum is a stepwise approach to HIV testing, diagnosis, linkage to care, ART initiation, treatment adherence, retention in care, and viral load suppression and maintenance. Considering the stigma that comes with aging and intersecting HIV-related stigmas described earlier in the chapter, tailored efforts to reduce stigma and advance Black women's health along the HIV care continuum throughout their life course is critical.

Longevity and quality of life of PLWH is connected to how soon they are linked to care, start ART, and achieve viral load suppression. As PLWH age, social support and comorbidities alongside use of multiple medications become growing concerns in addition to concerns about expertise of HIV specialists, who may or may not have been trained to care for an aging population (Sangarlangkarn et al. 2021). In addition, provider bias may lead to discriminatory clinical practice approaches that exclude older populations from sexual history taking and HIV testing, which necessitates a need to enforce current guidelines and move away from terms such as "sexual risk" (Ports et al. 2014; Tillman and Mark 2015). This is particularly true for women living with HIV whose sexuality is frequently problematized both within and outside of medical settings (Carter et al. 2017). Organizations like Older Women Embracing Life (www.owelinc.org), a network of Black senior women providing support for women living with and affected by HIV/AIDS, are also working to address this bias while also instilling a sense of community and hope for BWLH.

U=U: A New Hope

The HIV care continuum focuses on advancing individuals along the path to viral load suppression and maintenance. Viral load suppression, described as having fewer than 200 copies of HIV per milliliter of blood, is essential for improved quality of life and prolonged life expectancy (CDC 2022c). Viral suppression is also included as an indicator in the Ending the HIV Epidemic in the US initiative. In 2016, the Prevention Access Campaign initiated a campaign to increase the awareness of the benefits of viral suppression using the message "Undetectable equals Untransmittable (U=U)." The campaign aimed to create hope and reduce stigma by emphasizing that PLWH who are on treatment and virally suppressed cannot transmit HIV to their partners. This powerful message has gained global consensus throughout 102 countries, is supported by science that includes several clinical trials (e.g., HPTN052), and is endorsed by key US public health organizations (Cohen et al. 2016). However, Black women remain significantly underrepresented in this scientific research, especially within ART clinical trials in high-income countries such as the United States (Pepperrell et al. 2020).

Public health guidelines explicitly state that all people living with HIV should be informed that achieving and maintaining viral load suppression prevents sexual transmission of HIV. U=U messaging, which promotes a strengths-based and sex-positive approach to HIV care, has the potential to help to address HIV-related stigma and reduce HIV-related anxiety, and it incentivizes continued treatment adherence and engagement in care (Calabrese and Mayer 2020). Research found that awareness of U=U messaging decreased levels of anticipated sex-related HIV stigma and dating-related HIV stigma among PLWH (Hampton and Gillum 2022).

Although U=U messaging has shown to have clear benefits for PLWH, social determinants of health continue to be a barrier to access and inclusivity, creating circumstances that can limit the potential power of U=U messaging among BWLH. Thus, despite its potential to address HIV-related stigma, there remain gaps in U=U knowledge and awareness, especially among women and transgender women of color (Rivera et al. 2021). To maximize the benefits of U=U, tailored messaging and programs considering the needs of BWLH across the life course are needed to improve access to HIV testing and care. By considering the comprehensive sexual needs and desires of BWLH and improving access to care, the quality of life of BWLH can be improved while also potentially reducing stigma for those living with HIV.

CREATING HOPE THROUGH RESILIENCE AND HEALING

We have discussed how HIV/AIDS-related research, programming, and policies have often used deficit-based approaches to prevention and treatment, potentially further stigmatizing Black women living with and without HIV while also ignoring their sexual health needs and desires. A unidimensional focus on risk and behaviors linked to increased risk, such as people who engage in sex work or transactional sex or people who use substances, also ignores Black women who are successfully navigating systems along with those who are working to change systems to consider the sexual health of Black women through a more holistic lens. A growing number of researchers and community members have shifted to using strengths-based approaches and concepts to HIV prevention and care, emphasizing assets, community, and hope.

Resilience

Resilience is one strengths-based concept that has received more recent attention in the HIV/AIDS field, particularly as it relates to BWLH in the United States (Brown et al. 2021; Fletcher et al. 2020). Resilience can be defined as the multilevel processes that facilitate overcoming adversity. These processes can be psychological, but they also occur at the interpersonal and community level. As resilience processes occur at multiple levels, they can be influenced by context, as demonstrated in a study that explored African American adolescents' perceptions of resilience to HIV. In this study, adolescents conceptualized resilience to HIV as confidence, safe social activities, and innocence (Glenn and Wilson 2008).

Research has also explored how BWLH experience processes of resilience, via resources like social support, and how these processes help them overcome and cope with not only HIV-related stigma but also racism and trauma (Dale and Safren 2018; Dulin et al. 2021). A resilience-focused approach also offers opportunities to address HIV-related stigma faced by BWLH. Earnshaw et al. (2013) highlighted the potential of resilience to address HIV disparities by addressing stigma associated with race and ethnicity. While the role of resilience has been examined among BWLH in the United States, future research can help us to better understand how the concept can influence HIV prevention efforts among Black women across different contexts and developmental stages.

It is important to note that although resilience focuses more on strengths than other concepts, it can also benefit from a refocus on equity. An equity-based resilience approach focuses on changing the conditions that create disproportionate adversity for Black women to have and maintain safe, pleasurable sexual experiences and relationships. Furthermore, an equity-based approach moves beyond creating programs to build resilience among Black women to create systems and structures that do not require Black women to overcome adversity to live full, whole, healthy lives.

Healing

Like the concept of resilience, healing is a concept that has long been theorized and practiced by Black women. Healing is a process and incorporates important concepts such as repair, accountability, and justice. The concept of healing is rooted in Black feminist thought that has historically taken a more holistic and community-centered approach to the well-being of Black women. Black women community leaders working in the area of HIV/AIDS have connected their work and leadership practices with aspects of Black feminist thought, building upon historic movements of justice and healing (McLane-Davison 2016), and researchers have used Black feminist thought to guide the development of HIV interventions for low-income African American women (Gentry, Elifson, and Sterk 2005).

A holistic concept that considers the lived experiences of Black women in various life stages, healing can help to address root causes of disparities in HIV risk by focusing on recovering from trauma and breaking generational cycles of trauma and violence often cited as sexual risk factors. For example, organizations like Ballet After Dark (https://www.balletafterdark.com/about) use arts-based and somatic methods to create safe and healing spaces for Black women who have experienced sexual violence. Healing is also a concept that facilitates incorporation of culturally and developmentally relevant factors. One healing-focused intervention designed to reduce HIV risk among Black men and women is being developed and implemented with attention to cultural identity, relationships, and community (Jemal, Urmey, and Caliste 2021). Another HIV prevention program demonstrated significant changes among African American women in the United States by using an African-centered affirming and cultural approach (Nobles, Goddard, and Gilbert 2009). Black women living with and without HIV have unique needs and intersecting identities that are influenced by experiences that occur across all stages of life. Healing practices offer an opportunity to incorporate these important cultural and developmental approaches to not only end stigma related to HIV/AIDS but to also create hope for Black women.

CONCLUSION

Through individual actions, community building, organizing, and social movements, Black women have used the concepts of resilience and healing to create hope and address

HIV-related stigma. This work demonstrates what is possible when Black cis- and transgender women are given the resources and space to address the sexual health needs and desires of their communities. Black women have long understood the importance of using holistic and integrated approaches in HIV prevention and treatment, including those focused on strengths and those that consider how experiences throughout the life course affect sexual health and well-being. Research and community efforts have shown how addressing issues around safety, advocating for reproductive justice, and emphasizing pleasure can help prevent HIV through a less stigmatizing and more holistic lens. Recent work around treatment for those living with HIV has also highlighted the role of aging in HIV care and the promise of U=U in reducing HIV/AIDS-related stigma among Black women. As we look to the future, it will continue to be important to take the lead from Black women working to create hope and end stigma by using holistic and integrated approaches to HIV prevention and care.

REFERENCES

Adimora AA, Ramirez C, Poteat T, et al. HIV and women in the USA: what we know and where to go from here. *Lancet.* 2021;397(10279):1107–1115. https://doi.org/10.1016/S0140-6736(21)00396-2

Alexander KA, Willie TC, McDonald-Mosley R, Campbell JC, Miller E, Decker MR. Associations between reproductive coercion, partner violence, and mental health symptoms among young Black women in Baltimore, Maryland. *J Interpers Violence.* 2021;36(17–18):NP9839–NP9863. https://doi.org/10.1177/0886260519860900

Ball SC. Increased longevity in HIV: caring for older HIV-infected adults. *Care Manag J.* 2014;15(2):76–82. https://doi.org/10.1891/1521-0987.15.2.76

Brenick A, Romano K, Kegler C, Eaton LA. Understanding the influence of stigma and medical mistrust on engagement in routine healthcare among Black women who have sex with women. *LGBT Health.* 2017;4(1):4–10. https://doi.org/10.1089/lgbt.2016.0083

Brown MJ, Trask JS, Zhang J, Haider MR, Li X. Sociodemographic and psychosocial correlates of resilience among older adults living with HIV in the Deep South. *J Health Psychol.* 2021;26(11):2010–2019. https://doi.org/10.1177/1359105319897783

Calabrese SK, Mayer KH. Stigma impedes HIV prevention by stifling patient–provider communication about U = U. *J Int AIDS Soc.* 2020;23(7):e25559. https://doi.org/10.1002/jia2.25559

Carter A, Greene S, Money D, et al. The problematization of sexuality among women living with HIV and a new feminist approach for understanding and enhancing women's sexual lives. *Sex Roles.* 2017;77(11):779–800. https://doi.org/10.1007/s11199-017-0826-z

Catabay CJ, Stockman JK, Campbell JC, Tsuyuki K. Perceived stress and mental health: the mediating roles of social support and resilience among Black women exposed to sexual violence. *J Affect Disord.* 2019;259:143–149. https://doi.org/10.1016/j.jad.2019.08.037

Centers for Disease Control and Prevention. Diagnoses of HIV infection in the United States and dependent areas 2020: national profile. 2022a. Available at: https://www.cdc.gov/hiv/library/reports/hiv-surveillance/vol-33/content/national-profile.html

Centers for Disease Control and Prevention. HIV and Black/African American people in the US. 2022b. Available at: https://www.cdc.gov/nchhstp/newsroom/fact-sheets/hiv/black-african-american-factsheet.html

Centers for Disease Control and Prevention. HIV by age: viral suppression. 2022c. Available at: https://www.cdc.gov/hiv/group/age/viral-suppression.html

Chmielewski JF, Bowman CP, Tolman DL. Pathways to pleasure and protection: exploring embodiment, desire, and entitlement to pleasure as predictors of Black and white young women's sexual agency. *Psychol Women Q.* 2020;44(3):307–322. https://doi.org/10.1177/0361684320917395

Cohen MS, Chen YQ, McCauley M, et al. Antiretroviral therapy for the prevention of HIV-1 transmission. *N Engl J Med.* 2016;375(9):830–839. https://doi.org/10.1056/NEJMoa1600693

Crooks N, King B, Tluczek A. Protecting young Black female sexuality. *Cult Health Sex.* 2020;22(8):871–886. https://doi.org/10.1080/13691058.2019.1632488

Cruz C, Greenwald E, Sandil R. Let's talk about sex: integrating sex positivity in counseling psychology practice. *Couns Psychol.* 2017;45(4):547–569. https://doi.org/10.1177/0011000017714763

Dale SK, Dean T, Sharma R, Reid R, Saunders S, Safren SA. Microaggressions and discrimination relate to barriers to care among Black women living with HIV. *AIDS Patient Care STDS.* 2019;33(4):175–183. https://doi.org/10.1089/apc.2018.0258

Dale SK, Safren SA. Resilience takes a village: Black women utilize support from their community to foster resilience against multiple adversities. *AIDS Care.* 2018;30(suppl 5):S18–S26. https://doi.org/10.1080/09540121.2018.1503225

Davis SM, Green Montaque HD, Jackson CAB. Talking with my sistahs: examining discussions about HIV risk and prevention outcomes within Black women sistah circles. *Health Commun.* 2022:1–14. https://doi.org/10.1080/10410236.2022.2050006

Dehlin JM, Stillwagon R, Pickett J, Keene L, Schneider JA. #PrEP4Love: an evaluation of a sex-positive HIV prevention campaign. *JMIR Public Health Surveill.* 2019;5(2):e12822. https://doi.org/10.2196/12822

Dulin AJ, Earnshaw VA, Dale SK, et al. A concept mapping study to understand multilevel resilience resources among African American/Black adults living with HIV in the southern United States. *AIDS Behav.* 2021;25(3):773–786. https://doi.org/10.1007/s10461-020-03042-6

Earnshaw VA, Chaudoir SR. From conceptualizing to measuring HIV stigma: a review of HIV stigma mechanism measures. *AIDS Behav.* 2009;13(6):1160. https://doi.org/10.1007/s10461-009-9593-3

Earnshaw VA, Smith LR, Chaudoir SR, Amico KR, Copenhaver MM. HIV stigma mechanisms and well-being among PLWH: a test of the HIV stigma framework. *AIDS Behav.* 2013;17(5):1785–1795. https://doi.org/10.1007/s10461-013-0437-9

Fava NM, Fortenberry JD. Trauma-informed sex positive approaches to sexual pleasure. *Int J Sex Health.* 2021;33(4):537–549. https://doi.org/10.1080/19317611.2021.1961965

Fletcher FE, Sherwood NR, Rice WS, et al. Resilience and HIV treatment outcomes among women living with HIV in the United States: a mixed-methods analysis. *AIDS Patient Care STDS.* 2020;34(8):356–366. https://doi.org/10.1089/apc.2019.0309

Gentry QM, Elifson K, Sterk C. Aiming for more relevant HIV risk reduction: a Black feminist perspective for enhancing HIV intervention for low-income African American women. *AIDS Educ Prev.* 2005;17(3):238–252. https://doi.org/10.1521/aeap.17.4.238.66531

Geter A, Sutton MY, Hubbard McCree D. Social and structural determinants of HIV treatment and care among Black women living with HIV infection: a systematic review: 2005–2016. *AIDS Care*. 2018;30(4):409–416. https://doi.org/10.1080/09540121.2018.1426827

Glenn BL, Wilson KP. African American adolescent perceptions of vulnerability and resilience to HIV. *J Transcult Nurs*. 2008;19(3):259–265. https://doi.org/10.1177/1043659608317447

Goffman E. *Stigma: Notes on the Management of Spoiled Identity*. Englewood Cliffs, NJ: Prentice-Hall; 1963.

Hampton CJ, Gillum TL. "It changes everything": the impact of HIV-related stigma on sexual health and intimacy among African American women. *Cult Health Sex*. 2022;24(12):1619–1633. https://doi.org/10.1080/13691058.2021.1990411

Hargons CN, Dogan J, Malone N, Thorpe S, Mosley DV, Stevens-Watkins D. Balancing the sexology scales: a content analysis of Black women's sexuality research. *Cult Health Sex*. 2021;23(9):1287–1301. https://doi.org/10.1080/13691058.2020.1776399

Holliday CN, McCauley HL, Silverman JG, et al. Racial/ethnic differences in women's experiences of reproductive coercion, intimate partner violence, and unintended pregnancy. *J Womens Health*. 2017;26(8):828–835. https://doi.org/10.1089/jwh.2016.5996

Inelmen EM, Sergi G, De Rui M, Manzato E. Enhancing awareness to mitigate the risk of HIV/AIDS in older adults. *Aging Clin Exp Res*. 2014;26(6):665–669. https://doi.org/10.1007/s40520-014-0222-2

Jemal A, Urmey LS, Caliste S. From sculpting an intervention to healing in action. *Soc Work Groups*. 2021;44(3):226–243. https://doi.org/10.1080/01609513.2020.1757923

Jolly J. A reproductive justice response to HIV/AIDS and COVID-19. *Lancet*. 2021;398(10315):1958–1959. https://doi.org/10.1016/S0140-6736(21)02541-1

Kuh D, Ben-Shlomo Y, Lynch J, Hallqvist J, Power C. Life course epidemiology. *J Epidemiol Commun Health*. 2003;57(10):778–783. https://doi.org/10.1136/jech.57.10.778

Lilly MM, Graham-Bermann SA. Ethnicity and risk for symptoms of posttraumatic stress following intimate partner violence: prevalence and predictors in European American and African American women. *J Interpers Violence*. 2009;24(1):3–19. https://doi.org/10.1177/0886260508314335

McLane-Davison D. Lifting: Black feminist leadership in the fight against HIV/AIDS. *Affilia*. 2016;31(1):55–69. https://doi.org/10.1177/0886109915583545

Nobles WW, Goddard LL, Gilbert DJ. Culturecology, women, and African-centered HIV prevention. *J Black Psychol*. 2009;35(2):228–246. https://doi.org/10.1177/0095798409333584

Nydegger LA, Claborn KR. Exploring patterns of substance use among highly vulnerable Black women at-risk for HIV through a syndemics framework: a qualitative study. *PLoS One*. 2020;15(7):e0236247. https://doi.org/10.1371/journal.pone.0236247

Ojikutu BO, Amutah-Onukagha N, Mahoney TF, et al. HIV-related mistrust (or HIV conspiracy theories) and willingness to use PrEP among Black women in the United States. *AIDS Behav*. 2020;24(10):2927–2934. https://doi.org/10.1007/s10461-020-02843-z

Ojikutu BO, Bogart LM, Higgins-Biddle M, et al. Facilitators and barriers to pre-exposure prophylaxis (PrEP) use among Black individuals in the United States: results from the National Survey on HIV in the Black Community (NSHBC). *AIDS Behav*. 2018;22(11):3576–3587. https://doi.org/10.1007/s10461-018-2067-8

O'Malley TL, Hawk ME, Egan JE, Krier SE, Burke JG. Intimate partner violence and pre-exposure prophylaxis (PrEP): a rapid review of current evidence for women's HIV prevention. *AIDS Behav.* 2020;24(5):1342-1357. https://doi.org/10.1007/s10461-019-02743-x

Pepperrell T, Hill A, Moorhouse M, et al. Phase 3 trials of new antiretrovirals are not representative of the global HIV epidemic. *J Virus Erad.* 2020;6(2):70-73. https://doi.org/10.1016/S2055-6640(20)30019-4

Ports KA, Barnack-Tavlaris JL, Syme ML, Perera RA, Lafata JE. Sexual health discussions with older adult patients during periodic health exams. *J Sex Med.* 2014;11(4):901-908. https://doi.org/10.1111/jsm.12448

Poteat T, Reisner SL, Radix A. HIV epidemics among transgender women. *Curr Opin HIV AIDS.* 2014;9(2):168-173. https://doi.org/10.1097/COH.0000000000000030

Pyra M, Johnson AK, Devlin S, et al. HIV pre-exposure prophylaxis use and persistence among Black ciswomen: "women need to protect themselves, period." *J Racial Ethn Health Dispar.* 2022;9(3):820-829. https://doi.org/10.1007/s40615-021-01020-9

Reif S, Wilson E, McAllaster C. Perceptions and impact of HIV stigma among high risk populations in the US Deep South. *J HIV AIDS.* 2018;4(2). https://doi.org/10.16966/2380-5536.154

Rivera AV, Carrillo SA, Braunstein SL. Prevalence of U = U awareness and its association with anticipated HIV stigma among low-income heterosexually active Black and Latino adults in New York City, 2019. *AIDS Patient Care STDS.* 2021;35(9):370-376. https://doi.org/10.1089/apc.2021.0070

Ross LJ, Solinger R. *Reproductive Justice: An Introduction.* 1st ed. Oakland, CA: University of California Press; 2017. https://www.jstor.org/stable/10.1525/j.ctv1wxsth

Sangarlangkarn A, Yamada Y, Ko FC. HIV and aging: overcoming challenges in existing HIV guidelines to provide patient-centered care for older people with HIV. *Pathogens.* 2021;10(10):1332. https://doi.org/10.3390/pathogens10101332

Sharpless L, Kershaw T, Hatcher A, et al. IPV, PrEP, and medical mistrust. *J Acquir Immune Defic Syndr.* 2022;90(3):283-290. https://doi.org/10.1097/QAI.0000000000002956

Sharps PW, Njie-Carr VPS, Alexander K. The syndemic interaction of intimate partner violence, sexually transmitted infections, and HIV infection among African American women: best practices and strategies. *J Aggress Maltreat Trauma.* 2021;30(6), 811-827. https://doi.org/10.1080/10926771.2019.1667464

Smith TK, Larson EL. HIV sexual risk behavior in older Black women: a systematic review. *Womens Health Issues* 2015;25(1):63-72. https://doi.org/10.1016/j.whi.2014.09.002

Stockman JK, Hayashi II, Campbell JC. Intimate partner violence and its health impact on ethnic minority women. *J Womens Health.* 2015;24(1):62-79. https://doi.org/10.1089/jwh.2014.4879

Taggart T, Milburn NG, Nyhan K, Ritchwood TD. Utilizing a life course approach to examine HIV risk for Black adolescent girls and young adult women in the United States: a systematic review of recent literature. *Ethn Dis.* 2020;30(2):277-286. https://doi.org/10.18865/ed.30.2.277

Thompson TM, Young Y-Y, Bass TM, et al. Racism runs through it: examining the sexual and reproductive health experience of Black Women in the South. *Health Aff (Millwood).* 2022;41(2):195-202. https://doi.org/10.1377/hlthaff.2021.01422

Thorpe S, Malone N, Hargons CN, Dogan JN, Jester JK. The peak of pleasure: US southern Black women's definitions of and feelings toward sexual pleasure. *Sex Cult.* 2022;26(3):1115–1131. https://doi.org/10.1007/s12119-021-09934-6

Tillman JL, Mark HD. HIV and STI testing in older adults: an integrative review. *J Clin Nurs.* 2015;24(15–16):2074–2095. https://doi.org/10.1111/jocn.12797

Townes A, Thorpe S, Parmer T, Wright B, Herbenick D. Partnered sexual behaviors, pleasure, and orgasms at last sexual encounter: findings from a US probability sample of Black women ages 18 to 92 years. *J Sex Marital Ther.* 2021;47(4):353–367. https://doi.org/10.1080/0092623X.2021.1878315

Turan B, Hatcher AM, Weiser SD, Johnson MO, Rice WS, Turan JM. Framing mechanisms linking HIV-related stigma, adherence to treatment, and health outcomes. *Am J Public Health.* 2017;107(6):863–869. https://doi.org/10.2105/AJPH.2017.303744

Ware S, Thorpe S, Tanner AE. Sexual health interventions for Black women in the United States: a systematic review of literature. *Int J Sex Health.* 2019;31(2):196–215. https://doi.org/10.1080/19317611.2019.1613278

Whetten K, Reif S, Whetten R, Murphy-McMillan LK. Trauma, mental health, distrust, and stigma among HIV-positive persons: implications for effective care. *Psychosom Med.* 2008;70(5):531–538. https://doi.org/10.1097/PSY.0b013e31817749dc

Wilson EC, Arayasirikul S, Johnson K. Access to HIV care and support services for African American transwomen living with HIV. *Int J Transgend.* 2013;14(4):182–195. https://doi.org/10.1080/15532739.2014.890090

World Health Organization, UNDP/UNFPA/UNICEF/WHO/World Bank Special Programme of Research, Development and Research Training in Human Reproduction. Sexual health and its linkages to reproductive health: an operational approach. World Health Organization. 2017. Available at: https://apps.who.int/iris/handle/10665/258738

Wyatt GE. Enhancing cultural and contextual intervention strategies to reduce HIV/AIDS among African Americans. *Am J Public Health.* 2009;99(11):1941–1945. https://doi.org/10.2105/AJPH.2008.152181

22

Don't You Forget About Us: Sexuality and the Sexual and Reproductive Health of Black LGBTQ+ Women

Daphne Scott-Henderson, MS, RN

Sexual and reproductive health is but a portion of the health concerns for Black women who live at the intersection of gender, racial, and sexual marginalization in America. Studies have shown that lesbian, gay, and bisexual cisgender women visit gynecologists less than their heterosexual counterparts, and transgender women are even less likely to seek preventive health care and nonemergent medical care. A recent study on sexual and reproductive health of Black women in the American South revealed that Black women who also identify as a sexual minority (lesbian, same-gender-loving, queer, bisexual, and pansexual) are less likely to be tested for cervical cancer and HIV (Agénor et al. 2016). This is especially alarming because the virus that causes cervical cancer, the human papillomavirus (HPV), can be spread through skin-to-skin contact (Giles 2003). HPV vaccine awareness and uptake is significantly lower among Black women compared to white women (Ojeaga et al. 2019), and HIV infection affects more Black women than women in any other racial category in the United States (Agénor et al. 2016).

Black lesbian, gay, bisexual, transgender, and queer (LGBTQ+) women's fear of judgment and discrimination is as real and valid today as it was decades ago. Compounded with socioeconomic injustices in the United States that contribute to Black people being more likely to be underinsured or uninsured, this leaves scores of Black LGBTQ+ women unable to procure even the most basic health care needs without threat of financial ruin.

In addition, health literacy among Black LGBTQ+ women plays a significant role in health outcomes. As a Black cisgender woman who identifies as a lesbian, I have heard many erroneous health-related beliefs and misconceptions held by Black lesbian-identified women. I have met many Black lesbian-identified women who think that not having sex (not *regularly,* anyway) with cisgender men makes them exempt from the need for annual "well-woman" visits (pelvic examinations, Papanicolaou tests [pap smears], etc.). As a doctoral nursing student, these experiences and observed perspectives are my key reasons for making the sexual and reproductive health and health literacy of Black LGBTQ+ women my research priority.

Our transgender sisters, as gender minorities, also have unique perspectives and lived experiences. Research studies on the health care of Black transgender women reflect substandard or negative experiences, often directly related to disclosure and discrimination. A 2019 *Journal of General Internal Medicine* article details the experiences of various transgender persons of color navigating the health care system (Howard et al. 2019). The qualitative study presents participants' first-hand accounts of varying levels of discomfort seeking health care, fear of disclosing their transgender status to health care providers, and fear of facing discrimination based on their gender, racial, and ethnic identities (participants were African American and Latinx). Furthermore, according to a National Center for Transgender Equality and National Gay and Lesbian Task Force Survey, Black transgender women are at a disproportionate risk of being the victim of a violent crime and of experiencing extreme poverty, unemployment, and/or homelessness—all social determinants of poor health outcomes (Grant et al. 2011).

What is the driving force or forces behind these intraracial health care disparities? What are the main health concerns of LGBTQ+ Black women today? Just as Blackness is not a monolith, neither are Black women, nor Black women who identify as one or more of the categories covered by the ever-expanding LGBTQ+ acronym. This chapter seeks answers to these questions by going to the source to hear directly from Black LGBTQ+ women. One-on-one qualitative, semistructured interviews were conducted from May to December 2022 with a pansexual-identified Black woman and a transgender Black woman to provide additional context around their experiences and concerns regarding their general health, sexual health, and health care experiences. All interviews were conducted in confidentiality, and the names of the interviewees have been changed to protect their identities and health information, but their stories are authentic and compelling. By sharing their stories, they hope to shed light on these unique health care inequalities and help other Black women in the LGBTQ+ community reckon with the sometimes overwhelming barriers to living our best and healthiest lives. The author and interviewees hope that this chapter pushes us toward sexual and reproductive health equity and well-being for *all* Black women.

THE SOURCE (INTERVIEWS)

Interview #1: M.

M. is a bubbly 40-year-old woman from the South. She has long braids and impeccable makeup. She identifies as pansexual and states that a friend helped her reach this realization after noticing she had crushes on men, women, and transgender men and women .

> **M.:** For many years, I guess I identified as "I have no idea" [*chuckles*]. I was just, like, living life, and I always considered myself a strong ally to the LGBTQ+ community. Because I did not know what I—I just thought I was a free, loving person, and never put a title on what I

was. So, I just was like, "I love everybody," and, you know, I support everybody, and I fight for everybody.

Yeah, and not only am I from the South. I am from the South, *and* I am from a Christian pastor's home…

Interviewer: Oh, wow! Your daddy's a preacher?!

M.: My dad is the pastor of *two* churches. And I'm the only girl, and I grew up with Christian ideals of what is supposed to be.

Interviewer: So, what are your overall thoughts about your health and your personal health care? You've told me that you meditate. You do reiki. You take lots of vitamins and supplements. So, just, overall, like a blurb, of how you feel about your health and your personal health care.

M.: I would say, for my personal health, I would say the reason I feel good about it is because I am making steps to try to do better. I'm not saying that my health is great. I am saying that at 40, I am now saying out loud things that I probably wasn't comfortable with saying out loud or hearing from people. Like, I really gotta get my weight under control; let me get to a doctor to talk about what are my steps, you know. Like, a few months ago, I just went to my doctor, and I was like, look, what can I do? I've done this; I've done that; I've done this; I've done that. None of these things are working. Can you just wire my mouth shut, please? So I can stop eating. And then they were like, "Oh, my God!" And I was like, "Look, I ain't got time for this bullshit; I've done this. I've done keto. I've done weight calorie deficit. I've done all these things." I was just like—Argh!—help me, you know?

And, so, for that I am, like, patting myself on the back, that I'm like, really, like what can we do? Let's make an appointment. Let's talk about these things. And, so, I feel like I'm taking the right steps so that next year this time I won't be having the same complaints, so, you know? Like, literally, I'm like following up with the doctors. It's, like, I'm changing this. I'm pulling this out of my diet. I'm like, you know, cutting down on meat. I'm in my pescetarian stage right now.

I was just like, hey? Okay, what can I do to help myself until I can get a more permanent fix?

You know? And, so, especially because I know how doctors are. If I go in there, they're gonna be, like, what have you done for yourself? And, so, I could be, like, these are all the things that I've done. This does not work; this does not work…

So, how can you help me, mixed with the things that I've already done? What can you bring to this to help me? And, so, I would say that's why I feel good about where I'm at, even if physically, it's like, "Well you need to work on some things," and I'll be like, "I agree. That's what I'm working on."

Interviewer: Do you have any chronic or acute health conditions that you feel comfortable talking about?

M.: In 2006, I was diagnosed with congestive heart failure. I've had hypertension. I have macular degeneration, so I'm, like, going blind in one eye. Um, yeah, I think those are my, like, big hitters. And, so, I'm like, so good, because I wanna say when I was diagnosed with my congestive heart failure, they gave me like a year to live, so you know...[*chuckles and points index finger*].

I'm just consistent! I will say that, you know, medicine works. Especially for my heart condition. A particular medicine, that was like a trial pill that they put me on, like really reverted, like reversed things.

You know, I mentioned I had a hysterectomy, and everything that went along with me trying to get this hysterectomy was just very telling. I had been on my cycle for about nine months straight. I was iron deficient; you know, I was just...It was horrific. It was like the first two days of your cycle when it's just like cramps, and like just painful, and I was wearing all black, because that was the only thing—it was so many—you know...you understand what I'm saying.

It was very mentally draining and physically draining. And I had gone to the doctor so many times, like, begging them, like: "Please help me. Help me."

I was already, you know, mentally saying that I was okay with not having kids, you know. I was like 30 at the time. I had ended an engagement years prior because my fiancée at the time wanted to have kids, and I was like, I don't wanna have kids. That's not what I saw for my life.

And, so, I was 30 at this point, and I had never been pregnant, not even a pregnancy scare.

So, I was just like, I think I'm kind of adamant about kids not being for me. You know that's not something that people are always ready to hear. But I wish people would stay it out loud. You know, know your truth.

And I had a white male doctor, and he was just so dismissive of everything that was going on with me. I was going to the doctor so often. I'm like, "I'm on my period." I'm still on my period and, you know, it's month two, month three, four, you know. And I was like, "What is wrong?" Like, something must be wrong; like, check for something. Why? Why is this happening to me?

And, of course, my emotions are all over place, you know, 'cause I'm just, like, PMSing constantly. I'm, like, angry and crying, and, you know, just like a nerve of emotions. And I go on Monday, and he comes in and he's like, "Oh, hi, Miss D." Like, *you again?* And I'm like, "Tell me what's wrong. Pick something, do something." And he goes, "Why are you always in here crying?" And I was just like [*stares blankly*]. And then he says, "Never mind. My wife is like this as well."

And I was like, wow, I'm in pain and all they want to do is, like, do a biopsy. He's like, "We're just gonna do a biopsy." I was just like, "First thing first I'm already cramping, and when y'all do biopsy this crap, this is painful. You're gonna biopsy my freakin' vagina."

And he was just like, "Well I do see that you have endometriosis and fibroids." And I was like, "Okay, so if you fix that would that fix this?" And he's like, "Well, I'm not really sure."

And I'm like, tell me something. So, I just start, like, I'm like screaming, and I'm crying, like I'm profusely crying. And he's just like, "You know, you're such a pretty girl. If you would just stop crying so much, you know. Maybe wear some brighter colors—'cause you're always in here in black, and maybe you would feel a little better."

And I just lost it. I just started screaming and cussing. And the nurse practitioner for this particular office was a family friend. I had known her since I was a little girl. She used to be a member of my dad's church. And the doctor was like, "Okay, calm down. Calm down. We're gonna figure something out. I'm gonna write you something. I just need you to go and sit in this other room."

So, he removes me from the room and makes me sit in this other room. And, so, while I'm sitting there, I know that I have to go to the restroom because my body is like, *Girl, we gotta go*. And so, when I open the door, there's a security guard standing in front of my door. And he's like, "Oh, ma'am, could you please just go back in the room."

And I was like, "The fuck? Naw. I gotta go to the restroom." And he was like, "Ma'am…" [*raises hand in a "stop" gesture*]. "We need you to just wait."

And I'm like, "What the fuck?" You know? So, I'm, like, going off on him, and so he pulls the door, so you know, I have to stay in the room. So, I'm crying. I'm like having an accident, and I'm like, "I have to go now. I have to go to the bathroom."

They won't let me leave the room. because they won't, and I don't know what's going on. I have no clue what's happening. I'm just like in pain, and I'm sitting on the floor in the corner of this room, just crying and in pain, and confused, when the door opens, and the nurse practitioner that I know comes in, and she's like, "Get your purse. Let's go." And I'm like [*in a tearful tone*], "But, I gotta go to the bathroom."

She's like, "No, no, no, no. Get your purse. Let's go." And, so, I'm finally like, "Oh, okay," and so she walks me to my car, and she says, "I'm gonna call you and call your parents in a couple of days, and we're gonna figure out about getting you a new doctor."

And I said, "Well, what happened? What's going on?" And she said, "They were trying to put you on a mental psych hold."

And I was like, "*What*?" And she went, "Yes, they were trying to put you on a mental psych hold." Because I blew up in this office. And I was just like, "You have got to be kidding me."

Interview #2: G.

G. is Black transgender woman in her mid-30s who started transitioning in 2018 and is not looking back. She recently relocated from the Midwest to New York City for her job as deputy director in a nonprofit. In New York City, she feels she has more access to trans-specific health care options.

Interviewer: So, growing up, how was health and well-being viewed or addressed in your family, or in the environment where you grew up?

G.: Health and wellness in my family wasn't really addressed. If I'm being completely honest, wasn't really addressed at all. The first thing that comes to mind is, like, our eating habits and things like that, right? And, of course, there's multiple facets of health, but let's start there. So, we're eating a lot of unhealthy food, heavy foods. You know? I'm not seeing my family, my parents, really work out. So that wasn't something that was really introduced to me even—I would say—even recently in my life, I really haven't started to work out just from my upbringing. But, yeah, and even like to the mental aspect of health and wellness, in my family, like, that wasn't really addressed either.

I started once I transitioned and, mostly, I would say, within this last year and a half I started working out. So, I do cycle. I love cycling. I've always been tall and slender. I'm 5 feet 9 inches without heels. So, you know, people are like, yeah, you're pretty tall, you know, for the for the average woman. But I had a recent procedure to just kind of like give my body some curves and some shape. That was always very important to me as I transitioned; I wanted to make sure that I felt good about how I looked. And, so, I got Lipo 360, and they, basically, remove fat from certain areas to give you a nice womanly shape. I've done that. And, like, I think that what kicked that in high gear was seeing my body in a way that I loved it, and I felt comfortable, and I also felt safe. You know? And it made me say, *Okay, well, now I have to kick it up. I have to eat good. I have to work out in order to keep this body.* So, that was just the kickstart, and it's been an amazing, fun journey filled with a lot of learning, and trial and error, of course. And a lot of finding of self-love and self, too.

[G. mentions that she has an exercise cycle at home because she doesn't feel safe as a Black transgender woman walking alone in the city, or cycling in the city, or even walking to catch the subway. She states that no matter how "passable" she appears to the naked eye, there is still always a threat of being victimized simply for being who she is.]

My grandmother, when I started spending more time with her when my mother fell ill, started to really instill some of those values about, you know, mental health and its importance and things like that. But, yeah, I didn't grow up really leaning into that or being taught about it.

My mother has multiple sclerosis. I will be completely honest and transparent, like she and I are not close. So, that again falls into that health and wellness piece. You know, I came out, which was safe for me at the time, I just came out as queer or gay at the age of 13.

My mother was a single mother. Also, my father was incarcerated for most of my adolescent life. We do have a relationship now, though, if you're wondering. Me and my father do. But my mother took it really difficult when I came out and continuously pushed me away in various ways.

I see mainly, especially in the Black community, the mothers who have the hardest time with it, but I also see an influx of cis Black women, who identify as hetero, too, in the community. There's just a lot of like stigmas that they also perpetuate about the LGBTQ+ community.

Yes, there's violence from Black men, but I also feel that Black cis hetero women perpetuate the stereotypes and the stigma and kind of keep that cycle going.

Interviewer: Even as an RN, I don't know much about this, so could you speak to, are there specific health concerns you have related to transitioning and hormones? Are there any risks that you are concerned about?

G.: Yeah, I mean, so I will say there's nothing that *I'm* concerned about, but I can speak to some of those risks that we see as Black trans women. And I want to preface it with, I am not concerned due the sole fact that I also have a lot of privilege and that privilege lies in the fact that I had access to health care during my transition. And I also made sure that I had the right resources.

A lot of Black trans women, who live in poverty, don't have that access. So, they're taking hormones, administering estrogen shots themselves that they bought, like, on the black market. I've literally been in a club space out of town, traveling, and I literally heard someone saying, like, "Oh, you know, I've got estrogen for sale." Things like that.

But some of the risks are, like, once you decide to transition, be you trans feminine or trans masculine, you have to have your levels regulated—your hormone levels, your blood levels, you know. All of those things need to be regulated and checked. Especially for trans feminine people. We take testosterone blockers to block testosterone production in our bodies, and then we take, of course, estrogen to kind of kickstart or give us some of those more feminine features. And, really at baseline—I tell people all the time—what it really does for us…It doesn't change your bone structure, right? But it does distribute fat in various places on your body that helps you kind of achieve that feminine look that most are going for. So, you know, if those levels are unregulated—I'm sure you know, as an RN—that can be dangerous.

So, you wanna make sure that everything is on the up and up while you're going through HRT [hormone replacement therapy]. The second thing is hormone therapy is also very harmful to the liver. And, so, a lot of people have liver issues, you know, especially if you aren't taking care of yourself during your transition. I think that's another reason why I got into this health kick of eating healthy and working out and trying to be active.

I think, lastly, one of the things that comes to mind, too, is the lack of education around the things that we need while we transition. So, again, I'm speaking to Black trans women who don't have access to health care, don't have the resources. So, again, their levels are not being regulated. They have misinformation or don't have any information at all. So, like, one of the things they ask you—and this is going into like gender reassignment surgery—they ask you, "Before we do this surgery, or perform the surgery, do you want children?" But, also, you have to take into consideration how long you've been on testosterone blockers, or hormones, because your body will stop producing sperm. So, then you can't have children of your own. I've run into a lot of Black trans women who wanted children of their own and maybe wanted to take the opportunity to put sperm in a sperm bank and hold it but weren't given that information.

So then when it came time to say, "Hey, how am I gonna do this?" Then they're like, "Oh your body doesn't produce sperm anymore, because you've been on HRT for this amount of years"…and, yeah, then they're like, "I wish someone had told me this sooner."

Interviewer: So, you mentioned briefly about being concerned about riding the subway and things like that, being a Black trans woman. We definitely hear a lot about—I can't remember the exact statistics—but Black trans women are, it's some very high number, like 70%, more likely to be the victim of violence and violent crimes. Can you speak a little bit about that, whether it's from personal experience, or from friends' experiences, or things that you've heard?

G.: Yeah. In working with the marginalized community, and, again, one of the things where I'm always open and honest about is my privilege. I had the privilege of accessing HRT pretty quickly. So, I started my journey. I also have the privilege, of even pretransition, I was always a soft, androgynous figure, so my transition came a little bit more easy physically. So, I cannot say that I have personally been attacked, or you know, have experienced any violence. So, it's always important for me to tell why *I* have not. And those are the reasons: privilege and passability, and things like that.

But I have heard from the community in which I work for, and I'm dedicated to, and I have heard from friends and...You asked me, why do I think that is?

I believe that, again, it's a very layered answer, and I'll try to compartmentalize it to start from the beginning, to where we are with it. But statistics say that a lot of the violence against Black trans women comes from Black men, so from our own community and typically they are men—or historically and typically—they are men who have been involved with the trans woman, in some capacity, that they have harmed or murdered.

As we know, there's a lot of stigmas within the Black community. For one, to come out as gay, trans, queer, whatever. Due to what I believe is pressures of religion, and that's very, very...Religion is very prominent in the Black community, as I'm sure you know. I came from a very Catholic family that, you know, went to church—Well, it was also...it was Baptist and Catholic—but they were very strict on going to church. I was also baptized. But that's neither here nor there. But I think that translates into Black men being filled with shame and discomfort around their attractions. And that could be same-sex attractions, but in the spirit of what we are discussing, their attraction to Black trans women. And, I will scream it from the mountaintops: trans women are women. I think that, you know, that is just period point blank for me. That is something I will always fight for. But, yeah, there's a lot of shame and sigma placed on Black men for who they love, specifically Black trans women, and when it comes to...because a lot of them want to see us behind closed doors.

But when it comes to being outed, then they're filled with this fear, and rage. A fear that also then translates into rage, and it's a secret that you are rushing to...And I think...and I think...and I sat, and I thought about, and wrote about this myself. But I had to, like, really think about it at the height of violence against Black trans women. I think last year, I was just sitting there, thinking, and when I was writing, I was just like trying to really break it down and figure out the whys. You know? We can say, *Oh, because it is a Black trans woman, that person was murdered.*

But I always look at things, and I'm just like, there's so many layers. There's so much nuance around everything for me. To me, that's just the way my brain works. But, yeah, I think that due to that stigma and the way that Black men are brought up to be tough and strong, and the leaders of their families, and the community. Hypermasculine, and that easily turns into rage. That fear of being found out or being seen as *othered*. Yeah, that turns into rage, and so then that turns into harming a lover. Because, typically, again, like most of those situations, from the stories that I've read, these men have known those women that they've murdered. I think that's really the basis of it, is just the fear of getting found out, or your friends, or your homeboys finding out that you, you know, have feelings for this trans woman.

Interviewer: I know, sometimes, in the stories, they try to put a spin on it as, like, the Black cis man was fooled, right? He was tricked, and he got so mad about that and then he snapped. And I'm like, okay, this can't be the case all the time. Right? That this is the first time you were with this woman, you know what I mean?

G.: That always happens. They try to use language to twist and turn, and it then turns into… Oh, well, you know, I've seen the conversations on Twitter. And you know conversations, like, "Oh, she could've fooled me, too. So, I could see how he was fooled." And it's just like, no that wasn't like that; that's not the case of the story. Like, he knew very well who he was seeing, but something happened to where, you know…But yeah…

Interviewer: Do you think that people, like, you know, Laverne Cox and India Moore…Do you think of that more trans women of color being more visible has made any difference as far as how noncelebrity Black trans women are treated?

G.: I don't. I don't. Personally, I don't think so. I think it has given us hope that we can be in some of the same spaces as our sisters, like the India Moores and the Laverne Coxes, but it really doesn't do anything for us. We've still seen a rise in the numbers of violence against Black trans women, you know, despite the visibility of trans feminine actresses and also musicians.

I haven't seen any differences. I've seen maybe people becoming a little bit more inquisitive, a little bit more open, as far as media and TV is concerned. And, like, watching those people on it, on those shows. But I think, baseline, Black trans women need resources. You know, again, I work in the nonprofit sector, and that's what I hear and see all the time—they need funds, they need initial aid. So, visibility, while we thought at some point was the tipping point for us to be more accepted, it was really just kind of the tip of the iceberg.

I think the last thing I'll say about, you know, health as a Black trans woman that makes it difficult, is when you don't have any resources or money. You tend to lean on your community, right? But we're also such a disenfranchised community, and we lack so much that, there's just so much misinformation that's given, even from someone who you think of as, like, a trans elder…and it's really…I don't know, it's just really sad [*lowers her head*].

CONCLUSION

It sometimes feels as if Black LGBTQ+ women go in and out of fashion, and that society's acceptance of us is always teetering on the verge of collapse, like a Jenga game where the stakes are, literally, life or death (ours). Make no mistake that we are continually making progress, and, if we continue to advocate for our health care and to support and love each other, there is nothing we cannot accomplish. I hope I have done these women justice in amplifying their voices in these pages. As Black LGBTQ+ women, *we are all women*, and we all deserve to be as healthy and happy as possible.

REFERENCES

Agénor M, Austin SB, Kort D, Austin EL, Muzny CA. Sexual orientation and sexual and reproductive health among African American sexual minority women in the US South. *Womens Health Issues.* 2016;26(6):612–621. https://doi.org/10.1016/j.whi.2016.07.004

Giles S. Transmission of HPV. *Can Med Assoc J.* 2003;168(11):1391. https://www-cmaj-ca.ucsf.idm.oclc.org/content/168/11/1391.1.short

Grant JM, Mottet LA, Tanis J, Harrison J, Herman J, Kiesling M. Injustice at every turn: a report of the National Transgender Discrimination Survey. Washington, DC: National Center for Transgender Equality and National Gay and Lesbian Task Force; 2011: 228.

Howard SD, Lee KL, Nathan AG, Wenger HC, Chin MH, Cook SC. Healthcare experiences of transgender people of color. *J Gen Intern Med.* 2019;34(10):2068–2074. https://doi.org/10.1007/s11606-019-05179-0

Ojeaga A, Alema-Mensah E, Rivers D, Azonobi I, Rivers B. Racial disparities in HPV-related knowledge, attitudes, and beliefs among African American and white women in the USA. *J Cancer Educ.* 2019;34(1):66–72. https://doi.org/10.1007/s13187-017-1268-6

23

Wellness for Black Adolescent Girls and Young Women

Ndidiamaka Amutah-Onukagha, PhD, MPH, Vanessa Nicholson, DrPH, MPH, Telesha B. Zabie, MD, MBA, Lorraine J. Lacroix-Williamson, MPH, Elizabeth Bolarinwa, Aishwarya Amarnath, Michelle S. Jerry, Ruth Vigue, MS, and Yoann Sophie Antoine, MPH

This chapter highlights strategies that can be used by Black adolescent girls and young women to make better lifestyle decisions concerning their bodies, relationships, and sexual behaviors. There is a lack of research on the experiences and the life trajectory of young Black girls. This chapter seeks to highlight strengths-based and culturally specific approaches while also challenging the field to incorporate an intersectional framework to address the health inequities that impact Black girls and young women.

> It is time to identify and deconstruct social norms that have become acceptable forms of oppression for Black girls.

The public perceives Black girls as less innocent than their white peers of the same age. This lived experience, called "adultification bias," was documented in a Georgetown Law Center on Poverty and Inequality study that asked US Black girls and women aged 12 to 60 years questions about their real-world observations. The study revealed that Black women and girls are routinely affected by this form of discrimination and highlighted the generalized perception of how Black girls are seen today without reference to their individual behaviors. Respondents felt that change can only emerge through meaningful reforms such as training on gender responsiveness, in which the realities of Black girls' lives are understood and addressed effectively (Blake and Epstein 2019). As emerging Black women scholars and allies, we call for a narrative that is not only oppositional to this presumption but a narrative that also makes Black girls visible in a world that was designed to make us invisible.

"AT-RISK" BLACK GIRLS

The generalization and use of the term "at risk" to describe Black girls causes the same damaging effects of the adultification and oversexualization of Black girls and women. "Girlhood Interrupted: The Erasure of Black Girls' Childhood" provided—for the first time—data showing that adults view Black girls as less innocent and more adult-like than their white peers, especially in the age range of 5 to 14 years (Epstein, Blake, and González 2017). While data in this study are used to explain the overdiscipline of Black girls in comparison to their white peers, the same sentiments can be applied to the language used to describe Black girls in health care and policy settings.

At best, the term "at risk" is imprecise and fails to accurately describe the conditions in which Black girls need to be supported. Its use justifies the inaccurate notion that Black girls must be "saved," and its framing promotes bias and stigma. Education and awareness is a large part of the reframing of such damaging language, but it is not the only solution and is insufficient by itself. Given the dearth of health and wellness research about Black girls as a whole, Black girls must be listened to and have their voices and needs centered.

Across centuries and all over the world, Black girls continue to overcome a multitude of adversities. Black women researchers must be funded to accurately describe, investigate, and develop interventions that address "risks" Black girls may be exposed to. Despite battling both the systemic and structural effects of racism, sexism, and misogynoir, Black girls across the diaspora have shown resilience, tenacity, and advancement. Black girls do not need saving; they need support as they navigate their everyday lives.

THE EDUCATION OF BLACK GIRLS

Black women who do not receive a full high-school education have a higher risk for more negative health outcomes, including those related to sexual and reproductive health. A study conducted by Hinze, Lin, and Anderson (2012), which sought to understand intersections among race, gender, education, and health, affirmed this idea, finding that Black women who did not receive a complete high-school education had the lowest self-rated health outcomes.

In terms of sexual health, a lack of complete or adequate education correlates to a lack of education about sexual health and sexual behaviors, often taught in high-school curriculum, increasing likelihoods of unsafe sex, unplanned pregnancies, and risk of sexual violence. For those not in school-connected programs, self-deliverable interventions such as computer-delivered family-based programs or social media campaigns focused on educating youth about substance use and sexual health may be a strategy in lowering risks of poor health outcomes in Black women who are not able to receive a complete high-school education (Opara et al. 2022). In addition, public sexual health campaigns and research behind such campaigns must be culturally relevant and tailored toward young Black women and their health practices, as they are frequently overlooked and therefore may not have proper information about how to best practice safe sex in relation to their identity.

When a group of people is targeted, discriminated against, or oppressed over a period of time, they may internalize the damaging myths and misinformation society communicates to them about their group. There needs to be a shift in how sexual health and sexuality are perceived by Black women and girls to help shed the shame and stigma associated with sexuality (Thorpe et al. 2021). A means to this change would be moving from a fear-based conceptualization that supports using scare tactics in prevention efforts to a more affirming approach to improving outcomes and reducing disparities, such as comprehensive, sex-positive education and programming (Pratt et al. 2022).

Educating Black women and girls using an empowering, culturally appropriate, and medically informed framework has been shown to reduce risk, increase preexposure prophylaxis (PrEP) uptake, influence a later sexual debut, and improve mental and physical health and well-being (Taggart et al. 2020). Statistically, comprehensive sexuality education (CSE) leads to better sexual health outcomes for young people, from lower rates of sexually transmitted infections (STIs) to fewer unintended pregnancies (Harley 2022). To further help reduce shame and stigma, conversations must be open and welcomed in a variety of community-based and medical settings, such as within the Black church, during well-visits with pediatricians and health providers, and with trusted adults.

OVERSEXUALIZATION OF BLACK GIRLS

During adolescence, Black girls experience an earlier development of secondary sex characteristics and menarche compared to girls of other racial groups. While the reasons are inconclusive, the consequence of early development is the hypersexualization and fetishization of Black girls from a young age. Black adolescents are more likely to report an earlier sexual debut, which is associated with a higher STI and adolescent pregnancy rate than other racial groups (Biello et al. 2013).

The continual exploitation and objectification of Black women and girls is rooted in colonialism and the perception of Black people as sexually deviant. Thomas Jefferson, in *Notes on the State of Virginia* (1788), depicts Black women as "having an unlimited and undiscriminating sexual capacity" (Holmes 2016, p. 2). These ideas emphasize rape culture within the framework of American slavery, depicting Black women as sexual commodities rather than as human beings with sexual agency (Holmes 2016).

The stereotype of hypersexual Black women manifests in current society within the cultural fabric of mainstream media. This is further reflected in dating culture with white men purposefully seeking out Black women for their "exoticness" or the experience of sex. Statements such as, "I've never been with a Black girl before" or "I like to mess around with Black girls" are prominent examples of fetishization that is all too common within the current dating environment. This is especially apparent on online dating apps, where misogynoir runs rampant and users feel protected by a screen. Unfortunately, Black adolescent girls and young women must be cognizant of their partner's focus when dating. It is important to be aware of stereotypes, as it may lead to harmful situations.

CONSENT AS A DISMANTLING TOOL AGAINST OPPRESSION

Up to 60% of Black women report being subjected to coercive sexual contact by the age of 18 years (Hart 2018). CSE emphasizes bodily autonomy and is an effective strategy for teaching Black adolescent girls and young women that their voice needs to be respected. Providing consent to engage in sexual activity with a partner equips young Black women with knowledge, skills, attitudes, and values that can help them navigate sexual situations. It also empowers them to prioritize their health and well-being in a racially charged society. One in four Black girls will be sexually abused before the age of 18 years (American Psychological Association n.d.). This statistic showcases the need for effective education and allocation of resources to protect the mental and physical health of young Black girls. CSE, including education about consent, can be a powerful tool to dismantle systems of power and oppression. Black adolescent girls and young women need tools to navigate not only their physical health but also their personal relationships and boundaries. Consent is a skill that equips young people to articulate their needs and desires while respecting those of others.

It is important that CSE be implemented for all students over the course of K-12 education. More than half of adolescents engage in sexual activity before they graduate high school (Centers for Disease Control and Prevention 2018). Black girls are even more vulnerable to sexual exposure at a young age due to the oversexualization of Black bodies. It is important that they are given the tools to navigate and recognize predatory behavior and feel confident in reporting instances of sexual violence. In 2022, it was reported that Black women comprised 40% of sex trafficking victims (National Black Women's Justice Institute 2022; Hart 2018). Education and knowledge of trafficking tactics are important to protect against sexual violence. Many underage victims of human trafficking are students in the American school system. Human trafficking prevention curriculum should be incorporated into sex education to ensure that Black girls are not only equipped for harmful situations that they may be presented with but are able to recognize and report abuse they see in other Black girls. Young people who identify as a sexual or gender minority should also receive education in an environment that is affirming of their sexual orientation, gender identity, and racial identity. These identities intersect to place young Black youth at heightened risk of sexual violence.

Comprehensive sexual education can also support the development of sexual autonomy. Deciding when to have sex is a very personal decision, and it is important for Black girls and young women to confidently arrive at such a decision on their own terms. The appropriate time for each person may vary. They may choose to wait until they are an adult or until they, along with their partner, feel their relationship is ready. Some indicators for readiness may be when (1) one can be completely honest with their partner and there is mutual trust; (2) one feels they can talk with their partner about difficult topics such as feelings, other relationships, and STIs; (3) one can be responsible for protecting themselves and their partner against STIs and pregnancy; and, lastly, (4) one can respect the other person's decisions about not having sex and about using protection (American Academy of Pediatrics 2015).

Though PrEP is highly effective in preventing HIV infection, education increases positive behavior change. This intervention approach is still being studied in adolescent girls and young women, as there are many contextual social and biological factors to consider, including cognitive development, lack of experience with sustained medication use, identity formation, and experimentation, that place adolescents at an increased risk. Nonetheless, educating Black adolescent girls and young women about PrEP can lead to a sense of empowerment by arming them with available safeguards to prevent and reduce the possibility of HIV-related sexual risk (Opara et al. 2022).

SUBSTANCE USE INTERVENTIONS AND SEXUAL ASSAULT STRATEGIES

Though Black girls make up a fairly small portion of the overall substance-using population, they experience worse health and well-being outcomes. Adolescent pregnancy, substance use before or during sex, and history of sexual assault are all barriers to sexual health that Black girls face at disparate rates compared to their peers. Drug use among Black girls is beginning to rise, according to most recent statistics related to drug use among adolescent girls. Factors including perceived racial discrimination, sexism, low self-esteem, and poor mental health symptoms may explain the sudden rise in substance use among Black girls (Opara et al. 2022).

There are many structural and individual-level factors that can drive Black girls and young women toward substance use and subsequently increased risk of sexual assault. Factors include traumatic life experiences (e.g., sexual assault itself) or stressful environmental factors like poverty, violence, and exposure to others with substance use disorders. Substance use can be utilized as a coping mechanism for those who experience such adverse experiences frequently, some of whom may not have proper systems for emotional, financial, or other support, or who have not received proper education about the risks of substance use (Opara et al. 2022).

One stigmatized aspect of Black girls and their sexual health is the involvement and role of substances in sexual safety and how substance use can impact experiences with sexual assault. Though there is a gap in literature surrounding substance use in Black women in particular, existing research demonstrates a correlation between substance use and increased risk of sexual assault. One study by Opara et al. (2022) stated a correlation between substance use and sexual risk behaviors that opens young Black girls up to a higher risk of adverse sexual experiences, including sexual and reproductive health issues and sexual exploitation.

To support Black girls and young women in preventing adverse health outcomes related to substance use, asset-based programs that reduce drug use and promote positive sexual well-being, targeted specifically toward Black girls and their experiences, must be developed. Seeking support systems and mental health care for traumatic or adverse life experiences, through addiction counseling or community support groups, may help prevent tendencies toward substance use. For Black girls who are neither in school nor connected to schools or youth-serving organizations, incorporating interventions either in home settings or online may be beneficial. Because the most socially marginalized groups of adolescents, such as those in foster care, are more likely to contract STIs and HIV, have unintended pregnancies, and engage in drug use, it is imperative that interventions are coordinated and promoted within local child welfare agencies to reduce the likelihood and vulnerability for youth in out-of-home care (Opara et al. 2022).

STRENGTHS-BASED METHODS

Black girls and young women comprise a group that is hindered by sexual health inequities, and there continues to be a focus on individual risk factors, which paint a biased perception and narrative associated with poor outcomes (Mosher 2017). Sexual health is experienced within one's belief and value system, informed by culture, social norms, relationships, education, and behaviors. Therefore, it is imperative to focus on the positive aspects of Black girls' identities when conceptualizing programs and evaluation to improve sexual and reproductive health. Interventions can incorporate strategies around sexual self-efficacy, self-esteem, the family and community environment, and sexual agency within romantic relationships. For example, the original Sistas, Informing, Healing, Living, and Empowering/Sisters Informing Sisters About Topics on AIDS (SIHLE/SISTA) interventions incorporates sessions that highlight racial/ethnic identity and gender identity as a way to challenge negative view of self and increase confidence in Black girls (Opara et al. 2022).

We provide some proposed recommendations to assist Black adolescent girls and young women on their unique journeys as they develop and come of age. Best practices for health and wellness call for multilayered, comprehensive, culturally competent approaches that encompass intersectional identities shaped by lived experiences and commit to challenging social injustices Black girls often experience (Opara et al. 2022; Caldwell and Matthews 2016). Furthermore, there is a lack of sexual health interventions that focus on more holistic aspects of sexual health, including sex positivity and pleasure. We encourage researchers to test the effectiveness of such interventions in young Black women.

RADICAL SELF-LOVE

Acknowledging their identities as sources of power plays a large role in how Black girls exercise radical self-love and is imperative for maintaining personal well-being. Furthermore, self-love may act as a sexual wellness strategy that could empower Black girls and young women to practice safer sexual practices. Evidence suggests that body esteem is positively associated with inquiry regarding a partner's sexual history (Brown et al. 2014). This finding suggests that programs promoting body esteem for Black girls and young women may be useful in aiding them in healthy decision-making as it relates to sexual behaviors and relationships.

Learning to preserve oneself in a society that prevents us from being well, both physically and mentally, is the goal for any liberation movement. Through both online and social media programming, there is vast opportunity to encourage Black girls to practice radical self-love and be intentional about building self-esteem. It is time for Black girls and young women to prioritize self-care. This can include going for a walk or simply sitting in a quiet environment. Learning how to find joy and peace, making sure physical and mental health are in alignment with personal values, and researching ways to properly nourish one's body are all a part of wellness. Lastly, setting boundaries, extending ourselves the same grace and compassion we give to others, and finding friends, family, and communities to work together with toward personal and collective healing are essential in practicing self-love.

The trajectory of Black sexuality as it pertains to Black women and girls has weathered through colonization, white supremacy, and the Civil Rights Movement. With the proposed strategies, strides can continue to be made to improve the sexual and reproductive health of Black adolescent girls and young women. Reframing "at risk" language, providing accurate and comprehensive sexuality education, and conducting more research are all important means of promoting health and sexual well-being.

REFERENCES

American Academy of Pediatrics. For teens: how to make healthy decisions about sex. January 8, 2015. Available at: https://www.healthychildren.org/English/ages-stages/teen/dating-sex/Pages/default.aspx

Barlow JN. Black women, the forgotten survivors of sexual assault. American Psychological Association. February 2020. Available at: https://www.apa.org/pi/about/newsletter/2020/02/black-women-sexual-assault

Biello KB, Ickovics J, Niccolai L, Lin H, Kershaw T. Racial differences in age at first sexual intercourse: residential racial segregation and the Black-white disparity among US adolescents. *Public Health Rep.* 2013;128(suppl 1):23–32. https://doi.org/10.1177%2F00333549131282S103

Blake J, Epstein R. Listening to Black women and girls: lived experiences of adultification bias. Georgetown Law Center on Poverty and Inequality. 2019. Available at: https://www.law.georgetown.edu/poverty-inequality-center/wp-content/uploads/sites/14/2019/05/Listening-to-Black-Women-and-Girls.pdf

Brown D, Webb-Bradley T, Cobb P, Spaw D, Aldridge K. African American women's safer sexual practices: the influence of ethnic-racial socialisation and body esteem. *Cult Health Sex.* 2014;16(5):518–532. https://doi.org/10.1080/13691058.2014.891048

Caldwell K, Mathews A. The role of relationship type, risk perception, and condom use in middle socioeconomic status Black women's HIV-prevention strategies. *J Black Sex Relatsh.* 2016;2(2):91–120. https://doi.org/10.1353/bsr.2016.0002

Centers for Disease Control and Prevention. Over half of US teens have had sexual intercourse by age 18, new report shows. June 22, 2018. Centers for Disease Control and Prevention. Available at: https://www.cdc.gov/nchs/pressroom/nchs_press_releases/2017/201706_NSFG.htm

Epstein R, Blake JJ, González T. Girlhood interrupted: the erasure of Black girls' childhood. Georgetown Law Center on Poverty and Inequality. 2017. Available at: https://genderjusticeandopportunity.georgetown.edu/wp-content/uploads/2020/06/girlhood-interrupted.pdf

Harley CS. Sex ed is a vehicle for social change. Full stop. SIECUS. February 22, 2022. Available at: https://siecus.org/sex-ed-is-a-vehicle-for-social-change

Hart C. Black women and sexual assault. The National Center on Violence Against Women in the Black Community. October 2018. Available at: https://ujimacommunity.org/wp-content/uploads/2018/12/Ujima-Womens-Violence-Stats-v7.4-1.pdf

Hinze SW, Lin J, Andersson TE. Can we capture the intersections? Older Black women, education, and health. *Womens Health Issues.* 2012;22(1):e91–e98. https://doi.org/10.1016/j.whi.2011.08.002

Holmes CM. The colonial roots of the racial fetishization of Black women. *Black & Gold.* 2016;2. Available at: https://openworks.wooster.edu/cgi/viewcontent.cgi?article=1026&context=blackandgold

Jefferson T. *Notes on the State of Virginia.* 1788.

Mosher CM. Historical perspectives of sex positivity: contributing to a new paradigm within counseling psychology. *Couns Psychol.* 2017;45(4):487–503. https://doi.org/10.1177/0011000017713755

Opara I, Pierre K, Assan MA, et al. A systematic review on sexual health and drug use prevention interventions for Black girls. *Int J Environ Res Public Health.* 2022;19(6):3176. https://doi.org/10.3390/ijerph19063176

Pratt MC, Jeffcoat S, Hill SV, et al. "We feel like everybody's going to judge us": Black adolescent girls' and young women's perspectives on barriers to and opportunities for improving sexual health care, including PrEP, in the southern US. *J Int Assoc Provid AIDS Care*. 2022;21:1–11. https://doi.org/10.1177/23259582221107327

National Black Women's Justice Institute. Sex trafficking of Black women and girls. National Resource Center on Domestic Violence. 2022. Available at: https://vawnet.org/material/sex-trafficking-black-women-and-girls

Taggart T, Liang Y, Pina P, Albritton T. Awareness of and willingness to use PrEP among Black and Latinx adolescents residing in higher prevalence areas in the United States. *PLoS One*. 2020;15(7):1–13. https://doi.org/10.1371/journal.pone.0234821

Thorpe S, Tanner AE, Nichols TR, Kuperberg A, Foh EP. Black female adolescents' sexuality: pleasure expectancies, sexual guilt, and age of sexual debut. *Am J Sex Educ*. 2021;16(2):199–220. https://doi.org/10.1080/15546128.2021.1892005

24

How Much Longer? Exploring the State of Comprehensive Sexual and Reproductive Health Education for Black Girls in the United States

Aja Clark, MPH, Phoebe Wescott, MPH, and Joia Crear-Perry, MD

This chapter explores comprehensive sexuality education (CSE) as an overlooked but vital intervention to promote and support sexual and reproductive health experiences and outcomes for Black girls. We first discuss related health outcomes for Black women and girls, demonstrating the need for accessible CSE. Then, we briefly examine the history of school-based sex education in the United States. Next, we report on the current state of sexuality and reproductive health education in the United States. Finally, we explore the value and challenges associated with both community-based and school-based CSE. After engaging with this chapter, we hope that public health practitioners and stakeholders will urgently continue to develop and support the provision of equitable, culturally informed sexuality and reproductive health education across settings for Black girls in the United States.

REPRODUCTIVE AND SEXUAL HEALTH OF BLACK GIRLS AND WOMEN

Historically, cultural deficit theories and victim-blaming narratives were allowed to provide context for racialized health disparities (Apugo, Mawhinney, and Mbilishaka 2020). Today, partly due to the labor and greater visibility of racial- and gender-equity advocates, there is a more widespread understanding of the role that racism and sexism play in creating and sustaining disproportionate health outcomes.

Among several sexual, reproductive, and maternal health measures, compared to those of other races, Black girls and women fare worse (National Center for HIV/AIDS, Viral Hepatitis, STD, and TB Prevention 2019). For example, in 2020, the rate of chlamydia for Black females aged 15 to 19 years was almost five times that of their white counterparts (Centers for Disease Control and Prevention [CDC] 2022). In 2018, the rate of gonorrhea cases among Black females of this same age group was a staggering 6.9

times the rate for white females (CDC 2020a). According to the most recent report of maternal mortality rates in the United States, racial disparities persist and have grown (Hoyert 2023). Finally, the most recently published Department of Justice report on sexual violence in the United States noted that Black girls and women aged 12 years and older experienced higher rates of rape and sexual assault than white, Asian, and Latina girls between 2005 and 2010 (Planty et al., 2013).

Misogynoir, a term coined by Moya Bailey, describes the violence directed at Black women as a result of ingrained racism and sexism (Bailey 2021). This bias is familiar to many Black women and also significantly impacts the lived experiences of Black girls. A 2017 study conducted by the Georgetown Law Center on Poverty and Inequality found that Black girls were viewed by adults as more adult-like than their white counterparts and more knowledgeable about sex topics. The report also found that the same historical narratives (e.g., Sapphire, mammy, Jezebel) created and utilized to justify racialized and gendered oppression toward Black women contribute to the development of implicit and explicit bias against Black girls (Epstein, Blake, and González 2017; Hill Collins 2009).

The impact of this "age compression" experienced by Black girls can be illustrated in the ways that they are disproportionately impacted by disciplinary practices in school settings. Research also indicates that Black girls and adolescents are being sexualized by their peers and even the staff members charged with their care (Apugo, Mawhinney, and Mbilishaka 2020). Though it is clear that many of the health outcomes named previously cannot be solved solely through the provision of CSE, it is still an important factor in maintaining population health that must be addressed.

History of Comprehensive Sexuality Education

Data have repeatedly shown that the content, presence, and absence of sexual health education impact sexual and reproductive health-related outcomes (Goldfarb and Lieberman 2021). In 2018, the United Nations Education, Scientific, and Cultural Organization (UNESCO) reviewed sexual education curricula worldwide. Their research concluded that comprehensive sexual education programming could lead to health outcomes such as delayed sexual initiation, reduced sexual partners and frequency of sexual encounters, and increased use of contraceptives. Further research notes that a comprehensive sexual education curriculum could improve positive body image and knowledge of gender identity and reduce the risk of intimate partner violence (UNESCO et al. 2018).

Despite the promise of current trends in CSE toward evidence-based, culturally appropriate, gender-affirming curricula, sex education in the United States did not begin this way. Early attempts at sex education in this country were born from a hegemonic desire to quell the reproduction of populations that were not white and middle class and to stop the spread of sexually transmitted diseases (STDs; Sexuality Information and Education Council of the United States [SIECUS] 2021b). During this time, a powerful group of people known as social hygienists believed that teaching the population about the dangers of "promiscuous" sex would course-correct society's regression from traditional Victorian family ideals. They believed that sex should only belong within the confines of heterosexual marriage, that women were not interested in sex outside of its utility for reproduction, and that protection of women—white women—was best reached solely through the education of white men. Eugenics was central to this school of thought, as many social hygienists believed that people who were not middle class and white would be biologically incapable of adhering to the standards of morality and behavior that they regarded as acceptable (SIECUS 2021b).

Concurrent to the social hygiene movement were Progressive Era pushes to improve the public school system in the United States. As schools began focusing on the importance of health, social hygiene was a welcomed addition to the greater inclusion of health-related topics.

Chicago public schools were amongst the first in the country to begin teaching sex education in 1913. During this time, racism pervaded every structure of American society, including education. Therefore, the socialization led by white middle-class reformers that took place in schools related to sex education also reflected racist beliefs about deviance and biological differences between Black and white populations. As mentioned previously, sexual education efforts were chiefly focused on the education of white boys. Efforts to stop the spread of STDs and sexually transmitted infections (STIs) did not extend to the Black community, because people in power at the time believed that STIs and STDs in the Black community were inevitable. White girls were not included in sexual and reproductive health education to not offend the "reputation" and traditional roles of femininity ascribed to white, middle-class girls. Black girls were not considered (SIECUS 2021b). Black girls were denied access to sexual health education because of their social location: the intersection of Black and girl.

At the time, because of sex education's focus on STD and STI prevention, doctors served as primary sources of information related to sexual and reproductive health. Despite the growing Black doctor population at that time, many hesitated to push back or conduct their own programming for fear of reinforcing stereotypes about Black sexual deviance and hypersexualization (Shah 2015).

Over time, sexual education practices continued to reflect the culture and priorities of those with enough capital to set and operationalize educational programming. These practices often placed values on marriage from a heterosexist and racially concordant viewpoint while continuing to deny the presence and validity of nonwhite races and nonheterosexual behaviors and partnerships (SIECUS 2021b).

The information presented in this section is not intended to be an exhaustive history of sex education in the United States. However, we hope that it serves as context for some of the current shortfalls of sex education, particularly as it relates to Black girls. Today, many sexual health advocates in the United States are calling for nationwide CSE. The next section explores current programming and its impact.

State of Sexual and Reproductive Health Education in the United States

According to SIECUS, a leader in the field of sexuality and sex education, high-quality CSE includes "age, developmentally, and culturally appropriate, science-based, and medically accurate information on a broad set of topics related to sexuality, including human development, relationships, personal skills, sexual behaviors, including abstinence, sexual health, and society and culture." They also note that "CSE programs provide students with opportunities for learning information, exploring their attitudes and values, and developing skills" (Harley 2019).

Despite broad recognition of the need for widespread sex education, federal and state budgets and, therefore, the programming, do not reflect its importance (SIECUS 2022). As of December 2022, only 38 states mandate some form of sex education and/or HIV education in schools. Amongst these 38, requirements vary widely. For example, only two states mandate "sex education," while 11 mandate "HIV education." Twenty-five states and the District of Columbia mandate both "sex education" *and* "HIV education." To further complicate the landscape, of the states with mandates, only 17 require medically accurate programming, 13 require programming to be lesbian, gay, bisexual, transgender, queer, and questioning plus (LGBTQ+)-inclusive, and 10 states mandate that information be provided in a way that is appropriate for a student's cultural background without bias against a race, sex, or ethnicity (Guttmacher Institute 2022a; SIECUS 2021a).

A report released by In Our Own Voice: National Black Women's Reproductive Justice Agenda indicates that the current sexual and reproductive health programming has a true impact on Black adolescents. This harm is illustrated in racial disparities in exposure to information and sexual and reproductive health outcomes. While states and the federal government underfund contradicting streams of programming, advocates for Black youth call for the *inclusion* of additional programming components that speak to the unique cultural and social experiences of Black adolescents, such as media literacy, trauma-informed pedagogy, self-esteem, and empowerment (Williamson, Howell, and Batchelor 2017). The state of sex education in the United States is in disarray, to the detriment of young people who could benefit from these resources.

Only 30% of non-Hispanic Black adolescent females were reported to have learned where to obtain contraception before the first time they had sex (Lindberg and Kantor 2022). Data collected by the National Center for Health Statistics National Survey of Family Growth indicate that 47% of females in the United States did not receive sex education that met the minimum standards set by Healthy People 2030 (Guttmacher Institute 2022b). These data also reflect that adolescent females between 2015 and 2019 were less likely than adolescent females in 1995 to receive sex education on key topics such as sexual refusal (Guttmacher Institute 2022b). This demonstrates that today's adolescents are worse off than those 26 years ago.

Formal Sex Education in the United States

Federal funding for sex education in the United States indicates mixed priorities. While there have been some promising efforts to increase evidence-based programming, a significant amount of funding is also provided to abstinence-only-until-marriage programming, which has been proven to be incomplete, violent toward LGBTQ+ adolescents, stigmatizing toward students of color, and ineffective (SIECUS 2022; Guttmacher Institute 2021b). In addition to the patchwork of federal sex education-related programs, some states, such as California and New Jersey, have taken steps toward implementing CSE (Shapiro and Brown 2018). While steps in the right direction are promising, there is no indication that CSE for all Black girls and women in the United States will be possible in the near future. How much longer will we wait?

Federally Funded Evidence-Based Programs

There is no federal funding allocated to increase accessibility to comprehensive sex education as it is defined by SIECUS. There are, however, several programs funded by the federal government that incorporate some aspects of CSE, including utilizing evidence-based methods and medical accuracy. These programs include the Family Youth and Services Bureau's Personal Responsibility Education Program (PREP) and the Office of Population Affairs' Teen Pregnancy Prevention (TPP) program (Guttmacher Institute 2021a).

PREP supports programs seeking to prevent pregnancy and STIs by promoting abstinence and contraceptive use. Formula grant funding is available to states, tribes, and tribal organizations (Guttmacher Institute 2021a). In states that decline funding, competitive grants are awarded to local organizations to conduct innovative strategies and interventions in alignment with the program. (Family and Youth Services Bureau n.d.) Programs funded by PREP focus on at-risk youth, aged 10 to 19 years, who are homeless, in the foster care system, or soon to age out; those with HIV or AIDS; people pregnant or parenting; victims of human trafficking; and/or those living in communities with high adolescent birth rates (Guttmacher Institute 2021a). An evaluation of PREP performance measures found that between program years 2013 and 2017, PREP reached more than 100,000 students per year, most of which, 76% to 79%, were instructed in school settings (Murphy, Hulsey, and Zief 2021). For scale, according to the Centers for Disease Control and Prevention, school settings in the United States have direct contact with about 56 million students each year for at least six hours a day (CDC 2020b).

Despite limited reach, participants in PREP programming have reported that the program changed their intentions to participate in "risky behaviors" (Murphy, Hulsey, and Zief 2021).

The TPP program funds many organizations working on adolescent pregnancy prevention. It serves nearly 250,000 young people a year (US Department of Health and Human Services [HHS] n.d.). Ten percent of its funding goes to program support. Of the remaining funds, the program has a tiered funding structure where 75% is directed toward tier 1 grants that replicate effective adolescent pregnancy programming, and 25% is provided to tier 2 grants that test innovative strategies to reduce adolescent pregnancy rates (Guttmacher Institute 2021b). Funding is awarded to a wide range of private and public organizations (SIECUS 2022). Evaluations have demonstrated that many programs funded by the TPP program have met the criteria for program effectiveness in one or multiple outcomes of interest, such as reduced number of sexual partners, increased knowledge of sexual health in LGBTQ+ youth, and others (Guttmacher Institute 2021a; HHS n.d.).

Even when combined, these programs do not meet the need for youth sexual health education in the United States. As a consequence, many advocates have worked for the creation and passing of the Real Education and Access for Health Youth Act (REAHYA). Introduced in the House of Representatives by Barbara Lee (D-CA) and Alma Adams (D-NC) and in the Senate by Cory Booker (D-NJ) and Mazie Hirono (D-HI), the REAHYA, for the first time, offers federal funding for comprehensive, honest, and inclusive sex education programs in the United States (Diamondstein 2021). It would fund training for teachers and mandate medical accuracy and cultural responsibility. It would also mandate programs to be LGBTQ+-inclusive (Human Rights Campaign n.d.) If passed, the Act would also defund abstinence-only-until-marriage programs (Guttmacher Institute 2021a).

Abstinence-Only Until Marriage

Recently rebranded as sexual-risk-avoidance education (SRAE), abstinence-only-until-marriage sexual education is focused on teaching children and adolescents to delay sexual activity until marriage as the best way to avoid unintended pregnancies, STIs, and HIV. While doing so, it omits information on condom use and contraception (Kaiser Family Foundation 2018; Ott and Santelli 2007). The Family, Youth, and Services Bureau currently funds two abstinence-only programs: the Title V state SRAE program, created in 1996, which provides funding to states and territories across the nation, and the Title V Competitive SRAE program, created by a 2016 appropriations bill that provides discretionary funding to projects that solely implement sexual risk avoidance (Family and Youth Services Bureau, HHS n.d.). These programs typically focus on the potential risks and negative outcomes associated with premarital sexual activity (Stanger-Hall and Hall 2011).

These curricula tend to be incomplete and provide medically inaccurate information. They also tend to stigmatize and discriminate against marginalized students, including those that identify as LGBTQ+ (SIECUS 2021a). The continued use of this programming potentially increases adolescents' risk of other harmful outcomes and behaviors, such as STI/HIV infections, intimate partner violence, and suicide (The Society for Adolescent Health and Medicine 2017). A nine-year Congressional study by Mathematica Policy Research examined selected abstinence-only programs and found that federal programming had no constructive impact on adolescents' sexual behaviors (Trenholm et al. 2007).

Reputable medical organizations, including the Society for Adolescent Health and Medicine, the American Medical Association, and the American College of Obstetricians and Gynecologists, are clear in their opposition to abstinence-only programs and continue to support research proving their ineffectiveness (American College of Obstetricians and Gynecologists Committee on Adolescent Health Care 2020; American Medical Association 2022; The Society for Adolescent Health and Medicine 2017). Though the debate rages on over the favorable effects of comprehensive versus abstinence-only curricula, research shows that states promoting abstinence-only programming have higher rates of STIs, HIV, and adolescent pregnancy (The Society for Adolescent Health and Medicine 2017). In fact, states with the highest levels of adolescent pregnancy in 2020, such as Mississippi, Arkansas, and Louisiana, have required educational programming to teach that sex is only acceptable within marriage (Guttmacher Institute 2022a; Office of Population Affairs, HHS n.d.) Research has shown that abstinence-only education is not effective. Resources should be pulled from these programs and diverted toward interventions that can demonstrate their effectiveness over time.

WHEN WILL SCHOOL-BASED SEX EDUCATION MEET OUR NEEDS?

Earlier in the chapter, we detailed some of the sexual and reproductive health outcomes that demonstrate how Black girls have been failed due to a lack of CSE and other manifestations of structural racism. We have also reviewed mostly school-based sex education programming at the federal level and have detailed some of its successes and inadequacies. As advocates and practitioners who say we are interested in increasing the health, pleasure, and joy available to Black women and girls, we must hold systems accountable for their failure to steward our resources and power in ways that are life-affirming.

With each year and election cycle, we necessarily participate with the hope of creating policies and changes that would bring about health for all, including marginalized populations. It is the government's responsibility to ensure that young people have access to the information and care they need. It is also the government's responsibility to ensure that schools are a safe place for all students, including Black girls and other marginalized populations. Despite this, we have countless examples that point to an inability and possibly a lack of intention to correct the harms of the past and present quickly. After centuries of structural neglect, disrespect, and denials of access, how long will we, as public health practitioners, expect systems that perpetually harm the Black community to simultaneously provide them with the information and care they need and deserve?

How do we, as practitioners, reconcile the idea that schools are a viable setting for sex education for Black girls while attuning to the students and scholars that tell us that school is not a safe place for them? We know that there are social and cultural differences in how Black girls and adolescents are perceived relative to girls and adolescents of other races, particularly white girls. This knowledge is key to our collective understanding as public health practitioners and should broadly inform our calls for advocacy and the next steps related to sexual and reproductive health education. If we agree that schools are the most effective location for educating students about sexual and reproductive health, calls for CSE must be paired with calls for educational equity for all students. We must look at the settings in which health-protective behaviors are established and support them unceasingly. While we as advocates work to correct the violence taking place in school systems, let us consider the promise of community-based solutions that can be created to ensure Black girls have the support that they need.

Community-Based Sexuality Education

Community-based sexual and reproductive health education has the potential to impact the lives of Black women and girls significantly. According to McLeroy et al. (2003), "community-based" programming indicates that interventions are set in communities such as neighborhoods, schools, and community-based organizations. For this chapter, community-based sexuality education is discussed in juxtaposition with school-based programming.

In 2015, Cushman noted several beneficial characteristics of community-based sexuality programs. The author notes that because school-based sexuality education is required to follow structural guidelines and mandates enforced by state legislatures, school boards, and others, school-based sexuality programming is often limited in the topics that are allowed to be covered. School-based programs are also likely to face time constraints and are often required to provide information to a wide variety of students from different neighborhoods and cultural backgrounds, making the content offered naturally more generalizable to a wider audience.

On the contrary, community-based sexuality education programs are not confined by sometimes harmful or counterproductive governing structures that seek to limit what information adolescents have access to in school. Community-based programming also permits a level of specificity not available in school settings. It can be targeted to specific population groups, in this case, Black girls, allowing for cultural congruency with the values and experiences of the community being served (Cushman 2015).

An additional benefit of community-based sexuality programming includes incorporating families and parents in the educational process in ways that school-based programming cannot. Research has often noted parents and family members as primary sources for sex education. Literature also notes that some parents and family members do not feel equipped to talk about sexuality. They may unknowingly provide information that is counterintuitive to the development of knowledge and positive sexual and reproductive health behaviors or refrain from engaging in conversations related to these topics with their adolescents (Cooper and Koch 2007; Costos, Ackerman, and Paradis 2002; Dashiff and Buchanan 1995; Logan et al. 2021; Teitelman 2004). Programming that includes parents and family members may prove successful in delivering comprehensive sexual health information.

In 2014, a systematic review of the impact of parent-child communication programs on Black youth found that a preponderance of the 15 programs reviewed were successful in improving at least one sexual health outcome related to the uptake of condom usage, delayed sexual initiation, and sexual intentions, among others (Cushman 2015). Again, because community-based sexuality programs possess the flexibility to involve caregivers in programming efforts, these interventions, when effectively developed and implemented, stand as a very large source of potential for building community capacity and knowledge related to sexual and reproductive health.

In *Black Feminist Thought*, Dr. Patricia Hill Collins (2009) points to the fact that Black women have always served as safe spaces for one another and have done the work to create nurturing and life-affirming relationships where we can be seen, understood, and supported. In the realm of sexual and reproductive health education, how can we incorporate this knowledge? The Black feminist tradition encourages naming systems of oppression and, despite them, making choices to value oneself and other Black women and girls. It encourages a rejection of the idea that systems and people in power have the authority to name, define, or decide what is best for Black women and girls. Given this, we argue that it is Black women and girls who have the experience, tools, and ability to design and implement programming at the community level for ourselves. What systemic shifts must take place for this to be possible at scale?

Today, there are not many options for community-based sexuality education programs targeted toward Black women and girls. One community-based program called Get Smart B4U Get Sexy is based in Los Angeles, California, and offered by Black Women for Wellness (BWW). BWW is a Black woman-led, community-based organization specializing in a multigenerational approach to improving health outcomes in the Black community. The evidence-based, inclusive program focuses on Black adolescents and young adults (aged 12–30 years), especially those in the foster care system and in high-risk communities, to provide them with intervention and prevention resources.

The program provides abortion resources and health care information, descriptions of birth control methods, STD/STI-testing clinic locations, frequently asked questions about sex, and a downloadable curriculum to supplement school-based sex education. BWW also provides information on how to become a peer educator and how to host CSE workshops in local communities. Besides supporting training opportunities, BWW also has volunteer positions and internships for those interested in serving as peer advocates to help shift attitudes using CSE. While BWW's comprehensive programming is helping young Black people make healthy, responsible choices, we need more options. Black girls and women deserve sexuality education options that meet them where they are and can be safe, literally and figuratively. Based on the information presented about the program, the community-based model is an intervention we think deserves more attention and resources (Get Smart B4 U Get Sexy n.d.).

CONCLUSION

This chapter has discussed various topics as they relate to the provision of CSE for Black girls. We ask these questions: What would it mean for schools and communities to have the capacity to provide Black girls and adolescents with the knowledge, attitudes, behaviors, and skills that would lead to better sexual and reproductive health outcomes? How can we bring this vision into reality quickly?

A liberation mindset calls for us to have a long memory to contextualize contemporary systemic outcomes. While we recognize that in-school models for the provision of CSE have the potential to reach most students in the United States, the reality is that this pathway is not currently working at scale. We know that calls for CSE must be met with calls for reimagining what public education looks like in the United States. The transformation of this system will take time that we do not have to spare. Here is an opportunity for us to leverage cultural assets such as the legacy of black feminist thought and community-building!

While advocates push for state and federal action, it is important for us to be mindful that communities can also advocate, but need resources to concurrently do the work of obtaining and transmitting information to younger generations. We must do this so that Black girls may experience their rights to pleasure-filled, violence-free, and gender-, race-, and body-affirming sexual and reproductive health education. We know that messaging related to sexuality, sex, and relationships is constantly being offered to Black women and girls. In the traditions of Black Radical Teaching, Anti-Racist Public Health Praxis, and Black Systems of Care, practitioners should continue to find ways to provide educational, financial, and logistical support for communities to be self-sufficient in the provision of CSE while working to improve school environments for all students including, and especially, Black girls.

REFERENCES

American College of Obstetricians and Gynecologists' Committee on Adolescent Health Care. Comprehensive sexuality education. 2020. Available at: https://www.acog.org/en/clinical/clinical-guidance/committee-opinion/articles/2016/11/comprehensive-sexuality-education

American Medical Association. Sexuality education, sexual violence prevention, abstinence, and distribution of condoms in schools H-170.968. 2022. Available at: https://policysearch.ama-assn.org/policyfinder/detail/Sexuality%20Education,%20Sexual%20Violence%20Prevention,%20Abstinence,%20and%20Distribution%20of%20Condoms%20in%20Schools%20H-170.968?uri=%2FAMADoc%2FHOD.xml-0-993.xml

Apugo D, Mawhinney L, Mbilishaka A. *Strong Black Girls: Reclaiming Schools in Their Own Image*. New York, NY: Teachers College Press; 2020.

Bailey M. *Misogynoir Transformed*. New York, NY: New York University Press; 2021.

Centers for Disease Control and Prevention. Health disparities in HIV, viral hepatitis, STDs, and TB: African Americans/Blacks health disparities. September 14, 2020a. Available at: https://www.cdc.gov/nchhstp/healthdisparities/africanamericans.html

Centers for Disease Control and Prevention. Sexually transmitted disease surveillance 2020. August 22, 2022. Available at: https://www.cdc.gov/std/statistics/2021/default.htm

Centers for Disease Control and Prevention. Why schools? Adolescent and school health. September 21, 2020b. Available at: https://www.cdc.gov/healthyyouth/about/why_schools.htm

Cooper S, Koch P. "Nobody told me nothin'": communication about menstruation among low-income African American women. *Women Health*. 2007;6(1):57–78. https://doi.org/10.1300/J013V46N01_05

Costos D, Ackerman R, Paradis L. Recollections of menarche: communication between mothers and daughters regarding menstruation. *Sex Roles*. 2002;46:49–59. https://doi.org/10.1023/A:1016037618567

Cushman N. Community-based sexuality education. In: Ponzetti Jr JJ, ed. *Evidence-Based Approaches to Sexuality Education*. New York, NY: Routledge; 2015:169–184. Available at: https://www.taylorfrancis.com/chapters/edit/10.4324/9781315755250-20/community-based-sexuality-education-nicole-cushman?context=ubx&refId=0e4ff544-9d6b-4cb5-b529-db6d15b43f53

Dashiff CJ, Buchanan, LA. Menstrual attitudes among Black and white premenarcheal girls. *J Child Adolesc Psychiatr Nurs*. 1995;8(3):5–14. https://doi.org/10.1111/j.1744-6171.1995.tb00535.x

Department of Health and Human Services. TPP Innovation Grants show positive results. Available at: https://opa.hhs.gov/TPPTier2BEvaluation

Diamondstein M. Federal bill would promote youth sex education in US. Center for Reproductive Rights. May 26, 2021. Available at: https://reproductiverights.org/federal-bill-would-promote-youth-sex-education-in-u-s

Epstein R, Blake JJ, González T. Girlhood interrupted: the erasure of Black girls' childhood. *SSRN*. June 27, 2017. https://doi.org/10.2139/SSRN.3000695

Family and Youth Services Bureau. State Personal Responsibility Education Program. Available at: https://www.acf.hhs.gov/fysb/fact-sheet/state-personal-responsibility-education-program

Family and Youth Services Bureau, Department of Health and Human Services. Adolescent pregnancy prevention. Available at: https://www.acf.hhs.gov/fysb/adolescent-pregnancy-prevention

Get Smart B4 U Get Sexy. Get Smart Before You Get Sexy. Available at: https://getsmartb4ugetsexy.com

Goldfarb ES, Lieberman LD. Three decades of research: the case for comprehensive sex education. *J Adolesc Health*. 2021;68(1):13–27. https://doi.org/10.1016/j.jadohealth.2020.07.036

Guttmacher Institute. Federally funded abstinence-only programs: harmful and ineffective. April 28, 2021a. Available at: https://www.guttmacher.org/fact-sheet/abstinence-only-programs

Guttmacher Institute. Federally funded sex education: strengthening and expanding evidence-based programs. June 2, 2021b. Available at: https://www.guttmacher.org/fact-sheet/sex-education

Guttmacher Institute. Sex and HIV education. August 2022a. Available at: https://www.guttmacher.org/state-policy/explore/sex-and-hiv-education

Guttmacher Institute. US adolescents' receipt of formal sex education. February 2022b. Available at: https://www.guttmacher.org/fact-sheet/adolescents-teens-receipt-sex-education-united-states

Harley C. Sex ed is a vehicle for social change. Full stop. SIECUS. January 17, 2019. Available at: https://siecus.org/sex-ed-is-a-vehicle-for-social-change

Hoyert DL. Maternal mortality rates in the United States, 2021. NCHS Health E-Stats. March 16, 2023. https://dx.doi.org/10.15620/cdc:124678

Hill Collins P. *Black Feminist Thought: Knowledge, Consciousness, and the Politics of Empowerment*. New York, NY: Routledge; 2009.

Human Rights Campaign. Real Education and Access for Healthy Youth Act. Human Rights Campaign. Available at: https://www.hrc.org/resources/real-education-for-healthy-youth-act

Kaiser Family Foundation. Abstinence education programs: definition, funding, and impact on teen sexual behavior. June 1, 2018. Available at: https://www.kff.org/womens-health-policy/fact-sheet/abstinence-education-programs-definition-funding-and-impact-on-teen-sexual-behavior

Lindberg, LD, Kantor LM. Adolescents' receipt of sex education in a nationally representative sample, 2011–2019. *J Adolesc Health*. 2022;70(2):290–297. https://doi.org/10.1016/j.jadohealth.2021.08.027

Logan RG, Vamos CA, Daley EM, Louis-Jacques A, Marhefka SL. Understanding young Black women's socialisation and perceptions of sexual and reproductive health. *Cult Health Sex*. 2022;24(12):1760–1774. https://doi.org/10.1080/13691058.2021.2014976

McLeroy KR, Norton BL, Kegler MC, Burdine JN, Sumaya CV. Community-based interventions. *Am J Public Health*. 2003;93(4):529–533. https://doi.org/10.2105/ajph.93.4.529

Murphy L, Hulsey L, Zief S. The Personal Responsibility Education Program evaluation performance measures final report: 2013–2017. Mathematica. March 2021. Available at: https://www.mathematica.org/publications/prep-performance-measures-final-report-2013-2017

National Center for HIV/AIDS, Viral Hepatitis, STD, and TB Prevention. Sexually Transmitted Disease Surveillance 2018. Centers for Disease Control and Prevention. 2019. Available at: https://www.cdc.gov/std/stats18/STDSurveillance2018-full-report.pdf

Office of Population Affairs, Department of Health and Human Services. Trends in teen pregnancy and childbearing. Available at: https://opa.hhs.gov/adolescent-health/reproductive-health-and-teen-pregnancy/trends-teen-pregnancy-and-childbearing

Ott MA, Santelli JS. Abstinence and abstinence-only education. *Curr Opin Obstet Gynecol.* 2007;19(5):446–452. https://doi.org/10.1097/GCO.0b013e3282efdc0b

Planty M, Langton L, Krebs C, et al. Female victims of sexual violence, 1994–2010. In: US Department of Justice, Bureau of Justice Statistics. March 2013. Available at: https://www.bjs.gov/content/pub/pdf/fvsv9410.pdf

Shah CQ. *Sex Ed, Segregated: The Quest for Sexual Knowledge in Progressive-Era America.* New ed. Rochester, NY: Boydell & Brewer. 2015. http://www.jstor.org/stable/10.7722/j.ctt-13wzt5w

Shapiro, S, Brown C. Sex education standards across the states. Center for American Progress. May 9, 2018. Available at: https://www.americanprogress.org/article/sex-education-standards-across-states

SIECUS. Comprehensive sex education federal fact sheet. SIECUS. September 2021a. Available at: https://siecus.org/wp-content/uploads/2021/10/CSE-Federal-Factsheet-Sept-2021-Update-2.pdf

SIECUS. Federal funding overview: fiscal year 2022. SIECUS. March 2022: 21. Available at: https://siecus.org/wp-content/uploads/2022/05/FY22-Federal-Funding-Overview.pdf

SIECUS. History of sex education. SIECUS. 2021b. Available at: https://siecus.org/wp-content/uploads/2021/03/2021-SIECUS-History-of-Sex-Ed_Final.pdf

The Society for Adolescent Health and Medicine. Abstinence-only-until-marriage policies and programs: an updated position paper of the Society for Adolescent Health and Medicine. *J Adolesc Health.* 2017;61(3):400–403. https://doi.org/10.1016/j.jadohealth.2017.06.001

Stanger-Hall KF, Hall DW. Abstinence-only education and teen pregnancy rates: why we need comprehensive sex education in the US. *PLoS One.* 2011;6(10):e24658. https://doi.org/10.1371/journal.pone.0024658

Teitelman AM. Adolescent girls' perspectives of family interactions related to menarche and sexual health. *Qual Health Res.* 2004;14(9):1292–1308. https://doi.org/10.1177/1049732304268794

Townes A, Guerra-Reyes L, Murray M, et al. "Somebody that looks like me" matters: a qualitative study of Black women's preferences for receiving sexual health services in the USA. *Cult Health Sex.* 2022;24(1):138–152. https://doi.org/10.1080/13691058.2020.1818286

Trenholm C, Devaney B, Fortson K, Quay L, Wheeler J, Clark M. Impacts of four Title V, Section 510 abstinence education programs. Mathematica. April 2007. Available at: https://www.mathematica.org/publications/impacts-of-four-title-v-section-510-abstinence-education-programs

UNESCO, Joint United Nations Programme on HIV/AIDS, United Nations Population Fund, United Nations Children's Fund, United Nations Entity for Gender Equality and the Empowerment of Women, World Health Organization. International technical guidance on sexuality education: an evidence-informed approach. 2018. Available at: https://unesdoc.unesco.org/ark:/48223/pf0000260770

US Department of Health and Human Services. About the Teen Pregnancy Prevention program. Available at: https://opa.hhs.gov/grant-programs/teen-pregnancy-prevention-program-tpp/about-tpp

Williamson H, Howell M, Batchelor M. *Our Bodies, Our Lives, Our Voices: The State of Black Women and Reproductive Justice.* In Our Own Voice: National Black Women's Reproductive Justice Agenda. 2017. Available at: http://blackrj.org/wp-content/uploads/2017/06/FINAL-InOurVoices_Report_final.pdf

25

Sex Positivity and Culturally Affirming Sexuality Education

Ashley Townes, PhD, MPH, and Shemeka Thorpe, PhD

Sexuality education for Black communities is crucial given the disproportionate impact of sexually transmitted infections (STIs) and HIV among Black women (Centers for Disease Control and Prevention [CDC] 2022; CDC 2020; CDC n.d.). However, limited access to comprehensive sexuality education (CSE) across the United States only exacerbates these concerns. Historically, sexuality education took a sex-negative approach and was rooted in religious and moral judgements, which have become exacerbated for Black women. This chapter highlights sex-positive educational and research approaches for Black women and girls, while discussing the need for more culturally affirming sexuality education information that is comprehensive and shame free.

"BABIES HAVING BABIES": THE ABSTINENCE-ONLY PUSH

Sexuality education became more widespread in the early to mid-20th century through science, health, and physical education curricula focusing on reducing STIs and improving hygiene (Elia and Tokunaga 2015). Historically, sexuality education among Black communities has been rooted in racist stereotypes and pregnancy prevention and has focused primarily on abstinence-only–based education. The push of abstinence-only sexuality education reflects the history of controlling sexual myths and stereotypes about Black women's and girls' sexuality as their being overly promiscuous, having an insatiable sexual appetite, and being temptresses (Collins 2002; Rose 2004; Lamb, Roberts, and Plocha 2016). Slogans like "children having children" and "babies having babies" were repeated mostly for low-income Black urban girls and were used to push the agenda that Black girls were immoral for engaging in premarital sex.

The support for abstinence-only education, both presently and in the past, is usually supported by white women and men (Fields 2005; Habersham 2015). For example, white women who are members of school boards in primarily Black school districts promote and vote for abstinence-only education, despite the negative sexual health implications it will have on Black communities (Fields 2005). In 2011, Chris Perry reviewed Fields's research on social inequality and sexuality education among white educators, school board members, and Black students. Perry stated,

> In the case of the two public schools, Fields finds that the predominantly white and middle-class school had greater autonomy than the predominantly black and working-class school when it came to reconfiguring its sex education curriculum to address the abstinence-only education policy. The political firestorm that surrounded the predominantly black school's sex education curriculum is an example of how abstinence-only education advocates were able to adopt racist, sexist, classist, and overall paternalistic rhetoric to argue that the "crisis" of "babies having babies" (which is coded speech to refer to the predominantly black female student population) demanded that a stringent abstinence-only education curriculum be implemented in the predominantly black, lower-income school. (Perry 2011, pp. 164–165)

White people have made decisions about what they believe is appropriate for Black women and girls from slavery until the 21st century. The continued push for abstinence-only education requires us to acknowledge that Black girls have never been seen as moral or worthy of protection and that we have to understand the interactions between racism, sexuality, and who (what race) is seen as innocent in society (Fields 2005). Racial-gendered discrimination and stereotypes are all-pervading for Black women and girls and ultimately affect their overall access to CSE, resources, and supportive adults who will advocate for CSE in their communities.

COMPREHENSIVE SEXUALITY EDUCATION

CSE is recommended by leading public health organizations over abstinence-only education (American Public Health Association 2014). It moves beyond stigma and fear tactics and is founded on sexuality being a natural and healthy part of development. CSE provides positive messages about sex and sexuality expression, contraceptives, and making informed decisions based on individual, family, and community values. It encourages Black girls to recognize their bodily autonomy as well as develop skills to initiate and negotiate during sexual communication with partners. CSE has been proven to reduce sexual risk behaviors, adolescent pregnancy, and STIs (Kohler, Manhart, and Lafferty 2008; Rabbitte and Enriquez 2018). While CSE is certainly more effective than abstinence-only education, evidence-based CSEs are often not tailored for Black girls and femmes and are created through a white lens.

Unfortunately, Black girls' higher rates of STIs and adolescent births have influenced how educators approach curricula by focusing on preventing these outcomes versus building on their assets and strengths, and addressing important topics beyond pregnancy prevention (Brinkman et al. 2019; Ware, Thorpe, and Tanner 2019). To move the field of sexuality education forward and provide CSE that is tailored to Black women, professionals have to acknowledge the racial injustices that exist within sexuality education.

In 2014, The Women of Color Sexual Health Network (2014) developed the Solidarity Statement for Racial Justice in Sexuality Education to address the history of racial injustices in the field of sexuality education. In this statement, professionals were charged to address and undo racism on professional and institutional levels within the field of sexuality education so we can move forward toward racial justice. Part of this includes realizing that not all curriculums work for all races and that Black girls are worthy of sex-positive, affirming, culturally relevant sexuality education curricula.

Components of Comprehensive Sexuality Education for Black Women and Girls

The most important part of developing a CSE curriculum is focusing on what Black women and girls desire to learn more about. For example, Black women and girls in the Get Smart B4 U Get Sexy intervention and prevention resource program desired sexuality education topics and trainings that included exploration of queer culture, self-advocacy, body image, and self-love (Brinkman et al. 2019; LeMaistre 2022). In addition, they wanted opportunities to learn about the effects of mainstream media expectations and beauty ideals on Black women's sexualities. Leaders of Get Smart B4 You Get Sexy also highlight that community collaborations and building upon the leadership within government or community departments that focus on youth may be the best way to create a cycle of education.

In a systematic literature review on Black women's sexual health interventions, researchers found that most interventions only included individual-level assets such as lessons on ethnic and cultural pride and empowerment (Ware, Thorpe, and Tanner 2019). These interventions provided sessions and modules that allowed the participants to engage in culturally relevant activities (e.g., African rites of passage), incorporated the achievements of Black women, identified Black women role models, empowered Black sexuality, and provided feedback on how to achieve goals set by the women. Community-level assets focused on religious cohesion and social networks in prevention efforts (Ware, Thorpe, and Tanner 2019).

Researchers emphasize that focusing on individual-level assets is not enough, and there must be a focus on protective factors such as the resilience and collectivism of Black women and communities (Ware, Thorpe, and Tanner 2019). CSE should also recognize and embrace queer bodies and relationships, and ethically nonmonogamous relationship structures. Currently, discussion of lesbian, gay, bisexual, transgender, and queer or questioning (LGBTQ) identities varies based on states, political structures, and communities. Given what we know about how sexuality education has been taught in schools, there have been systematic and ongoing ways in which individuals, communities, and sexualities have been othered. CSE has the opportunity to embrace queer Black girls and acknowledge the contributions of queer Black women in the field of sexuality education.

Beyond the lessons in and approaches to interventions, developers must think critically about the theoretical and social justice underpinnings of their curricula. CSE curricula for Black women should be rooted in intersectionality, reproductive justice, and social justice. Due to the unique experiences of Black women, girls, and femmes living in the United States, intersectionality is an appropriate way to frame their experiences. Given the history of violence, injustice, and reproductive trauma and coercion in the United States, the reproductive justice framework argues that people must examine the sociocultural contexts in which Black women make reproductive health decisions including the right to have or not have children and to parent children in safe and sustainable communities (SisterSong 2022; Ross et al. 2016).

Reproductive justice principles are very important for Black women and girls because their challenges and cultures were not considered when older forms of sex education were created. In addition, because of the previously mentioned dark history of racism in sexuality education, CSE must be rooted in racial and social justice. Using asset-based approaches for Black women and girls, addressing systems of oppression that are a detriment to their sexual health, increasing access to care, and ensuring that Black bodies are represented in textbooks and curricula are keys to advocating for racial and social justice.

In a review of anatomical images in eight collegiate human sexuality textbooks, only 1.1% represented dark skin tones while 83.5% represented light skin tones. Skin colors commonly associated with Black people were underrepresented compared to skin tones associated with white or white-presenting people, which comprised 42.3% of anatomical images (Rosenstock Gonzalez, Williams, and Herbenick 2022). Historically, images of Black bodies have been used to model surgeries, experimentations, and STIs. Black women and girls deserve to see their bodies represented in positive ways; therefore, medical illustrations of Black bodies are needed.

Although components, approaches, and frameworks are critical to the advancement of CSE for Black women and girls, one of the most important aspects is that the curriculum is taught by other Black women and femmes. For decades, the voices of Black sexuality educators have been silenced by society and by their white peers. However, Black women sexual health educators tend to utilize intersectional frameworks and have a shared understanding of historical experiences of oppression and culture that allows them to combine their personal experiences with their professional expertise to be the ideal educator to build rapport and meaningful relationships with other Black women and girls. In addition, they are more empowered and aware of how to adapt evidence-based curricula that resonate with Black women and girls more clearly (Flowers 2018). Hiring Black women educators is essential to moving the field of sexuality education forward and creating meaningful experiences and safer spaces for Black women to learn about their sexuality and sexual health.

SEX RESEARCH FOR BLACK WOMEN: FROM DATA TO EDUCATION
Why Is It Important That We Have These Data?

Sexuality research and educational materials tend to be focused on the experiences of majority populations (i.e., white experiences), with the exception of adverse sexual and reproductive health outcomes. These data and messages often center the sexual lives of minority populations, with an emphasis on Black adolescents and adult women. Sex research on Black women often focuses on identifying what types of sexual behaviors they are engaging in, promoting messages of sexual risk and the prevention of health-related outcomes (e.g., unintended pregnancy, STIs, and HIV), and investigating health disparities that exist between Black women and other racial/ethnic groups. This view of Black women and their sexual lives is problematic for various reasons:

1. It perpetuates negative stereotypes and myths about Black sexuality (Wyatt 1982; Stephens and Phillips 2003; Staples 2006; Rosenthal and Lobel 2016).
2. It exacerbates stigma and discrimination (Cunningham et al. 2002).
3. It fails to highlight pleasure, intimacy, and other aspects of sexuality (Hargons et al. 2018).

In general, the imagery and depiction of Black women in mainstream media and early research brought on a portrayal of Black women that impacts the way Black women are viewed by society, how Black women view themselves, and Black women's sexual behaviors and experiences.

Early Sex-Positive Research for Black Women

The earliest evidence of sex research on Black women was conducted by Alfred Kinsey and his colleagues (1953); however, the data were excluded from analyses in *Sexual Behavior in the Human Female* due to the small sample size. The analyses also excluded women with a history of being incarcerated in prison. The subsequent analysis among Black women presented statistics about their sexual experiences, including age of sexual debut, number and characteristics of partners, prevalence of sexual behaviors, views and attitudes toward sex, use of contraceptives, and reported sexual abuse during childhood. While informative, especially for the time period, much of that research was compared to data from the white women in the original report and had several data limitations. The Kinsey study was prefaced as an exploratory sexuality survey among all Americans and reported the data as such; however, the vast majority of interviewees were middle-class and college-educated.

Furthermore, the study did not use random or probability sampling and, whether intended or unintended, led to a misguided view of Black sexuality. Subsequent studies investigating the sexual experiences of Black women (and adolescents) since the Kinsey study have sought to provide sexual behavior prevalence and trend updates; however, most have been comparative in nature—to white women or to a previous time period (Wyatt, Peters, and Guthrie 1988). Moreover, the data are reflective of Black women from clinic-, college-, or community-based samples rather than probability samples. It therefore provides a limited scope to understand Black women, especially as it relates to the cultural and social factors that impact their sexual lives. As a result, the majority of sex research portrays Black women as being sexually experienced or as having engaged in sexual risk-taking behaviors rather than being sexually responsible or having sexual autonomy.

Looking Ahead: Sex-Positive Research for Black Women

Sexuality research and education should present a holistic view of Black women's experiences. These are the data that Black women want and need so that they feel seen, heard, and represented. While there has been a shift toward promoting sexual exploration, knowledge, and sexual agency among Black women, there is a significant need for more sex-positive research. The data should encompass all aspects of sexual and reproductive experiences from pain to pleasure, including both qualitative and quantitative studies that capture the joys and sorrows of Black womanhood. The research should embrace and communicate the lived experiences that will drive sexuality education, policy, and clinical practice. When sex-positive research is made available, comprehensive sexuality educators are better equipped to educate and support Black women. Moving from theory to practice involves both researchers and educators.

SEX-POSITIVE AND CULTURALLY RELEVANT SEXUALITY EDUCATION

What Does It Look Like and Who Teaches It?

The Professional Learning Standards for Sex Education were developed and released in 2018 by the Sex Education Collaborative (SEC; 2018), a collaboration of 20 national, regional, and state-based organizations with extensive experience training educators to deliver school-based sex education. However, there remained significant gaps in quality of sex education that youth of color received. In 2020, members of the SEC formed the Racial Justice and Equity Task Team, and later released Centering Racial Justice in Sex Education: Strategies for Engaging Professionals and Young People (Dixon et al. 2021). The authors provided suggested content for racially just sex education, qualities of racially just sex educators, administrative and management practices that support sex educators of color, and measurement and evaluation practices to enhance sex education for youth of color. The strategies and guidelines were developed with the perspective and expertise of Black and Brown sex educators, with the intent to give Black and Brown youth opportunities to learn about sexuality that speak to their lived experiences and offer guidance to celebrate youth of color.

Are There Any Curricula Available?

There is a significant gap in the availability of sexuality textbooks or curricula developed specifically for Black women. The Resiliency in Sexuality Education Model consists of six practical steps to develop a curriculum for Black women (R. Davis Moss, PhD, MPH, A. Townes, PhD, and D. I. Brown, MEd, written communication, March 31, 2021):

1. Check yourself: The first step involves cultural humility. It is important to recognize one's biases when aiming to provide ethical and competent sexuality education. Sex educators must work toward shifting their thoughts and biases to respect and understanding.
2. Check with the community: The second step is engagement. Acknowledge that experts need to be brought to the table when developing a curriculum, and meaningful community involvement is necessary. Asking the community for input and feedback is a great way to engage the target population.
3. Incorporate the community: The third step is inclusion. Once the community is engaged, outreach and inclusion of Black sexuality researchers and educators is paramount. Incorporate their experiences and expertise. Find and reference Black authored publications using the principles of the Cite Black Women Critical Praxis (Smith et al. 2021).
4. Highlight the community: The fourth step is representation. Funding to support development and implementation should include hiring Black women in various capacities (e.g., educators, researchers, evaluators). Utilize community members for implementation and support.
5. Address and honor subcultures: The fifth step is understanding micro-communities within communities. Acknowledge that Black women are not monolithic, and, therefore, it is important to understand the needs of the specific community being served and who will be facilitating the curriculum.
6. Be authentic: The last step is recognizing that who you are matters. Being a change agent does not mean individuals (including you) need to change who you are to meet the needs of the community. Change happens when integrity and honesty are embedded in the work.

Following are additional suggestions:

- Make a list of Black-authored publications.
- Read Black women's work.

- Attend presentations by Black sex educators and researchers.
- Incorporate sex-positive images and illustrations of Black women.
- Seek personal and professional development opportunities.

REFERENCES

American Public Health Association. Sexuality education as part of a comprehensive health education program in K to 12 schools. Policy number: 20143. November 18, 2014. Available at: https://www.apha.org/policies-and-advocacy/public-health-policy-statements/policy-database/2015/01/23/09/37/sexuality-education-as-part-of-a-comprehensive-health-education-program-in-k-to-12-schools

Brinkman BG, Garth J, Horowitz KR, Marino S, Lockwood KN. Black girls and sexuality education: Access. Equity. Justice. Black Girls Equity Alliance. 2019. Available at: https://www.gwensgirls.org/wp-content/uploads/2019/10/BGEA-Report2_v4.pdf

Centers for Disease Control and Prevention. HIV Surveillance Report, vol. 33, 2020. May 2022. Available at: https://www.cdc.gov/hiv/library/reports/hiv-surveillance.html

Centers for Disease Control and Prevention. How STDs impact women differently from men. Available at: https://www.cdc.gov/nchhstp/newsroom/docs/factsheets/STDs-Women.pdf

Centers for Disease Control and Prevention. National overview of STDs. 2020. Available at: https://stacks.cdc.gov/view/cdc/125947/cdc_125947_DS1.pdf

Collins PH. *Black Feminist Thought: Knowledge, Consciousness, and the Politics of Empowerment.* New York, NY: Routledge; 2022.

Cunningham SD, Tschann J, Gurvey JE, Fortenberry JD, Ellen JM. Attitudes about sexual disclosure and perceptions of stigma and shame. *Sex Transm Infect.* 2002;78(5):334–338. https://doi.org/10.1136/sti.78.5.334

Dixon R, Gilbert T, Soto M, Gathings J, DiPonio S. Centering racial justice in sex education: strategies for engaging professionals and young people. White paper. Sex Education Collaborative. 2021.

Elia J, Tokunaga J. Sexuality education: implications for health, equity, and social justice in the United States. *Health Educ.* 2015;115(1):105–120. https://doi.org/10.1108/HE-01-2014-0001

Fields J. "Children having children": race, innocence, and sexuality education. *Soc Problems.* 2005;52(4):549–571. https://doi.org/10.1525/sp.2005.52.4.549

Flowers SC. Enacting our multidimensional power: Black women sex educators demonstrate the value of an intersectional sexuality education framework. *Meridians.* 2018;16(2):308–325. https://doi.org/10.2979/meridians.16.2.11

Habersham R. Beyond the basics: why Black girls need comprehensive sex ed. For Harriet. May 21, 2015. Available at: http://www.forharriet.com/2015/05/beyond-basics-why-black-girls-need.html

Hargons CN, Mosley DV, Meiller C, et al. "It feels so good": pleasure in last sexual encounter narratives of Black university students. *J Black Psychol.* 2018;44(2):103–127. https://doi.org/10.1177/0095798417749400

Kinsey AC, Pomeroy WB, Martin CE, Gebhard PH. *Sexual Behavior in the Human Female.* Philadelphia, PA: W.B. Saunders; 1953.

Kohler PK, Manhart LE, Lafferty WE. Abstinence-only and comprehensive sex education and the initiation of sexual activity and teen pregnancy. *J Adolesc Health.* 2008;42(4):344–351. https://doi.org/10.1016/j.jadohealth.2007.08.026

Lamb S, Roberts T, Plocha A. *Girls of Color, Sexuality, and Sex Education.* New York, NY: Springer; 2016.

LeMaistre V. BWWLA: Centering reproductive justice in sex ed. Planned Parenthood. March 21, 2022. Available at: https://www.plannedparenthood.org/blog/bwwla-centering-reproductive-justice-in-sex-ed

Perry G. *Risky Lessons: Sex Education and Social Inequality* (review). *Feminist Teacher.* 2011;21(2):164–165. Available at: https://www.muse.jhu.edu/article/462007

Rabbitte M, Enriquez M. The role of policy on sexual health education in schools: review. *J Sch Nurs.* 2018;35(1):27–38. https://doi.org/10.1177/1059840518789240

Rose T. *Longing to Tell: Black Women Talk About Sexuality and Intimacy.* New York, NY: Farrar, Straus, and Giroux; 2004.

Rosenstock Gonzalez YR, Williams D, Herbenick D. Skin color and skin tone diversity in human sexuality textbook anatomical diagrams. *J Sex Marital Ther.* 2022;48(3):285–294. https://doi.org/10.1080/0092623X.2021.1989533

Rosenthal L, Lobel M. Stereotypes of Black American women related to sexuality and motherhood. *Psychol Women Q.* 2016;40(3):414–427. https://doi.org/10.1177/0361684315627459

Ross L, Gutierrez E, Gerber M, Silliman J. *Undivided Rights: Women of Color Organizing for Reproductive Justice.* Chicago, IL: Haymarket Books; 2016.

Sex Education Collaborative. Professional learning standards for sex education. 2018. Available at: https://siecus.org/resources/professional-learning-standards-for-sex-education

SisterSong. What is reproductive justice? 2022. Available at: https://www.sistersong.net/reproductive-justice

Smith CA, Williams EL, Wadud IA, Pirtle WN, Cite Black Women Collective. Cite Black women: a critical praxis (a statement). *Feminist Anthropol.* 2021;2(1):10–17. https://doi.org/10.1002/fea2.12040

Staples R. *Exploring Black Sexuality.* Oxford, UK: Rowman and Littlefield Publishers; 2006.

Stephens DP, Phillips LD. Freaks, gold diggers, divas, and dykes: the sociohistorical development of adolescent African American women's sexual scripts. *Sex Cult.* 2003;7(1):3–49. https://psycnet.apa.org/doi/10.1007/BF03159848

Ware S, Thorpe S, Tanner AE. Sexual health interventions for Black women in the United States: a systematic review of literature. *Int J Sex Health.* 2019;31(2):196–215. https://doi.org/10.1080/19317611.2019.1613278

Women of Color Sexual Health Network. Solidarity statement on racial justice in sexuality education. Delivered at: 2014 National Sex Ed Conference. 2014. Available at: https://sexedconference.com/solidarity-statement-on-racial-justice-in-sexuality-education

Wyatt GE. Identifying stereotypes of Afro-American sexuality and their impact upon sexual behavior. In: Bass BA, Wyatt GE, Powell GJ, eds. *The Afro-American Family: Assessment, Treatment, and Research Issues.* New York, NY: Grune and Stratton; 1982:333–346.

Wyatt GE, Peters SD, Guthrie D. Kinsey revisited, part II: comparisons of the sexual socialization and sexual behavior of Black women over 33 years. *Arch Sex Behav.* 1988;17(4):289–332. https://doi.org/10.1007/BF01541810

26

A Lifespan Approach to Black Women's Mental Health and Sexuality: Kellye's Story

Kisha B. Holden, PhD, MSCR, Sharon Rachel, MA, MPH, Rhonda Reid, MD, Allyson S. Belton, MPH, and Folashade Omole, MD

Mental health, like sexual health, is a lifelong process. Mental health is indispensable to personal well-being and is defined as "a state of successful performance of mental function, resulting in productive activities, fulfilling relationships with other people, and the ability to adapt to change and cope with adversity" (US Department of Health and Human Services [HHS] 1999, p. 4). In general, Black women are disproportionately exposed to stressors across multiple domains that adversely affect their mental health (Holden et al. 2012). These stressors may include racism, gender discrimination, and stressful or traumatic life events and can lead to detrimental health behaviors and outcomes such as lack of help seeking and poor treatment adherence (Sporinova et al. 2019; Lake 2017). Mental health is inextricably linked to physical and sexual health. At each stage of the lifespan, Black women's experiences can be affirming of or harmful to sexual health.

This chapter covers some of what is understood about sexual and reproductive attitudes, behaviors, and well-being in Black girls and women. It takes us on a journey with "Kellye" through the stages of her life, beginning in pre-adolescence and continuing through old age. It follows her sexual development and explores the mental health implications associated with different life stages: childhood and adolescence, late adolescence and early adulthood, middle adulthood, and older adulthood.

CHILDHOOD AND ADOLESCENCE

Kellye struggled with self-esteem in middle school and high school. Health and physical education classes at her predominantly white school were not culturally competent and made no mention of any developmental differences and disparities between white people and people of color. Kellye first got her period when she was in the fifth grade. She did not feel comfortable talking to her friends about it, even when they started getting their periods in the sixth grade. By the time she was 13, Kellye was taller than most of her peers, had fully developed breasts and hips, and was often mistaken for someone much older. The unwanted attention she got from well-meaning adults ("You're putting on weight in all the right places!"), strangers on the street ("Baby, you fine!"), and kids at her school giggling when they saw her made her feel ashamed of her body. Looking at images of beautiful women on Instagram made her feel even worse, and she buried her feelings in food. As an overweight adolescent, Kellye found herself feeling extreme emotions of anger and sadness, particularly in the days leading up to her period, making it difficult for her to concentrate on school. She longed to have a "normal" body like her peers and felt like if she fit in better, she would not have so many problems.

Identity

Establishing identity is an important part of adolescence. Adolescents often struggle with self-esteem and feeling accepted by their peers. Black girls who believe that their bodies are different from their peers' bodies are more likely to engage in maladaptive behaviors such as arguing with adults, defying behavioral expectations, and intentionally provoking others (Carter et al. 2011). Research has also found associations between body surveillance—preoccupation with physical appearance and attractiveness—and depression and hostility in Black girls (Butkowski, Dixon, and Weeks 2019; Grower, Ward, and Rowley 2021). A Black girl at a predominantly white school may also have to navigate through peer groups that have yet to develop an appreciation for cultural diversity. This may exacerbate anxieties over belonging, lead to feelings of shame and insecurity, and cause schoolwork to suffer (Bécares and Priest 2015).

Puberty and Physical Development

Black girls tend to reach developmental milestones earlier than girls of other racial and ethnic backgrounds. Generally, growth of reproductive organs in girls starts with breast development (thelarche) around age 9 and continues with onset of menstrual periods (menarche) at approximately age 11. Over the past several decades, however, the age of thelarche has decreased for all ethnic groups (Aksglaede et al. 2009), with Black girls experiencing an earlier age of thelarche compared to other groups (Biro et al. 2013). The age of menarche has also been decreasing across demographic groups, with increased body mass index, food insecurity, and exposure to stressors and trauma commonly associated with this phenomenon. Girls of color have been found to have the most prominent changes (Krieger et al. 2015; Burris and Wiley 2021; Stenson et al. 2021).

While sexual education starts as early as elementary school in some states, there are marked disparities in access, timing, and content (Goldfarb and Lieberman 2021, Lindberg and Kantor 2022). Many states' sexual education curricula are not required to be medically accurate or culturally appropriate, often addressing sexuality solely through a white, cisgender, heterosexual lens (Sexuality Information and Education Council of the United States [SIECUS] 2020). At the same time, earlier development may also account for premature socialization of Black girls, a phenomenon known as adultification in which Black girls are overly sexualized and perceived as maturing at a faster rate (e.g., Epstein, Blake, and González 2017). Sexual objectification of Black girls can range from lewd comments and harassment to sexual assault, and has been associated with psychological distress, anxiety, and disordered eating among those targeted by objectification (Watson et al. 2012; University of Southern California 2009). It has also been demonstrated that Black girls are often dismissed by authority figures when they bring forth harassment concerns at school (Wilmot, Migliarini, and Ancy Annamma 2021).

LATE ADOLESCENCE/EARLY ADULTHOOD

Kellye's family moved when she was in her second year of high school. Her new school was very diverse, Kellye had more peers who looked like her, and she finally felt like she fit in more. She found a close set of friends and became involved in a mentoring program. Kellye's pediatrician, Dr. Jackson, referred her to the practice's embedded licensed clinical psychologist who diagnosed her with premenstrual dysphoric disorder, or PMDD, which got Kellye connected with the right treatment. Dr. Jackson also referred Kellye to an endocrinologist who diagnosed her with polycystic ovary syndrome, or PCOS, which had been partially responsible for her difficulties controlling her weight. Once she had her physical and mental health under control, Kellye thrived in her new environment. However, the stresses of young adulthood remained ever present. Kellye's best friend came out as nonbinary, and their mental health suffered as they felt rejected by their family and faith community. Another close friend became pregnant because her boyfriend refused to use a condom, and Kellye supported her as she agonized over whether or not to continue the pregnancy. When Kellye was 26 and out of college, her family began asking her when she was planning on getting married and having children. Kellye wondered the same thing herself.

Reproductive Health

In addition to early puberty and social stressors contributing to mental health concerns, there are also reproductive disorders that include mental health symptomatology. For instance, PCOS is a hormonal disorder characterized by irregular periods, development of cysts (fluid-filled sacs) on the ovaries, and weight gain, and is highly associated with depression and anxiety during the lifespan (Cooney et al. 2017; Greenwood et al. 2019). PMDD is another mental health concern in which women and girls experience predictable shifts in mood in accordance with their menstrual cycles (Mayo Clinic 2020). Few studies have investigated racial disparities in mental health symptoms related to PCOS, and results have been mixed. One study found no difference in depression scores and lower anxiety symptoms among Black female participants with PCOS (Alur-Gupta et al. 2021), while another found increased depressive symptoms in Black women compared with white women (Greenwood et al. 2019).

Sexual Orientation and Gender Identity

When considering mental health symptomology among sexual minority youth (SMY)—youth who identify as lesbian, gay, bisexual, transgender, queer, etc.—multiple studies have found that SMY are more likely to report depression, suicidal ideation, and self-injury behaviors compared to heterosexual individuals (e.g., Bostwick et al. 2014; Fox et al.

2020) and more likely to report being bullied compared to their heterosexual counterparts (Fox et al. 2020; Webb et al. 2021). With regard to behaviors, one study found that Black SMY have higher rates of risky sexual behavior and exposure to physical and sexual violence compared to white heterosexual youth (Gattamorta, Salerno, and Castro 2019). A study investigating behaviors of Black youth found that sexual minority females were more likely to use substances before sex, to have a higher number of oral sex partners, and to expect negative consequences from engaging in safe sex discussions compared to their heterosexual female counterparts (Norris et al. 2019). Another study found that Black and Latina females who identified as bisexual or "unsure" had a decreased likelihood of condom and contraceptive use compared to those who identified as heterosexual (Pollitt and Mallory 2021).

Some studies have explored ways to protect against traumatic events or development of mental health symptoms. For example, healthy relationships may act as a protective factor for SMY. In one study of SMY between the ages of 16 and 20 years, Black individuals who identified as gay or lesbian who were in romantic partnerships were less likely to report mental health symptoms compared to white gay or lesbian individuals in partnerships (Whitton et al. 2018). Resilience and spirituality may also protect against symptoms of depression in African American adolescents (Freeny et al. 2021). Parental control has also been hypothesized to be preventive of future instances of interpersonal violence among adolescents, but this was not observed in African American families (East and Hokoda 2015).

Adolescent Pregnancy

While adolescent birth rates have been steadily declining from their peak in 1991, there are still marked racial disparities. Moreover, research shows strong associations between adolescent pregnancy and poor mental health outcomes, both concurrent with the pregnancy and later in life. Patel and Sen (2012) also suggested that not only can adolescent pregnancy lead to poor mental health outcomes but so can the conditions and factors that lead to adolescent pregnancy. For example, adverse childhood experiences (ACEs) are traumatic events that occur in childhood, including witnessing or experiencing violence or living in a household with the presence of mental health and substance use disorders (Felitti et al. 1998). ACEs are associated with negative health outcomes, and numerous studies have shown that ethnic minorities experience an increased number of ACEs compared to their white counterparts (e.g., López et al. 2017; Zhang and Monnat 2021). Research has found that Black adolescents and young adults also experience more interpersonal violence compared to their white counterparts (Min et al. 2021). Sexual trauma has been linked to multiple poor mental health outcomes (Chen et al. 2010) as well as sexual risk behaviors (Senn, Carey, and Vanable 2008; Hill et al. 2018).

MIDDLE ADULTHOOD

Kellye met Wes on a dating app when she was 39 and the two quickly became serious. A year into their relationship, Kellye discovered she was pregnant. While the pregnancy came as a surprise, Kellye and Wes were overjoyed at the thought of becoming parents. At her 11-week ultrasound, however, it was discovered that the baby had a severe deformity, and a week later she lost the pregnancy. Though her doctor assured Kellye that she had done nothing wrong, Kellye blamed herself for the loss of her baby and became severely depressed. With the help of individual and couples counseling, Kellye and Wes eventually found themselves ready to try to conceive again and a year later welcomed a baby girl that they named Maya. As a new mom, Kellye experienced an array of emotions ranging from elation to exhaustion. She figured this emotional roller coaster was normal, but Maya's pediatrician screened Kellye positive for postpartum depression at one of their well-baby visits. With few mental health professionals—particularly African Americans—where Kellye and Wes now lived, Kellye struggled to get the help she needed from a provider with whom she felt comfortable.

Pregnancy and Motherhood

Mental, emotional, and behavioral health issues are significant for women during pregnancy and motherhood at any phase of life. Lucas et al. (2019) conducted a study that indicated that younger adolescent mothers face mental health challenges during and after pregnancy, including increased rates of depression compared to older mothers. While the prevention of adolescent pregnancy in countries such as the United States and the United Kingdom has been a focus for policy and research in recent decades, the need to understand young women's own experiences was highlighted in a meta-ethnography. During middle adulthood, pressures related to professional and career interests that may intersect with family expectations, risks for chronic health conditions, and competing life demands are realities. Generally, it is extremely important that women embrace social support and approaches to access to mental health care if needed.

Sexuality and Mental Health in Midlife

In a study conducted with midlife women, it was indicated that sexuality incorporated women's desires, appearance, sexual feelings, and expression, and four concerns were indicated centered on (1) the changing body, (2) meeting the needs of others, (3) loneliness, and (4) effectively communicating sexual interests and needs (Reed et al. 2022; Kralik, Koch, and Telford 2001). In another study about personal conceptions of sexuality and mental health realities among women aged 30 to 60 years living with a chronic medical condition, it was proposed that constructions of sexuality encompassed physical sexual responses, perceptions of appearance and attractiveness to self and others, self-image, and self-esteem. In addition, this study revealed that, often, sexual activity was placed on hold as other aspects of living with a chronic illness intervened and enumerated a close relationship to shifts in self and identity (Schick et al. 2010; Koch, Kralik, and Eastwood 2002). Utilizing a feminist framework, a qualitative study of women suggested that understanding the nexus of sexuality and emotional well-being, particularly during midlife, was critical (Davidson and Huntington 2010).

Sexual health problems common in middle-aged women have the potential to affect all aspects of their lives. These issues can include diminished or lack of desire for sex, difficulty with arousal and sexual pleasure, inability to orgasm, and pain with sex. Causes of sexual health issues can be complex and multifaceted; therefore, a holistic perspective, in which all potential factors are considered, is warranted. Despite the prevalence of women's sexual health issues, discussion by providers is often absent or limited to avoidance of sexually transmitted infections (STIs) or unwanted pregnancies (Zielinski 2013). Sexual health issues may be further exacerbated among midlife women that may not be facing pregnancy or STI-related issues. Thus, there is a need for health care professionals and providers to account for psychosocial and sociocultural influences from a holistic and comprehensive perspective.

OLDER ADULTHOOD

After finally identifying a counselor that was a good fit for both Kellye and Wes as individuals and as a couple, they were able to address their issues. Though they had been a couple for several years and were raising a daughter together, Kellye and Wes eventually decided to "make it official" and get married. At 45, Kellye reflected on having found balance in her life. She was pursuing an exciting career and had grown as a professional. Despite being diagnosed with diabetes in her early 50s and learning to navigate through living with a chronic condition, she felt like she was where she wanted to be physically, emotionally, and spiritually. As Maya grew up, Kellye noticed both similarities and differences between her and her daughter's experiences as a child and adolescent. Though she was now well into her 50s, Kellye felt like it was not that long ago that she was an insecure fifth grader and then a "typical teenager." Shortly after Kellye turned 60, she and Wes became "empty nesters" when they sent Maya off to college out of state. However, after enjoying a year and a half of empty nest life, Wes tragically died of a heart attack at age 62. With her husband gone and her daughter away, Kellye struggled with grief. As her counselor from decades ago had long since retired, Kellye again found herself struggling to find a mental health provider. She engaged with a psychiatrist who recommended pharmacotherapy. Though reluctant to use medications at first due to potential side effects from her diabetes medication, Kellye noticed a marked improvement in her mental health. She also had a strong social support network through her friends, a diverse assortment of married, divorced, and other widowed women. Three years after Wes passed away, Kellye met Steven and learned what it was like to date later in life.

Bodily Changes

Older adulthood is a life phase characterized by several unique developmental transitions that are relevant for experiencing one's sexuality (Infurna, Gerstorf, and Lachman 2020). For example, the menopausal transition may constitute a challenge for sexual functioning (Avis et al. 2017). In a similar vein, late midlife is assumed to be the period of life of increasing risks of health problems (e.g., disease onset), and poor health has been repeatedly shown to be related to poor sexual functioning among adults aged 50 years and older (Lee et al. 2016). On the other hand, sexuality remains for many adults a valuable aspect of life until old age, and a fulfilling sex life in older age is linked with indicators of successful aging (Buczak-Stec, König, and Hajek 2019; Štulhofer et al. 2018).

Sexuality is lifelong. Older adulthood sexuality is a central aspect of being human. Studies have shown that sexuality extends well into the ninth decade of life. However, menopause and other aging chronic diseases such as dementia and arthritis may limit sexual desire (Omole et al. 2014). Low estrogen in the later years results in vaginal mucosa thinning and dryness, resulting in vaginal irritation during sexual activity. The expression of sexuality is not always penetrative; it can be through touch and stimulation (National Institute on Aging 2022). Simultaneously, it is important to remember that the elderly are not exempt from contracting HIV and other STIs (HHS, Office on Women's Health 2021).

CONCLUSION

Mental health, like sexual health, is indeed a lifelong journey. Kellye's story takes us through some of the interwoven mental health and sexual health issues experienced by some Black girls and women across the lifespan. External influences such as peers, family, and media are important factors that can enhance or harm mental health. Understanding sexual health through a culturally competent lens is critical for children, adolescents, and young adults to develop positive attitudes about themselves and grow into mentally and sexually healthy adults.

Unfortunately, our society sends many negative messages about Black women's sexuality, resulting in disparities in both mental and sexual health. More research is needed to understand causes for earlier physical development in Black girls, given the psychological and social impact of early puberty. Education regarding physical development, recognition and identification of mental health symptoms, and promotion of sexual health strategies may also be a source of empowerment. More research is also needed to understand the effects of trauma on Black adolescent girls, as well as potential clinical, familial, and community-based strategies to mitigate the risk of developing psychological symptoms.

REFERENCES

Aksglaede L, Sørensen K, Petersen JH, Skakkebaek NE, Juul A. Recent decline in age at breast development: the Copenhagen puberty study. *Pediatrics.* 2009;123(5):e932–e939. https://doi.org/10.1542/peds.2008-2491

Alur-Gupta S, Lee I, Chemerinski A, et al. Racial differences in anxiety, depression, and quality of life in women with polycystic ovary syndrome. *F S Rep.* 2021;2(2):230–237. https://doi.org/10.1016/j.xfre.2021.03.003

Avis NE, Colvin A, Karlamangla AS, et al. Change in sexual functioning over the menopausal transition. *Menopause.* 2017;24(4):379-390. https://doi.org/10.1097/gme.0000000000000770

Bécares L, Priest N. Understanding the influence of race/ethnicity, gender, and class on inequalities in academic and non-academic outcomes among eighth-grade students: findings from an intersectionality approach. *PLoS One.* 2015;10(10):e0141363. https://doi.org/10.1371/journal.pone.0141363

Biro FM, Greenspan LC, Galvez MP, et al. Onset of breast development in a longitudinal cohort. *Pediatrics.* 2013;132(6):1019-1027. https://doi.org/10.1542/peds.2012-3773

Bostwick WB, Meyer I, Aranda F, et al. Mental health and suicidality among racially/ethnically diverse sexual minority youths. *Am J Public Health.* 2014;104(6):1129-1136. https://doi.org/10.2105/AJPH.2013.301749

Buczak-Stec E, König H-H, Hajek A. The link between sexual satisfaction and subjective well-being: a longitudinal perspective based on the German Ageing Survey. *Qual Life Res.* 2019;28(11):3025-3035. https://doi.org/10.1007/s11136-019-02235-4

Burris ME, Wiley AS. Marginal food security predicts earlier age at menarche among girls from the 2009-2014 National Health and Nutrition Examination Surveys. *J Pediatr Adolesc Gynecol.* 2021;34(4):462-470. https://doi.org/10.1016/j.jpag.2021.03.010

Butkowski CP, Dixon TL, Weeks K. Body surveillance on Instagram: examining the role of selfie feedback investment in young adult women's body image concerns. *Sex Roles.* 2019;81(5-6):385-397. https://doi.org/10.1007/s11199-018-0993-6

Carter R, Caldwell CH, Matusko N, Antonucci T, Jackson JS. Ethnicity, perceived pubertal timing, externalizing behaviors, and depressive symptoms among Black adolescent girls. *J Youth Adolesc.* 2011;40(10):1394-1406. https://doi.org/10.1007/s10964-010-9611-9

Chen LP, Murad MH, Paras ML, et al. Sexual abuse and lifetime diagnosis of psychiatric disorders: systematic review and meta-analysis. *Mayo Clin Proc.* 2010;85(7):618-629. https://doi.org/10.4065/mcp.2009.0583

Cooney LG, Lee I, Sammel MD, Dokras A. High prevalence of moderate and severe depressive and anxiety symptoms in polycystic ovary syndrome: a systematic review and meta-analysis. *Hum Reprod.* 2017;32(5):1075-1091. https://doi.org/10.1093/humrep/dex044

Davison J, Huntington A. "Out of sight": sexuality and women with enduring mental illness. *Int J Ment Health Nurs.* 2010;19(4):240-249. https://doi.org/10.1111/j.1447-0349.2010.00676.x

East PL, Hokoda A. Risk and protective factors for sexual and dating violence victimization: a longitudinal, prospective study of Latino and African American adolescents. *J Youth Adolesc.* 2015;44(6):1200-1300. https://doi.org/10.1007/s10964-015-0273-5

Epstein R, Blake JJ, González T. *Girlhood Interrupted: The Erasure of Black Girls' Childhood.* Washington, DC: Georgetown University Law Center, Center on Poverty and Inequality; 2017:1-19.

Felitti VJ, Anda RF, Nordenberg D, et al. Relationship of childhood abuse and household dysfunction to many of the leading causes of death in adults. *Am J Prev Med.* 1998;14(4):245-258. https://doi.org/10.1016/s0749-3797(98)00017-8

Fox KR, Choukas-Bradley S, Salk RH, Marshal MP, Thoma BC. Mental health among sexual and gender minority adolescents: examining interactions with race and ethnicity. *J Consult Clin Psychol.* 2020;88(5):402-415. https://doi.org/10.1037/ccp0000486

Freeny J, Peskin M, Schick V, et al. Adverse childhood experiences, depression, resilience, & spirituality in African-American adolescents. *J Child Adolesc Trauma*. 2021;14(2):209–221. https://doi.org/10.1007/s40653-020-00335-9

Gattamorta KA, Salerno JP, Castro AJ. Intersectionality and health behaviors among US high school students: examining race/ethnicity, sexual identity, and sex. *J School Health*. 2019;89(10):800–808. https://doi.org/10.1111/josh.12817

Goldfarb ES, Lieberman LD. Three decades of research: the case for comprehensive sex education. *The J Adolesc Health*. 2021;68(1):13–27. https://doi.org/10.1016/j.jadohealth.2020.07.036

Greenwood EA, Yaffe K, Wellons MF, Cedars MI, Huddleston HG. Depression over the lifespan in a population-based cohort of women with polycystic ovary syndrome: longitudinal analysis. *J Clin Endocrinol Metab*. 2019;104(7):2809–2819. https://doi.org/10.1210/jc.2019-00234

Grower P, Ward LM, Rowley S. Beyond objectification: understanding the correlates and consequences of sexualization for Black and white adolescent girls. *J Res Adolesc*. 2021;31(2):273–281. https://doi.org/10.1111/jora.12598

Hill DC, Stein L, Rossi JS, Magill M, Clarke JG. Intimate violence as it relates to risky sexual behavior among at-risk females. *Psychol Trauma*. 2018;10(6):619–627. https://doi.org/10.1037/tra0000316

Holden KB, Hall SP, Robinson M, et al. Psychosocial and sociocultural correlates of depressive symptoms among diverse African American women. *J Natl Med Assoc*. 2012;104(11–12):493–504. https://doi.org/10.1016/S0027-9684(15)30215-7

Infurna FJ, Gerstorf D, Lachman ME. Midlife in the 2020s: opportunities and challenges. *Am Psychol*. 2020;75(4):470–485. https://doi.org/10.1037/amp0000591

Koch T, Kralik D, Eastwood S. Constructions of sexuality for women living with multiple sclerosis. *J Adv Nurs*. 2002;39(2):137–145. https://doi.org/10.1046/j.1365-2648.2002.02253.x

Kralik D, Koch T, Telford K. Constructions of sexuality for midlife women living with chronic illness. *J Adv Nurs*. 2001;35(2):180–187. https://doi.org/10.1046/j.1365-2648.2001.01835.x

Krieger N, Kiang MV, Kosheleva A, Waterman PD, Chen JT, Beckfield J. Age at menarche: 50-year socioeconomic trends among US-born Black and white women. *Am J Public Health*. 2015;105(2):388–397. https://doi.org/10.2105/AJPH.2014.301936

Lake J. Urgent need for improved mental health care and a more collaborative model of care. *Perm J*. 2017;21:17–024. https://doi.org/10.7812/TPP/17-024

Lee DM, Nazroo J, O'Connor DB, Blake M, Pendleton N. Sexual health and well-being among older men and women in England: findings from the English Longitudinal Study of Ageing. *Arch Sex Behav*. 2016;45(1):133–144. https://doi.org/10.1007/s10508-014-0465-1

Lindberg LD, Kantor LM. Adolescents' receipt of sex education in a nationally representative sample, 2011-2019. *J Adolesc Health*. 2022;70(2):290–297. https://doi.org/10.1016/j.jadohealth.2021.08.027

López CM, Andrews AR, Chisolm AM, de Arellano MA, Saunders B, Kilpatrick DG. Racial/ethnic differences in trauma exposure and mental health disorders in adolescents. *Cult Divers Ethn Minor Psychol*. 2017;23(3):382–387. https://doi.org/10.1037/cdp0000126

Lucas G, Olander EK, Ayers S. et al. No straight lines—young women's perceptions of their mental health and wellbeing during and after pregnancy: a systematic review and meta-ethnography. *BMC Womens Health*. 2019;19(1):152. https://doi.org/10.1186/s12905-019-0848-5

Mayo Clinic. Polycystic ovary syndrome (PCOS). *Symptoms and causes*. 2021. Available at: https://www.mayoclinic.org/diseases-conditions/pcos/symptoms-causes/syc-20353439

Min J, Faerber J, Skolnik A, Akers AY. Racial/ethnic disparities in female sexual health from adolescence to young adulthood: how adolescent characteristics matter? *J Pediatr Adolesc Gynecol*. 2021;34(3), 404–411. https://doi.org/10.1016/j.jpag.2020.11.005

National Institute on Aging. Sexuality and intimacy in older adults. April 18, 2022. Available at: https://www.nia.nih.gov/health/sexuality-and-intimacy-older-adults

Norris AL, Brown LK, DiClemente RJ, et al. African-American sexual minority adolescents and sexual health disparities: an exploratory cross-sectional study. *J Natl Med Assoc*. 2019;111(3):302–309. https://doi.org/10.1016/j.jnma.2018.11.001

Omole F, Fresh EM, Sow C, Lin J, Taiwo B, Nichols M. How to discuss sex with elderly patients. *J Fam Pract*. 2014;63(4):E1–E4.

Patel PH, Sen B. Teen motherhood and long-term health consequences. *Matern Child Health J*. 2012;16(5):1063–1071. https://doi.org/10.1007/s10995-011-0829-2

Pollitt AM, Mallory AB. Mental and sexual health disparities among bisexual and unsure Latino/a and Black sexual minority youth. *LGBT Health*. 2021;8(4):254–262. https://doi.org/10.1089/lgbt.2020.0374

Reed S, Carpenter J, Larson J, Mitchell C. Toward a better measure of midlife sexual function: pooled analyses in nearly 1,000 women participating in MsFLASH randomized trials. *Menopause*. 2022;29(4):397–407. https://doi.org/0.1097/GME.0000000000001940

Schick V, Herbenick D, Reece M, et al. Sexual behaviors, condom use, and sexual health of Americans over 50: implications for sexual health promotion for older adults. *J Sex Med*. 2010;7:315–329. https://doi.org/10.1111/j.1743-6109.2010.02013.x

Senn TE, Carey MP, Vanable PA. Childhood and adolescent sexual abuse and subsequent sexual risk behavior: evidence from controlled studies, methodological critique, and suggestions for research. *Clin Psychol Rev*. 2008;28(5):711–735. https://doi.org/10.1016/j.cpr.2007.10.002

SIECUS. Sex ed state law and policy chart. May 2020. Available at: https://siecus.org/wp-content/uploads/2020/05/SIECUS-2020-Sex-Ed-State-Law-and-Policy-Chart_May-2020-3.pdf

Sporinova B, Manns B, Tonelli M, et al. Association of mental health disorders with health care utilization and costs among adults with chronic disease. *JAMA Netw Open*. 2019;2(8):e199910. https://doi.org/10.1001/jamanetworkopen.2019.9910

Stenson AF, Michopoulos V, Stevens JS, Powers A, Jovanovic T. Sex-specific associations between trauma exposure, pubertal timing, and anxiety in Black children. *Front Hum Neurosci*. 2021;15:636199. https://doi.org/10.3389/fnhum.2021.636199

Štulhofer A, Hinchliff S, Jurin T, Carvalheira A, Træen B. Successful aging, change in sexual interest and sexual satisfaction in couples from four European countries. *Eur J Ageing*. 2018;16(2):155–165. https://doi.org/10.1007/s10433-018-0492-1

University of Southern California. Black girls are 50 percent more likely to be bulimic than white girls, study finds. *ScienceDaily*. March 25, 2009. Available at: https://www.sciencedaily.com/releases/2009/03/090318140532.htm

US Department of Health and Human Services. *Mental Health: A Report of the Surgeon General*. Rockville, MD: Substance Abuse and Mental Health Services Administration, National Institute of Mental Health; 1999.

US Department of Health and Human Services, Office on Women's Health. Menopause and sexuality. 2021. Available at: http://womenshealth.gov/menopause/menopause-and-sexuality

Watson LB, Robinson D, Dispenza F, Nazari N. African American women's sexual objectification experiences: a qualitative study. *Psychol Women Q.* 2012;36(4):458-475. https://doi.org/10.1177/0361684312454724

Webb L, Clary LK, Johnson RM, Mendelson T. Electronic and school bullying victimization by race/ethnicity and sexual minority status in a nationally representative adolescent sample. *J Adolesc Health.* 2021;68(2):378-384. https://doi.org/10.1016/j.jadohealth.2020.05.042

Whitton SW, Dyar C, Newcomb ME, Mustanski B. Romantic involvement: a protective factor for psychological health in racially-diverse young sexual minorities. *J Abnorm Psychol.* 2018;127(3):265-275. https://doi.org/10.1037/abn0000332

Wilmot JM, Migliarini V, Ancy Annamma S. Policy as punishment and distraction: the double helix of racialized sexual harassment of Black girls. *Educ Policy.* 2021;35(2):347-367. https://doi.org/10.1177/0895904820984467

Zhang X, Monnat SM. Racial/ethnic differences in clusters of adverse childhood experiences and associations with adolescent mental health. *SSM Popul Health.* 2021;17:100997. https://doi.org/10.1016/j.ssmph.2021.100997

Zielinski RE. Assessment of women's sexual health using a holistic, patient-centered approach. *J Midwifery Womens Health.* 2013;58:321-327. https://doi.org/10.1111/jmwh.12044

27

Well-Educated: Culturally Centered Sexual Wellness With and by Sex Educators

Davondra I. Brown, MEd, and Tiffany L. Reddick, MEd, LPC

While sex is intrinsically a natural process, the current nature of sex and sexuality is extremely complex. Due to socialization, religiosity, objectification, and many other societally imposed layers, most are not experiencing sexuality in a genuine, free, and pleasurable manner. Sexuality is a complicated and often unattended part of health and wellness practices, and with the multiple marginalizations of Black women, the lack of attention to such an important part of life has significant and far-reaching effects. Even the documented positive disparity that Black women report greater occurrence of having sexual health discussions with their health care provider than white women (Townes et al. 2020) is not rooted in positive intent. Black women have been associated with sexual risk taking, and their sexual lives are believed to be riddled with adverse sexual and reproductive health issues (Bond et al. 2021). Therefore, their reporting of more sexual health conversation is actually rooted in bias and a lack of cultural competence on the part of providers approaching the conversation from a disease prevention perspective instead of with a sexual wellness, pleasure and satisfaction, or personal decision-making lens.

Almost every modern healing practice functions within a medical model, which is to systematically isolate a problem and treat it accordingly. Preventive care, behavioral health, nutrition, and fitness are all rooted in separate frameworks and modalities that result in parts of the body and its functions being compartmentalized for that specific discipline. For example, an examination of the clitoris, an important body part in terms of sexual pleasure, is not usually included in a well-woman's examination and may only be conducted if the patient requests it (Aerts et al. 2018). Likewise, some sexual topics may be avoided during therapy as mental health has an uncomfortable history around sex, sexuality, and stigma, specifically among Black women and those who are not heterosexual. Even when attempts have been made to adjust, such as incorporating community health, interdisciplinary, or population health models, interventions have still failed to adequately affirm or address the sexual health of the Black female. A shift from health to *wellness* is needed.

Wellness incorporates pleasure, which is more than a mere sensory event, but, rather, conceptualized as a complex, multiform experience involving memory, motivation, homeostasis, and, sometimes, negative effects (Moccia et al. 2018). It is the positively supported processing of these factors that allows people to explore and define their own sexuality. With no well-known or well-accepted place to do so, people are at a sexual disadvantage. There is no health care doctrine that systematically integrates into current practice appropriate, accurate, and affirming sexual health information and certainly not any that is culturally aware enough to encompass the intersectionality of Black female sexuality. This chapter articulates the need for intentional patient-provider sexuality and sexual wellness education geared toward Black women and their heritage, allowing them to take control of their own sexual narrative and find more authentic ways to engage in their sexuality. The authors of this chapter honor all womanhood as intersectional. When using the term women, it is inclusive of all those who identify as women, femme, girls, and gender-expansive.

SOCIAL CONDITIONING, SEXUALITY, AND SHAME

There is a reason the nature-versus-nurture debate will never end. The two are inextricably intertwined into the core of who we are. From birth until the moment of our death, we are being influenced by millions of sexual messages. Not only are we bombarded with messages but we also create and hold our own sexual constructs and internalize how others perceive us. This socialization is how we become who we are, so why is it such an immense challenge to acknowledge and address it when it is related to sexuality?

The major issue is the absence of a foundational context to frame these messages, constructs to support positivity in sex or sexuality along the life cycle, and, subsequently, the education by sexual health professionals promoting that positivity. For instance, there are varying messages for pursuing a college education. Yet, in the debate of higher-educational attainment, there is mutual agreement that "learning" is positive, and what or how to learn is what is argued. However, with sexuality education, there seems to be no agreement on what is "positive" to learn or discuss at any age. For young children, there is very limited information that is considered age-appropriate and even less that is universally agreed upon. Among aging adults and elders, sex is considered something older people are not *supposed* to have and viewed with disgust. Sex for adults between ages 21 and 40 is only acceptable for reproductive and/or phallocentric purposes. There is no universal acceptance or promotion of healthy sexuality.

When there are neither consistent, positive messages nor cultural connectedness, it is human nature to create meaning from available sources. Qualitative analyses reveal that race-based sexual stereotypes may cause Black women to adopt more traditional gender stereotypes and be less likely to feel empowered in the sexual decision-making process (Bond et al. 2021). Research using objectification and social learning theories suggests Black women experience negative cognitions and harmful behaviors after exposure to a variety of objectifying experiences and media (Fredrickson and Roberts 1997). In westernized society, where many people of the African diaspora arrived through the mediums of white supremacy and chattel slavery, objectification perpetuates a dehumanized view of Black folks where personal value is primarily determined by their body parts' output. While gains have been made in political, social, and economic power, the capitalist-born, legislation-supported ideology of devaluing individuation persists, based on Black females' bodies being used by others and for what their parts produce. This belief system is perpetuated through media and misguided means of familial socialization, as they become internalized and projected by Black folks themselves (Leath and Mims 2021).

Social cognitive theory asserts that people can learn behaviors through repeated exposure via media (Fritz et al. 2021). Some studies find that digital media's overrepresentation of exaggerated, aggressive, and hypersexualized imagery featuring Black women impedes development of full expressions of healthy sexual selves (Benard 2016). The negative impact is compounded by Black women's consumption of media at higher rates than their peers of other races (Nielsen 2017). Therefore, objectification and socialization mimic the nature-versus-nurture conundrum when there is a missing context of positive sexual socialization.

As a result of socialized objectification, erroneous teachings of personal and communal protection through respectability dynamics as a survival mechanism to avoid white violence emerged, which was essentially assimilation. Assimilation inherently forces the denial of self, including any culturally indigenous beliefs, practices, or values. This survival mechanism is employed hoping to avoid harm, but unavoidably harming their relationship to the sexual self by not pursuing pleasure. This trauma-rooted experience often creates feelings of guilt and shame around the development of secondary sex characteristics, age-appropriate social interactions, and rites of passages such as crushes on peers, desire to wear makeup, and healthy sexual curiosity (Kendall 2021). The underlying theme of the body's urges as disrespectful, morally damning, unhealthy, and even dangerous stunts a healthy view of the sexual self from an early age and negatively impacts ability to experience pleasure, a significant component of sexual wellness (Nagoski 2015). Promoting sexual wellness through the pursuance and acceptance of pleasure, and not by avoiding harm, can assist Black women with developing their own concepts of sexuality.

LACK OF ACCESS TO ACCURATE SEXUAL WELLNESS EDUCATION

The study and practice of medicine, psychology, and most health professions continue to be largely rooted in a white, cisgendered, male normative perspective, despite the growing diversity in the United States. The focus on individual pathology and treatment ignores not only systemic influences on well-being but also any racial prejudice Black women may face from health care workers when engaging with the American health care system (Stallings 2018). When health care, patient education, and, by extension, delivery of sexuality-related health education is provided from this flawed frame of reference, consumers, particularly the most marginalized, are at a deficit. According to the Centers for Disease Control and Prevention, there is an increasing body of work on the disparity in health outcomes due to inequities in the American health care system (2021). Inaccessibility to quality, culturally affirming care and sexuality education leaves Black women hesitant to seek treatment and services to inform sex-related decisions and actions. This results in them ignoring their needs or accessing grossly inaccurate, harmful content without validated, individualized, positive context to analyze and apply it.

Thus, it is the responsibility of the health or healing provider (e.g., physician, therapist, nurse practitioner), to provide an environment where the patient or client feels comfortable asking sexuality-related questions and confident that they will receive unbiased, accurate information. As a part of provider preparation, engaging and establishing a relationship with a sex educator should be encouraged. The deep knowledge and experience provided by a certified sexuality educator creates a professional partnership that promotes and prioritizes a sexually healthier world (Coleman 2002). Furthermore, sexual wellness–related interventions have been found to be enriching, complementary, and compatible with many existing health-related interventions (Satcher, Hook, and Coleman 2015).

The field of sexology uplifts organizations such as the American Association of Sexuality Educators, Counselors, and Therapists and The Society for the Scientific Study of Sexuality as industry standards for the most professional and accurate information. However, both are much less notable in the public eye. Due to the lack of an established, widely used standard for sexuality education in the United States, misinformation is abundant and pervasive. People often use alternative and unqualified sources for information, turning to those most easily accessible, such as online searches, social media, self-proclaimed experts, and other social connections. These resources do not always have the most accurate information; thus, there is a need for accurate, age-appropriate sexuality education delivered by and/or in conjunction with a certified, professional sex educator in community, medical, therapeutic, and all health and healing environments and practices.

When it relates to sexuality, both pleasure and desire are indicators of wellness as well as sources of individual, social, and political empowerment (Lorde 1978). However, patient services provided for sexual health often focus on disease and pregnancy prevention, mimicking the medical model and the risk and harm focus (Nagoski 2015). As stated previously, sexual wellness shifts away from merely harm avoidance and turns toward fullness, pleasure, and personal decision-making. Essential topics such as the spectrum of sexuality, boundaries, consent, intimacy, and self and relational awareness are included in the World Health Organization's position on sexual health but absent in medical-model-driven curricula. In countries where comprehensive sexuality education is the norm, participants report less sexual shame, increased sexual responsibility, and more pleasurable sexual experiences (Weaver, Smith, and Kippax 2005). Our prevailing pedagogy is incomplete and potentially harmful, particularly for young women belonging to marginalized communities (Fine 2013).

THE PURSUIT OF SEXUAL WELLNESS

Social conditioning, media messaging, and inadequate health education services have an impact on physical and emotional health, threatening components of safety that are necessary to navigate the pursuit of sexual wellness. Pleasure and desire are interwoven with the mental, physical, emotional, and spiritual aspects of an autonomous self. Centering components of sexuality and sexual wellness, such as pleasure and desire, is not always related to sexual intercourse and its related activities. When we purposefully encourage people to seek, find, and explore what makes them feel good and then empower them to express the need for these things, it has positive effects on how they experience sex, sexuality, and overall well-being (Fine and McClelland 2006). For Black women, a focus on creating deeply satisfying sexual experiences in a society dependent on their perpetual labor is a radical act of reclaiming power and freedom (Brown 2019). This not only sets the tone for prevention and treatment but also creates potential for individual and generational healing across all aspects of wellness.

In an attempt to respond to this need, we provide considerations for holistic collaboration between providers, their patients or clients, and sex educators, framed by the patient's or client's self-identified cultural community and grounded in modern approaches to African worldview–centered principles.

CULTURALLY CENTERED SEXUAL WELLNESS EDUCATION

Without the rigor of a longitudinal research study with proven outcomes, this chapter stops short of providing a single, definitive model. There is also a purposeful avoidance of a formulaic structure so as to not promote rigidity. Such prescriptive attempts have consistently caused undue harm, stress, and personal frustration by not centering individual differences, cultural expression, or general feelings of not being heard. What is offered are necessary considerations to use in any sexual health education model or curriculum that aims to reflect the positive health values toward which the intended population strives. The following considerations give way to systemic thinking, cultural humility, varied epistemological stances, and person-centered practices as crucial components of sexual wellness education, specifically for Black women.

Bias Identification and Resolution

Sexual Attitude Reassessment workshops have been used to train American sexologists and other helping professionals to be sensitive to sexual diversity and the sexual behavior of others. The purported outcome is a change in attitude and, therefore, a change in action in how the professional interacts with their clients. However, there is an argument that the development of a professional's sexological worldview would be a more accurate construct than attitude change (Sitron and Dyson 2012).

Addressing one's own biases for sex, gender, sexual acts, and their intersectionality with race and ethnicity would expand both a general and sexological worldview. It is also recommended and a best practice that this kind of reflective and internal awareness work be done with sex educators who are well versed on and a part of the population as well as educated, if not certified, in sexual health and wellness.

Culturally Aware Comprehensive Assessment and Intervention

Comprehensive assessment and intervention involves bridging disciplines to gain a more holistic appreciation for a group's situation and experience (James and Prilleltensky 2002). This concept of an integrative and interdisciplinary modality has historical precedent, dating back to the work of cyberneticians and social scientists such as Gregory Bateson. Collaborative methods have been developed, debated, and matured through the years, with an obvious missing component of cultural awareness. Majority narratives continue to lack attention to the Black experience.

Provider awareness and attention to intersectionality is critical to taking a holistic approach when working with Black women. Scholar activists like Patricia Hill Collins and bell hooks introduced and elevated the Black feminist epistemology (BFE) model, which articulates the need of Black female voices in knowledge discovery, identification, and theory development. BFE was never successfully integrated into mainstream ideology. Components of BFE, however, are more indicative of the strengths and collective experience of Black women, including sexuality; thus, sexuality education with the Black female in mind should include tenets like caring and personal accountability, shared agents of knowledge, validation processes, and power relations (Reola 2018).

For those not trained in sex education, comprehensive assessment and intervention should involve collaborating with sex educators to gain a fuller scope for addressing topics and presenting conversations. Sexuality educators provide positive and supportive methods and a subject expertise that providers (e.g., doctors, therapists, nurse practitioners) may not possess without specialized training. Utilizing a co-therapy model with sex educators addresses the negative impacts of socialization, which improves self-esteem, increases self-awareness, and challenges feelings of guilt and shame in a nonjudgmental and holistic way.

Autonomy and Self-Awareness of the Whole Body

Creation of a service delivery model that includes practices and policies that honor the cultural experiences of the population we serve and acknowledges the oppressive systems

Black women navigate daily will optimize sexual wellness in the Black community. There is a growing recognition of the need for wellness indicators that respect and reflect the Black community's worldview. Most importantly, wellness indicators should be developed, informed, and monitored with, by, and for that community.

Looking to longitudinal programs and research conducted in Indigenous communities, sexual wellness education for Black women should include benchmarks and attributes found in the Indigenous wellness indicators (Heggie 2018):

- Education
  - The teachings: The community maintains the knowledge, values, and beliefs important to them.
  - Elders: The knowledge keepers are valued and respected, and able to pass on the knowledge.
  - Youth: The community's future is able to receive, respect, and practice the teachings.
- Self-determination
  - Healing/restoration: Members of the community have availability of and access to healing opportunities, as well as the freedom to define and enact their own chosen health programs.
  - Development: The community has the ability to determine and enact their own chosen community enrichment activities without detriment from externally imposed loss of resources.
  - Trust: The community trusts and supports its government.
- Resilience
  - Self-esteem: The beliefs and evaluations community members hold about themselves are positive, providing an internal guiding mechanism to steer and nurture people through challenges and improving control over outcomes.
  - Identity: Community members are able to strongly connect with who they are as a community in positive ways.
  - Sustainability: The community is able to adapt in response to changes.

Prioritizing and conducting sexuality education in this manner encourages the introduction of culture. By definition, culture includes shared historical, ideological, social, and spiritual characteristics of a racial, religious, or social group. While we acknowledge Black women are not monolithic, when it comes to science and healing, there are themes that well align with an Afrocentric worldview. However, Afrocentricity has been purposefully suppressed through years of slavery, oppression, survival assimilation, and indoctrination into a contrived society. To make progress in the health and wellness of Black women, re-igniting embodied ancestral knowledge and practices such as expression of comfortable body exposure (e.g., exposed breast of indigenous Africans), free body movement (e.g., tribal dances), and matriarch-led social hierarchy systems that resonate with Black women is important. Each may have a personal connection to different aspects of known or reclaimed history and want to include that in their whole-health, sexual wellness journey.

Encouraging individualized attachments makes the education more personal. Clients' autonomy should be respected and collaborative engagement fostered (Ryan et al. 2011).

Empowerment and Elevation

Afrocentric themes include strong interpersonal relationships with others, as well as harmony, peace with nature, communalism, embodied movement, and spirituality. These practices also align with modern theory and frameworks such as liberation psychology and healing justice work (Bakari 1997).

Liberation psychology is an approach that aims to actively understand the psychology of oppressed and impoverished communities by conceptually and practically addressing the oppressive sociopolitical structure in which they exist (Bryant-Davis and Moore-Lobban 2020). Healing justice is a framework that identifies how we can holistically respond to and intervene on generational trauma and violence, to bring collective practices that can impact and transform the consequences of oppression on our bodies, hearts, and minds (Page 2010). Healing that occurs in communal settings with the incorporation of spirituality and rituals can be cathartic and liberating. Group practice and rituals also build confidence and assertiveness and empower a person to take an active role in their sexual health and wellness. Having a healthy and pleasurable relationship with sex is no longer seen as impossible to attain or only prescribed by society's standards. After rejuvenating exercises such as ritualistic baths and breathwork, sex and sexuality can be seen as a self-defined journey of exploration, active learning, and, most importantly, belonging.

There is evidence that communal, safe, and well-supported groups that center around reclaiming and redefining sexuality may be beneficial. Studies show they offer women a space they find lacking in society to heal, nourish, and empower themselves. Women-only spaces, or "women's circles," are indicative of women's heightened participation in the realm of subjective well-being culture, including both elements of spirituality and more secular "personal growth" (Longman 2018). Convening in this nature provides an opportunity to engage in a community of reciprocal contribution and begin the process of distancing from restrictive and objectifying representations of femininity and female sexuality.

Also well documented are all-female retreats geared toward helping women reconnect with their vital sexual energy. They have reportedly assisted participants in rediscovering the sacredness of their female bodies and healing from damaging and even traumatic experiences regarding their femininity and sexuality (Plancke 2005). Developers of such retreats also report having participants take part in "goddess" rituals as a way to give cultural expression to women's capacity and desire to engage with their fully embodied, sexual selves (Plancke 2020).

What is even more impressive are the reports from attendees of newfound ability to better appraise sensations (Plancke 2005), development of a more positive self-image, and an improved sexual identity. These seminars, retreats, and groups emerge out of a desire to "re/connect" with each other, their bodies, their inner selves, and sometimes with the sacred (Longman 2018). They conclude with an attachment to new, cultural rituals; a strong circle of positive influence; the freedom to explore; and the connection to feel what comes naturally to bodies when layers of shame, guilt, and oppression are shed.

Finally, following Friere's Theory of Freeing, marginalized populations should be elevated to the rightful place of experts of their own existence. The three-phase approach (Romas and Sharma 2010) holds the audience as the leader and the facilitator is simply there as a humble resource. Most current sex education frameworks teach from a didactic posture. A cooperative learning environment is the preferred sexuality education model for the facilitator.

A Co-Therapy Case Study

Kia presents to a therapist with the feeling of being "stuck" or ineffective in her ability to lose weight. At 19, she reports that she is sexually active and starting to realize how small other girls her age are compared to her and that she is feeling down.

The therapist focuses on psycho-analytics such as thought processing and symptoms of depression. The sex educator, with whom the therapist regularly collaborates, facilitates awareness of media literacy, body positivity, and cultural perspective. Sexual wellness education also focuses on exercises to identify positive sexual messages and empower self-expression, which may not come up in the clinical session. Because the sex educator shares race/ethnicity with Kia, the sex educator provides cultural context with representation and possibly shared experience.

Sex educators are uniquely equipped to approach sensitive topics with strategies that complement behavioral therapies. Utilizing the following components, the sex educator addresses the following:

- Bias: The sex educator informs Kia that studies find that national policies on sex education in schools have an inequitable impact on young people and disproportionately place the burden on girls, youth of color, youth with disabilities, and lesbian/gay/bisexual/transgender youth (Fine and McCelland 2006).
- Cultural awareness: The sex educator discusses how modern, hypersexualized, and degrading imagery of the Black female body exists in opposition to sexual wellness and sexual rights by focusing on existing representations of Black female eroticism as a legacy of colonialism (Benard 2016).

- Autonomy and self-awareness: The sex educator provides exercises to explore body autonomy and awareness of ownership as well as self-control over the body and facilitates body consciousness and its association with kinetic skills and various aspects of well-being (Virtanen et al. 2022).
- Empowerment and elevation: The sex educator encourages engagement with various women's empowerment tools and ones that embody the values Kia has expressed (Kabeer 1999) and encourages use of voice with her therapist and her partner about her sexual thoughts and body perception.
- Impact: The sex educator checks in often to gauge if it "feels" right or is resonating, and pivots when necessary.

CONCLUSION

This chapter presents the case for the need for intentional and integrated positive sexuality and sexual wellness education in established health and healing models that is centered on the bodies, minds, and lives of Black women. Through the exploration of social context and institutional shortcomings in care delivery, a list of considerations is offered. These considerations are essential first steps in disrupting the status quo and perpetuation of oppressive attitudes and strategies antithetical to the healing and recovery promised by current models. By continuously de-centering Black women's sexuality, health care continues to contribute to disparate outcomes, prolonging healing and thwarting efforts to achieve whole health. Comprehensive sexual well-being remains deprioritized in the health care domain despite its many benefits to overall well-being. Sexual wellness is central and paramount to improving the lives of Black women, and the sex educator is an integral component.

REFERENCES

Aerts L, Rubin R, Randazzo M, Goldstein S, Goldstein I. Retrospective study of the prevalence and risk factors of clitoral adhesions: women's health providers should routinely examine the glans clitoris. *Sex Med.* 2018;6(2):115–122. https://doi.org/10.1016/j.esxm.2018.01.003

Bakari RS. Epistemology from an Afrocentric perspective: enhancing Black students' consciousness through an Afrocentric way of knowing. *Different Perspectives on Majority Rules.* April 1997:20. Available at: https://digitalcommons.unl.edu/cgi/viewcontent.cgi?article=1019&context=pocpwi2

Benard AAF. Colonizing Black female bodies within patriarchal capitalism: feminist and human rights perspectives. *Sexualization Media Society.* 2016;2(4). https://doi.org/10.1177/2374623816680622

Bond KT, LeBlanc NM, Williams P, Gabriel CG, Amutah-Onukagha NN. Race-based sexual stereotypes, gendered racism, and sexual decision making among young Black cisgender women. *Health Educ Behav.* 2021;48(3):295–305. https://doi.org/10.1177/10901981211010086

Brown AM. *Pleasure Activism: The Politics of Feeling Good.* Chico, CA: AK Press; 2019.

Bryant-Davis T, Moore-Lobban SJ. Black Minds Matter: Applying liberation psychology to Black Americans. In: Comas-Diaz L, Torres Rivera E, eds. *Liberation Psychology: Theory, Method, Practice, and Social Justice*. 20th ed. American Psychological Association. 2020:189–206. Available at: https://psycnet.apa.org/record/2020-47579-011

Centers for Disease Control and Prevention. Racism and health. 2021. Available at: https://www.cdc.gov/minorityhealth/racism-disparities/index.html

Coleman E. Promoting sexual health and responsible sexual behavior: an introduction. *J Sex Res*. 2002;39(1):3–6.

Fine M. Sexuality, schooling, and adolescent females: the missing discourse of desire. *Harvard Educ Rev*. 2013;58(1):29–53. https://doi.org/10.17763/haer.58.1.u0468k1v2n2n8242

Fine M, McClelland S. Sexuality education and desire: still missing after all these years. *Harvard Educ Rev*. 2006;76(3):297–338. https://doi.org/10.17763/haer.76.3.w5042g23122n6703

Fredrickson BL, Roberts TA. Objectification theory: toward understanding women's lived experiences and mental health risks. *Psychol Women Q*. 1997;21(2):173–206. https://journals.sagepub.com/doi/pdf/10.1111/j.1471-6402.1997.tb00108.x

Fritz N, Malic V, Paul B, Zhou Y. Worse than objects: the depiction of Black women and men and their sexual relationship in pornography. *Gender Issues*. 2021;38(1):100–120. https://doi.org/10.1007/s12147-020-09255-2

Heggie K. Indigenous wellness indicators: including urban Indigenous wellness indicators in the health city strategy. Greenest City Scholars Program. 2018. Available at: https://tinyurl.com/IndWellInd

James S, Prilleltensky I. Cultural diversity and mental health: towards integrative practice. *Clin Psychol Rev*. 2002;22(8):1133–1154. https://doi.org/10.1016/s0272-7358(02)00102-2

Kabeer N. Resources, agency, achievements: reflections on the measurement of women's empowerment. *Dev Change*. 1999;30(3):435–464. https://doi.org/10.1111/1467-7660.00125

Kendall M. *Hood Feminism: Notes From the Women That a Movement Forgot*. New York, NY: Penguin Publishing Group; 2021.

Leath S, Mims L. A qualitative exploration of Black women's familial socialization on controlling images of Black womanhood and the internalization of respectability politics. *J Fam Stud*. 2023;29(2):774–791. https://doi.org/10.1080/13229400.2021.1987294

Longman C. Women's circles and the rise of the new feminine: reclaiming sisterhood, spirituality, and wellbeing. *Religions*. 2018;9(1):9–26. https://doi.org/10.3390/rel9010009

Lorde A. *Uses of the Erotic: The Erotic as Power*. Freedom, CA: Crossing Press; 1978.

Moccia L, Mazza M, Di Nicola M, Janiri L. The experience of pleasure: a perspective between neuroscience and psychoanalysis. *Front Hum Neurosci*. 2018;12:359. https://doi.org/10.3389/fnhum.2018.00359

Nagoski E. *Come as You Are: The Surprising New Science That Will Transform Your Sex Life*. New York, NY: Simon and Schuster; 2015.

Nielsen. Reaching Black women across media platforms. 2017. Available at: https://www.nielsen.com/us/en/insights/article/2017/reaching-black-women-across-media-platforms

Page C. Reflections from Detroit: transforming wellness & wholeness. INCITE! August 5, 2010. Available at: https://incite-national.org/2010/08/05/reflections-from-detroit-transforming-wellness-wholeness

Plancke C. Bodily intimacy and ritual healing in women's tantric retreats. *Anthropol Med*. 2005;27(3):285–299. https://doi.org/10.1080/13648470.2019.1702774

Plancke C. Yoni touch and talk: sacralizing the female sex through tantra. *Sexualities*. 2020;23(5–6):834–848. https://doi.org/10.1177/1363460719861832

Reola K. Black feminist epistemology. 2018. Available at: https://prezi.com/p/nwd1pnxschl7/chapter-11-Black-feminist-epistemology

Romas J, Sharma M. *Theoretical Foundations of Health Education and Health Promotion*. Burlington, MA: Jones & Bartlett Learning LLC; 2010.

Ryan RM, Lynch MF, Vansteenkiste M, Deci EL. Motivation and autonomy in counseling, psychotherapy, and behavior change: a look at theory and practice. *Counsel Psychol*. 2011;39(2):193–260. https://doi.org/10.1177/0011000009359313

Satcher D, Hook EW, Coleman E. Sexual health in America: improving patient care and public health. *JAMA*. 2015;314(8):765–766. https://doi.org/10.1001/jama.2015.6831

Sitron J, Dyson D. Sexuality Attitudes Reassessment (SAR): historical and new considerations for measuring its effectiveness. *Am J Sex Educ*. 2009;4(2):158–177. https://doi.org/10.1177/2158244012439072

Sitron J, Dyson D. Validation of sexological worldview: a construct for use in the training of sexologists in sexual diversity. *Sage Open*. 2012;2:1–16. https://doi.org/10.1177/2158244012439072

Stallings E. The article that could save Black women's lives. October 2018. *The Oprah Magazine*. Available at: https://tinyurl.com/oprahref

Townes A, Rosenberg M, Guerra-Reyes L, Murray M, Herbenick D. Inequitable experiences between Black and white women discussing sexual health with healthcare providers: findings from a US probability sample. *J Sex Med*. 2020;17:1520–1528. https://doi.org/10.1016/j.jsxm.2020.04.391

Virtanen N, Tiippana K, Tervaniemi M, Poikonen H, Anttila E, Kaseva K. Exploring body consciousness of dancers, athletes, and lightly physically active adults. *Sci Rep*. 2022;12(1):1–9. https://doi.org/10.1038/s41598-022-11737-0

Weaver H, Smith G, Kippax S. School-based sex education policies and indicators of sexual health among young people: a comparison of the Netherlands, France, Australia and the United States. *Sex Educ*. 2005;5(2):171–188. https://doi.org/10.1080/14681810500038889

28

Perinatal Health Care With Sexual Abuse Survivors in Mind: Trauma-Responsive Care as a Reproductive Justice Strategy

Inas K. Mahdi, MPH

Considerations for sexual abuse and its related mental and physical consequences are often relegated to a lower priority within the American health care system. Often, sexual, reproductive, and perinatal health policies and practices do not incorporate awareness of sexual trauma and the potential for retraumatization in these settings. In the United States, Black women and girls experience sexual victimization at rates significantly higher than their peers (Breiding et al. 2014). It is critical to understand that this reality is counter to societal notions that suggest Black women are not entitled to victimhood and, thus, not entitled to receive responsive treatment, prevention, and mitigation of these harms.

This chapter describes the urgent need for trauma-responsive services for Black sexual violence and abuse survivors in the provision of maternal and perinatal health services. It also highlights the social context that shapes Black women and birthing people's[1] experiences with sexual victimhood and racialized health care services and encourages the consideration of potential solutions utilizing reproductive justice and trauma-responsive care to improve provision of perinatal services.

PERPETUATION OF SEXUAL VIOLENCE AGAINST BLACK WOMEN AND GIRLS

National statistics state that 25% or one in four women have experienced sexual abuse victimization by age 18 (Finkelhor et al. 1990). By contrast, in studies conducted by Black women with Black women, 60% of respondents report having experienced sexual assault or abuse before age 18, eclipsing rates of their peers (Tanis, Tanis, and Brown 2019). Black women are experiencing violence at levels that are substantially higher their peers, with the exception of the rates of sexual abuse among Indigenous women and girls (US Department of Justice 2018). These statistics necessitate public health and health care delivery systems take a more intentional approach to designing holistic and responsive

---

[1] Birthing people refers to individuals with the capacity for birth without regard for gender identity.

sexual, reproductive, and perinatal health programming. Why, then, is this substantial violence ignored and/or minimized in communities, society, and care facilities?

SOCIAL CONTEXT SHAPING BLACK WOMEN'S SEXUAL VICTIMHOOD

Black women's and girls' sexual abuse herstories have been frequently erased from mainstream consciousness. As early as the capture and kidnapping of enslaved African women and girls, sexual abuse and violence perpetration against Black women in the United States has been minimalized and disregarded as a critical issue in societal concerns (Roberts 1999). Narratives that view Black women as incapable of being raped extended well beyond slavery, into post-emancipation and the present day, with many survivors finding difficulty in making their sexual abuse claims heard by law enforcement, local authorities, and society at large. Recent research on Black female college students' sexual abuse incidents identified that Black women's stories are frequently disregarded and victimhood denied by law enforcement and campus authorities (Kane 2018).

Undergirding victimhood narratives are white supremacist ideas that contrast supposed white female sexuality of purity and virtue with Black sexuality as essentially lascivious, wanton, and promiscuous by nature (Mgadmi 2009; Washington 2006). In addition, stereotypes of Black women as combative, unwomanly, domineering, and lacking in morality flooded the American consciousness as a result of racialized tropes painted before and following the abolition of slavery (Mgadmi 2009). This narrative directly contributes to ongoing harm to Black women and girls in their quest for human rights, dignity, respect, and appropriate medical care responsive to sexual abuse.

Racialization in Health Care Settings

To understand African Americans' experience with quality and provision of care, one must understand their interactions with medical systems and experiences of medical racism, the racialized perceptions of Black patients that impact corresponding treatments, speed of diagnostic decisions, dismissal of patients' concerns or challenges to clinicians, and punishing consequences for requesting participation in decision-making. The impact of each component of medical racism coalesces into poor quality of care and poor outcomes for Black people (Davis 2019; Washington 2006).

Within care settings, fictitious narratives around Black women's domineering presence and perceived lack of docility particularly impact the provision of sexual, reproductive, and maternal health care (Davis 2019). Harmful stereotypes in conjunction with poor treatment place Black pregnant women in the crosshairs of substandard maternal health care and obstetric racism. Birthing people can also be subjected to obstetric violence, the larger system of institutional and gender-based violence women experience during their pregnancy, birth, and postpartum periods of care (Davis 2018). Obstetric violence, primarily discussed and documented in a global setting, is characterized by degrading and harmful medical mistreatment and abuse facilitated by clinicians during periods of women's medical care. In the United States, obstetric violence has been less explored. However, Davis asserts that medical racism and obstetric violence synergize to create the larger phenomenon of obstetric racism, thus contributing to significant targeted harms to Black birthing people in care.

Black women report experiencing mistreatment at higher rates across their maternity care continuum, throughout pregnancy and birthing experiences (Vedam et al. 2019). These harms and mistreatment may manifest as neglect, unnecessary medical interventions, failure to obtain consent, and coercion in the white-dominated maternal care spaces (Davis 2019).

The United States has the highest rate of maternal mortality among all high-income industrialized countries, with Black birthing people bearing the brunt of the impact (World Health Organization [WHO] et al. 2012; WHO 2014; WHO 2019). Additional indicators of widespread poor quality of care for Black women is evidenced by the prevalence of severe maternal morbidity, the unexpected birth and labor complications that lead to long-term maternal health consequences (Creanga et al. 2014; Geller, Cox, and Kilpatrick 2006). Like maternal mortality, severe maternal mortality has increased over the last 20 years and is often preventable and correlated with quality of care provided to birthing women (Geller, Cox, and Kilpatrick 2006).

In McLemore and D'Efilippo's article describing differences in maternal mortality rates across industrialized countries, growing evidence suggested that variability in care and outcomes are related to the quality of care and experiences that Black women receive in comparison to their counterparts (2019). This care is riddled with stereotypes regarding Black women's racial and obstetric hardiness. For hundreds of years, Black women were considered simultaneously physically inferior and superior, and categorized as a "medical superbody" able to withstand extreme physical hardship and serve as a representative body for racist medical experimentation (Owens 2017). Black women and birthing people's complaints of pain and discomfort are so mired in racist ideology that these symptoms render prompt interventions and diagnoses impossible (Davis 2019).

Pregnancy as a Period of Sexual Trauma Reactivation

Sexual violence and assault survivors often suppress their sexual assault-related trauma as a coping strategy. During pregnancy, childbirth, and breastfeeding periods, suppressed sexual trauma can be activated by the physiological processes of these periods (Simkin and Klaus 2004). While the literature tells us that where there is reactivation of suppressed trauma, hypervigilance and anxiety about invasive medical procedures are normal among survivors, the pervasive ideas about Black people's behaviors within medical care settings indicate that any behavior deemed "undesirable" is an act of aggression, noncompliance, or a safety concern (Simkin and Klaus 2004; Davis 2019).

These underlying beliefs inevitably contribute to the practices, health sciences research, and intervention development present across the public health landscape. Despite persistent inequities in sexual violence victimization and perinatal care outcomes, there are limited resources to dismantle biased practices and policies, guide clinical practice and clinician behavior, and develop the skills necessary to respond to the needs of the population.

CALLS FOR MORE RESPONSIVE CARE

In the field of perinatal health, interventions to address outcomes for Black women are beginning to look toward improving patient experiences. As calls to restructure health systems and care provision are amplified, incorporating more responsive care structures must include not only culturally competent care but also trauma-responsive care. There is a clear need for models of care and interventions to address both structural racism and the prevalence of sexual trauma within care systems to improve perinatal outcomes.

Despite the application of some feminist approaches in clinical nursing care research, the lack of critical response surrounding the compounded oppression experienced by Black women highlights the need for an intersectional approach in perinatal health service design and evaluation (Barbee 1994). Understanding the complexities that continue to impact the valuation and devaluation of Black women's lives in America suggests that there must be new frameworks to support equitable outcomes. Sadiya Hartman (1997) describes a concept of the "afterlife of slavery" whereby the US system of valuation of lives follows the lineage of slavery and continues to value white bodies over Black bodies. Hartman describes the "afterlife of slavery" as a phenomenon of limited access to health information and education, increased premature death, incarceration, and impoverishment that impact health outcomes and "life chances" that Black people continue to face.

In June 1994, 12 Black women attending a national prochoice conference created a reproductive justice as a human rights- and Black feminist theory-based framework to view and center conversations about reproductive health and well-being inside the context of the environmental, social, and political conditions that dictate reproductive outcomes (Ross et al. 2017). Utilizing a lens of reproductive justice as a theoretical paradigm shift increases the possibility for care that centers the most marginalized and lays the foundation for developing responsive care services that mitigate previous and ongoing harms to Black women.

Importance of Trauma-Responsive Care Shaped by Reproductive Justice

As a framework for redesigning care, utilizing a trauma-responsive approach also highlights the typically unseen needs of a population. Trauma-responsive maternal and perinatal health care has the ability to recognize the lived experiences of patients and respond to the impact of traumatic stress on those birthing people and those who interact with them (e.g., their care providers). Programs and agencies operating within a trauma-responsive health system ensure that at every level of care provision, awareness of trauma, the pervasiveness of trauma, and the knowledge and skills to address trauma are incorporated into the organization's culture, praxis, and policies.

In a trauma-responsive system, each element of care, planning, and execution acts in conjunction with all who interact and engage with the birthing person, to maximize physical and psychological safety; facilitate the recovery of the person, their families, and communities; and support their ability to thrive (The Trauma-Informed Care Implementation Resource Center 2022).

Trauma-informed care seeks to

- realize the widespread impact of trauma and understand paths for recovery;
- recognize the signs and symptoms of trauma in patients, families, and staff;
- integrate knowledge about trauma into policies, procedures, and practices; and
- actively avoid re-traumatization (Substance Abuse and Mental Health Services Administration [SAHMSA] 2014).

The principles of a trauma-informed approach (SAHMSA 2014; Figure 28-1) include incorporation of

- cultural, historical, and gender issues;
- safety;
- trustworthiness and transparency;
- peer support;
- collaboration and mutuality; and
- empowerment and choice.

Ingrained in the tenets of reproductive justice is the concept of bodily autonomy, indicating the mothers of the movement understood the importance of bodily integrity and the full control of one's body as a critical factor for achieving reproductive justice. Not apparent in its operationalization is how programs and initiatives further this concept with regard to sexual trauma where threats of retraumatization and victimization are possible. Further consideration for how reproductive justice can shape trauma-responsive care

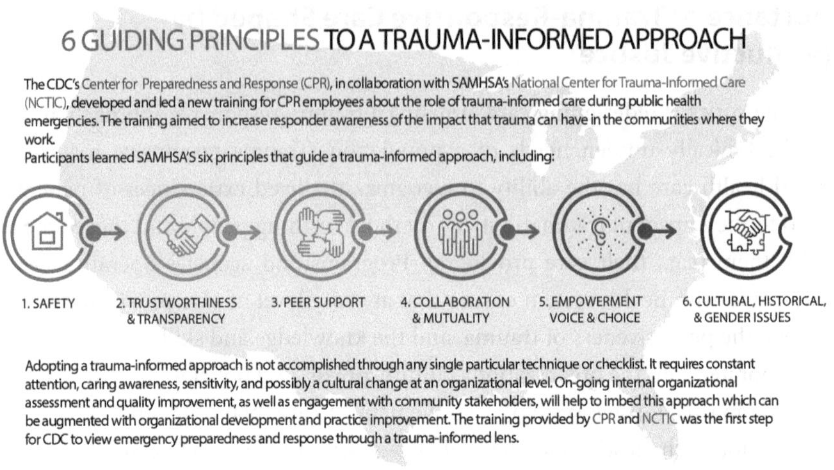

6 GUIDING PRINCIPLES TO A TRAUMA-INFORMED APPROACH

The CDC's Center for Preparedness and Response (CPR), in collaboration with SAMHSA's National Center for Trauma-Informed Care (NCTIC), developed and led a new training for CPR employees about the role of trauma-informed care during public health emergencies. The training aimed to increase responder awareness of the impact that trauma can have in the communities where they work.

Participants learned SAMHSA'S six principles that guide a trauma-informed approach, including:

1. SAFETY
2. TRUSTWORTHINESS & TRANSPARENCY
3. PEER SUPPORT
4. COLLABORATION & MUTUALITY
5. EMPOWERMENT VOICE & CHOICE
6. CULTURAL, HISTORICAL, & GENDER ISSUES

Adopting a trauma-informed approach is not accomplished through any single particular technique or checklist. It requires constant attention, caring awareness, sensitivity, and possibly a cultural change at an organizational level. On-going internal organizational assessment and quality improvement, as well as engagement with community stakeholders, will help to imbed this approach which can be augmented with organizational development and practice improvement. The training provided by CPR and NCTIC was the first step for CDC to view emergency preparedness and response through a trauma-informed lens.

Source: Reprinted from CDC (n.d.).
Note: CDC = Centers for Disease Control and Prevention; SAMHSA = Substance Abuse and Mental Health Services Administration.

Figure 28-1. Six Guiding Principles to a Trauma-Informed Approach.

provides an opportunity for service providers and care design teams to develop expansive care that seeks to protect the right to bodily autonomy; reduce the likelihood of retraumatization within care; understand the context and environments from which birthing people live, work, and play; and connect clients to their desired services, interventions, and outcomes.

Reconfiguring Care

By understanding the linkages between sexual abuse trauma, related mental health consequences, reproductive justice, and subsequent redesign of health systems, we can begin to create solutions that emphasize the health and well-being of Black birthing persons in perinatal care settings. To begin restructuring services, staff must be trained in the necessary skills, reflect awareness of the pervasiveness of sexual trauma and denied victimhood, and respond to signs and symptoms of trauma in a manner that does not do further harm. In addition, there must be true collaboration and leveling of power differences. Care should be informed by the end users of services. Black birthing people with histories of sexual assault, abuse, and other trauma and violence should lead the charge in developing care that considers the nature of care provision in the United States, incorporates opportunities for healing and treatment, and supports birth and well-being outcomes, from initial entry to care to postpartum.

CONCLUSION

Perinatal health systems must reconfigure to incorporate understanding of how obstetric racism, negative perceptions of Black women and girls, and the prevalence of sexual trauma impact how health systems synergize to predict Black birthing people's experiences in perinatal care. In the evolution of care design, we must be reminded of what reproductive justice leaders insist on as a guidepost; by constantly shifting the center to communities that face intersecting oppression, we have a more comprehensive view of the strategies to end all forms of violence (INCITE! Women of Color Against Violence 2016). Advancing reproductive justice–informed trauma-responsive care practices must acknowledge historical legacy, intersecting oppressions, and strategies derived from affected communities to see movement toward a more just and equitable health care system.

REFERENCES

Barbee EL. A Black feminist approach to nursing research. *West J Nurs Res.* 1994;16(5):495–506. https://doi.org/10.1177/019394599401600504

Breiding MJ, Smith SG, Basile KC, Walters ML, Chen J, Merrick MT. Prevalence and characteristics of sexual violence, stalking, and intimate partner violence victimization—National Intimate Partner and Sexual Violence Survey, United States, 2011. *MMWR Surveill Summ.* 2014; 63(8):1–18.

Centers for Disease Control and Prevention. Six guiding principles to a trauma-informed approach. Available at: https://www.cdc.gov/cpr/infographics/6_principles_trauma_info.htm

Creanga AA, Berg CJ, Ko JY, et al. Maternal mortality and morbidity in the United States: where are we now? *J Womens Health.* 2014;23(1):3–9. https://doi.org/10.1089/jwh.2013.4617

Davis D. Obstetric racism: the racial politics of pregnancy, labor, and birthing. *Med Anthropol.* 2018;38(7):560–573. https://doi.org/10.1080/01459740.2018.1549389

Davis DA. *Reproductive Injustice: Racism, Pregnancy, and Premature Birth.* New York, NY: NYU Press; 2019.

Finkelhor D, Hotaling G, Lewis IA, Smith C. Sexual abuse in a national survey of adult men and women: prevalence, characteristics, and risk factors. *Child Abuse Negl.* 1990;14(1):19–28. https://doi.org/10.1016/0145-2134(90)90077-7

Geller SE, Cox SM, Kilpatrick SJ. A descriptive model of preventability in maternal morbidity and mortality. *J Perinatol.* 2006;26(2):79–84. https://doi.org/10.1038/sj.jp.7211432

Hartman SV. *Scenes of Subjection: Terror, Slavery, and Self-Making in Nineteenth-Century America.* New York, NY: Oxford University Press; 1997.

INCITE! Women of Color Against Violence, ed. *Color of Violence: The INCITE! Anthology.* Durham, NC: Duke University Press; 2016. https://doi.org/10.1215/9780822373445

Kane O. The denial of victimhood: exploring the attitudes surrounding collegiate Black women and rape. 2019 National Conference of Black Political Scientists Annual Meeting; November 13, 2018. Available at: https://ssrn.com/abstract=3283963

McLemore M, D'Efilippo V. To prevent women from dying in childbirth, first stop blaming them. *Scientific American.* May 1, 2019. Available at: https://www.scientificamerican.com/article/to-prevent-women-from-dying-in-childbirth-first-stop-blaming-them

Mgadmi M. Black women's identity: stereotypes, respectability and passionlessness (1890-1930). *Revue LISA.* 2009;7(1):40–55. https://doi.org/10.4000/lisa.806

Owens DC. *Medical Bondage: Race, Gender, and the Origins of American Gynecology.* Athens, GA: University of Georgia Press; 2017. https://doi.org/10.2307/j.ctt1pwt69x

Roberts D. Killing the Black body: race, reproduction, and the meaning of liberty. *Isis.* 1999;90(1):101–102. https://doi.org/10.1086/384248

Ross L, Roberts L, Derkas E, Peoples W, Bridgewater P. *Radical Reproductive Justice: Foundation, Theory, Practice, Critique.* New York, NY: The Feminist Press; 2017.

Simkin P, Klaus P. *When Survivors Give Birth: Understanding and Healing the Effects of Early Sexual Abuse on Childbearing Women.* Seattle, WA: Classic Day Publishing; 2004.

Substance Abuse and Mental Health Services Administration. *SAMHSA's Concept of Trauma and Guidance for a Trauma-Informed Approach.* HHS Publication No. (SMA) 14-4884. 2014.

Tanis F, Tanis C, Brown S. *The Sexual Abuse to Maternal Mortality Pipeline: Unifying Sexual Assault and Reproductive Justice Advocates.* Brooklyn, NY: Black Women's Blueprint; 2019.

Trauma-Informed Care Implementation Resource Center. What is trauma-informed care? 2022. Available at: https://www.traumainformedcare.chcs.org/what-is-trauma-informed-care

US Department of Justice, Office on Violence Against Women. Tribal affairs. January 5, 2018. Available at: https://www.justice.gov/ovw/tribal-affairs

Vedam S, Stoll K, Taiwo TK, et al. The Giving Voice to Mothers study: inequity and mistreatment during pregnancy and childbirth in the United States. *Reprod Health.* 2019;16(1):77. https://doi.org/10.1186/s12978-019-0729-2

Washington HA. *Medical Apartheid: The Dark History of Medical Experimentation on Black Americans From Colonial Times to the Present.* New York, NY: Doubleday Books; 2007.

World Health Organization. Maternal mortality: evidence brief. 2019. Available at: https://apps.who.int/iris/handle/10665/329886

World Health Organization. Maternal mortality: fact sheet: to improve maternal health, barriers that limit access to quality maternal health services must be identified and addressed at all levels of the health system. 2014. Available at: https://apps.who.int/iris/handle/10665/112318

World Health Organization, World Bank, United Nations Population Fund, United Nations Children's Fund (UNICEF). Trends in maternal mortality: 1990 to 2010: WHO, UNICEF, UNFPA and The World Bank estimates. Geneva, Switzerland: World Health Organization; 2012.

29

An Approach to Applying an Intersectional Lens to Research on Black Women's Reproductive and Sexual Health

Maranda C. Ward, EdD, MPH, Bailey Moore, and Anna Barickman

While the concept of intersectionality is not new, its interpretation and translation across research remain inconsistent. Often, intersectionality is used as a theoretical framework to explain study findings without applying it as a lens to the study design or how data are collected (Bowleg 2012). These oversights contribute to how the complex sexualities of Black women get flattened and how structural barriers to reproductive health remain overlooked (Prather et al. 2018). Given that research informs policy and practice, it is important that intersectional approaches to Black women's reproductive and sexual health research are more robustly interrogated and uniformly understood.

Using the Silences Framework (Serrant 2020), we assessed how open-access, peer-reviewed articles published on Black women's reproductive and sexual health operationalized and integrated this concept into their research question(s), study design, discussion of findings, and practice or policy implications. By identifying themes that cut across how researchers define and apply the concept of intersectionality, we offer recommendations that better capture the richness of, and ongoing threats to, Black women's reproductive and sexual wellness. The intersections of race, class, and gender in research, policy, and practice serve as sites of oppression and strength in the analysis of Black women's health. Reframing how we talk, research, and write about the reproductive health and sexuality of Black women is necessary to advance health equity.

WHO ARE WE?

The first author of this chapter only knows her Black racial identity as a cisgender woman and cannot disentangle race and gender in the ways that research and data are often collected and reported. Attending Spelman College allowed her to deliberately draw upon the contributions of Black people across the African diaspora to affirm her own sense of self, identity, and agency. Her training in sociology, anthropology, public health, education, and participatory action research allows her to center those who often go unrecognized: youth and young adults. She thinks intently about whom she works with, why, and how these choices reflect her own social positions and webs of power and privilege.

The second author identifies as an unapologetic Black woman who sees the world as her classroom. As an undergraduate public health student with a focus in health equity, human services, and social justice who is interested in medical school, she is passionate about taking advantage of the path to education and opportunities paved for her to fight for Black maternal/reproductive health and justice, health equity, informed health education, and decolonizing what is known about Black birth/birthwork in America. Through her fierce determination, she aims to (1) live a life of service, advocacy, and leadership to eliminate the systems that have plagued her people for far too long and (2) advance the efforts of all the incredible Black women who came before her.

The third author identifies as a White cisgender woman. She is a recent public health graduate with a focus in health equity and psychology. Through her undergraduate education, she discovered a passion for child health and women's reproductive and sexual health. She is interested in eliminating health disparities within these areas and believes it is crucial to acknowledge her privilege both in her studies and beyond. She is inspired by the diverse identities associated with womanhood and believes that an intersectional lens is a valuable tool to amplify marginalized voices within research.

THE CONVERGENCE OF MULTIPLE IDENTITIES

We cannot afford to treat the simultaneous identities that Black women perform as confounding variables in research. In fact, the sociocultural and geopolitical terrain that Black women navigate shape their opportunities for health. What we know about Black women's sexualities and reproductive possibilities reflects the legacies of Black mommas, doulas, midwives, and community health workers that have long informed how medical providers and scholars treat and theorize the subject matter to date.

Kimberlé Williams Crenshaw (1989) coined the term "intersectionality" to explain how Black women experienced their Blackness, womanhood, and socioeconomic position in ways that either granted or denied them power, privilege, and rights. According to the conceptual framework of intersectionality, race and gender experiences cannot be dichotomized because these categories are mutually constituted and cannot be simply added. Specifically, it asserts that the intersection of multiple identities and forms of discrimination are not merely additive, but instead are multiplicative, meaning that they are experienced and interpreted at multiple levels within the social context of African American women's lives (Jackson, Rowley, and Curry Owens 2012; Collins 2000). We rely on this framing to guide our own work. In this chapter, we name the taken-for-granted research processes that undermine attempts for intersectional research to reflect the complexities of Black women's reproductive and sexual health.

We performed a Boolean search of MEDLINE using the following keywords: intersectional AND Black OR African American AND women OR female AND reproductive health OR sexual health. This search resulted in 12 articles dated 2016 to 2022 that included primary and secondary studies, as well as literature reviews, on the reproductive and sexual health of Black women in the United States, United Kingdom, and Brazil (often compared to white and/or Hispanic women).

One of the articles we located from this search described the Silences Framework by Serrant (2020). This intersectional framework was created by a Black woman professor in the United Kingdom who is clear on the positionalities she brings to her intersectional research. She names the "silences" that exist in public health research when scholars write about Black women. These silences result from what Serrant describes as unshared beliefs, values, and experiences about the lives of Black women.

We used her framework as a lens to review the remaining 11 articles and organize a set of recommendations for conducting intersectional research. After creating a coding matrix with excerpts to catalog and compare if, and how, each author defined and applied intersectionality to their research conceptualization, design, interpretation, and dissemination, we color-coded the four stages of the Silences Framework (Serrant 2020) to align with supporting evidence to determine cross-cutting themes. In the sections that follow, we describe each stage of Serrant's Silences Framework, our analysis, and recommendations.

STAGE 1. WORKING IN "SILENCES" (CONTEXTUALIZATION)

The first stage of the framework focuses on "what is known about the subject and how that information is acquired" (Serrant 2020, p. 5). We must question the structures that shape Black women's social positions. Otherwise, the assumptions and biases we bring to the literature we read, collect, and report in our work will go unchecked and silenced. This stage allows us to answer this question: How can I contextualize my research on the experiences of Black women in a way that avoids gaps and misinformation?

We are seldom taught to make explicit how we conceptualize the population(s) of interest to our lines of inquiry. We recognize that race, gender, and other identities are frequently used in research yet seldomly defined. Of the 11 studies we reviewed, two offered a clear definition of race (Alson et al. 2021; Burger, Evans-Agnew, and Johnson 2022). While another six studies mention or define concepts—such as intimate partner violence, gender-based violence, and theories of gender and power (Bagwell-Gray, Jen, and Schuetz 2020); gendered racism (Rosenthal and Lobel 2020); sexual self-concept (Logan et al. 2021); sexual health (Opara et al. 2021); racism (Goes et al. 2021); and ethnic-racial socialization, sexual assertiveness, and gender roles (Brown, Blackmon, and Shiflett, 2017)—they did not operationalize their use of race, sexuality, and/or gender.

Often, we *are taught* to rely on white women as the reference group in disparities research among Black and Brown women. Of the 11 studies we reviewed, six of them applied this unspoken analytic method. Agénor et al. (2021) name white heterosexual women as their reference group, and Logan et al. (2021) report phenomenological reflections of 22 Black women ages 18 to 29 who felt like "a 'white girl' in Black spaces, or a 'hood' or 'ghetto' girl in white spaces" (p. 5). This demonstrates how whiteness contributes to the othering of Black women across racialized spaces. Relying on white women as the comparison group for every health indicator furthers the idea that white womanhood is the standard for reproductive and sexual health. This untruth leads to anti-Black practices and policies that run counter to our aims for health and racial equity.

Among the researchers that did not use white women as the baseline for reproductive and sexual health, Goes et al. (2021) name institutional racism as the barrier that Black and Brown women face, and Opara et al. (2021) extend the discussion of how institutional racism contributes to the lack of rigorous and longitudinal research on sexually transmitted infection among Black girls and women. Both scholar teams insist that viewing Black women through a white gaze—perceptions of reality held by white people—leads to frameworks and theories that exclude or incorrectly contextualize the varied experiences of Black girls and women. In sum, metrics that maintain whiteness as the norm decontextualize research.

For research reflecting the experiences of Black women, Serrant (2020) calls for researchers to shift our units of analysis to the conditions, histories, and structures that frame Black women as hypersexual, intimidating, and lacking. Doing so will allow our research to address the webs of capitalism, colonialism, and misogynoir as the culprits of unfair outcomes. For instance, Rosenthal and Lobel (2020) describe the need to address stereotypical media images and tropes alongside historical medical abuse and experimentation. This historical trauma has contributed to disparities among Black women in nearly all domains of reproductive health for as long as Black women have advocated for their rights, dignity, and bodily autonomy (Alson et al. 2021). Articles such as these offer balanced narratives in describing how Black women are positioned in relation to their sexual and reproductive selves.

Several scholars critique how and why race, gender, and other social identities are used in research. Jenkins Hall and Tanner (2016) review how race and gender in research are often approached as interdependent and mutually constitutive factors. Gender also gets conflated with sex, as Agénor et al. (2021) point out in a national data set, which leads to misgendering of transgender respondents. In a secondary analysis of qualitative data, Crooks, Singer, and Tluczek (2020) assess how all socially constructed categories are based on stereotypes of privileged groups that compare power and privilege, oppression and discrimination, and positions within hierarchies of social status. To strengthen these valid arguments, these scholars must ensure readers have a shared understanding of how they apply the very social categories they critique in their research. In an attempt to move away from race-based medicine, there are calls for clinicians to begin rationalizing why they need to collect racial data so that we can maintain guidelines on how race gets clinically treated (Cerdeña, Plaisime, and Tsai 2020; Crear-Perry et al. 2020). We argue that this questioning should become standard research practice.

Recommendations

To make visible the silences in intersectional research, researchers should consider the following:

- Defining the social identities collected to assist in key comparisons and to normalize this practice.
- Comparing Black women to other Black women in research samples to elucidate the diversity within this subpopulation. Black women live across the African diaspora and have a range of experiences with education, finances, family, sex, and relationships.
- Addressing the sociopolitical histories that protect and harm Black women's reproductive and sexual health outcomes.

STAGE 2. HEARING "SILENCES" (LOCATION)

This stage is about exposing or locating silences in research. If researchers want to conduct intersectional Black women's research, we must seek out and highlight their voices. To center their stories, we need to take a closer look at who we are as researchers. Our own identities determine and guide our topics of interest, research questions, data points, and study design. This stage allows us to answer this question: Whose voices are amplified within my research with Black women?

To locate the silences, we reviewed whether the subjectivities of the authors were openly shared. Of the 11 studies we reviewed, two of the authors included positionality statements for how their biographies impact their work. To unsilence the role of privilege, three scholars who identify as white women shared their job titles, topics of interest, and research experiences to date (Burger, Evans-Agnew, and Johnson 2022). Similarly, Crooks, Singer, and Tluczek (2021) made explicit how the social categories of data in their study of 20 Black women reflected their own racial, gender, and educational identities. We believe that this reflexive practice enhances the integrity of intersectional research.

We continued to locate silences by reviewing how the research questions and/or hypotheses were framed. Of the 11 studies we reviewed, seven of the authors refer to intersectionality theory to apply as a lens to the research design itself (Agénor et al. 2021; Burger, Evans-Agnew, and Johnson 2022; Crooks, Singer, and Tluczek 2021; Goes et al. 2021; Jenkins Hall and Tanner 2016; Logan et al. 2021; Rosenthal and Lobel 2020). In a study on contraceptive use and counseling of 25,473 US Black, white, and Latina women between the ages of 15 and 44 years, Agénor et al. (2021) reference an intersectionality framework to address gaps in existing literature. Similarly, Jenkins Hall and Tanner (2016) examine the utility of applying an intersectional approach to existing literature on college hook-up culture, with the specific aim of centering the voices of Black women. Across these studies, they collected multiple interdependent identities or social characteristics related to either a research question, a hypothesis, or a statement of purpose.

An intersectional lens is key to locating silences when representing the voices or experiences of diverse Black women. For instance, in the study of 28 woman survivors of intimate partner violence (IPV) from various racial backgrounds, Bagwell-Gray, Jen, and Schuetz (2020) posed the following research question: "In the context of past or present IPV, how do women describe their sexual risks and resiliencies?" (p. 350). Despite recruiting a diverse group of women between the ages of 22 and 60 years, this question suggests a uniform experience of womanhood and silences experiences across intersecting identities.

To locate additional silences, we reviewed the language the authors used to narrate the lived experiences of Black women in their scholarship. We must take care to not flatten the experiences that Black woman have of their reproductive and sexual selves when naming the structural inequities they face. For example, Alson et al. (2021) acknowledge self-advocacy among Black women throughout history, but compare negative lived experiences of Black women to positive lived experiences of white women, which may de-amplify collective strengths.

Critical race theory (Crenshaw 1989) tells us that we can use counter-storytelling to disrupt the often pathologizing, dominant narratives about Black women. Of the 11 studies we reviewed, 5 authors presented counter-narratives (Agénor et al. 2021; Brown, Blackmon, and Shiflett 2017; Burger, Evans-Agnew, and Johnson 2022; Crooks, Singer, and Tluczek 2021; Opara et al. 2021). Opara et al. (2021) discuss how framing language that primarily focuses on disparities and individual risk behavior is harmful, particularly when discussing Black women's and girls' sexuality. In a literature review of existing intersectional research on reproductive justice for Black women, Burger, Evans-Agnew, and Johnson (2022) construct a compelling counter-narrative by citing the works of Black women and organizations advocating for their own reproductive justice, including Loretta Ross, Toni Bond Leonard, Sistersong, and the Black Mamas Matter Alliance. Crooks, Singer, and Tluczek (2021) provide key examples of Black women "content experts" such as the Combahee River Collective Statement and Patricia Hill Collins's *Black Sexual Politics* (2005).

Recommendations

To make visible the silences in intersectional research, researchers should consider the following:

- Identifying how the identities and personal experiences of the researchers and research participants shape the research.
- Applying an intersectional framework to the research question, hypothesis, or study aims.
- Using framing language that recognizes the complexities of social strata among subgroups of Black women.
- Normalizing how Black laywomen and professional women co-create knowledge.

STAGE 3. VOICING "SILENCES" (VERBALIZATION)

The third stage is dedicated to verbalizing the unsaid in the data collection phase of a research study. In particular, Serrant (2020) invites us to validate the lived experiences of Black women. This stage allows us to answer this question: Am I actively seeking out the direct knowledge and experiences of Black women by Black women?

For this stage of the framework, researchers are invited to engage in more than just "member-checking" to report internal consistency. Serrant (2020) writes that any aims to report intersectional findings among Black women should undergo a more rigorous review by a range of Black women beyond the study alone. Among the 11 studies we reviewed, the authors did not share whether they validated their results through seeking out the knowledge of Black women scholars.

To voice silences in intersectional research on Black women's reproductive and sexual health, we should actively seek out the collective voices of Black women. This is especially important because the voices of Black women are historically muted and overlooked in empirical research. While Black women experience their Blackness and their womanhood differently at the axes of many other simultaneous identities, there does remain a collective consciousness and shared understanding that has a significant influence on what it means to be a Black woman (Durkheim 2014; Serrant 2020). By actively working to verbalize the voices of Black women, researchers can work to ensure that "silences" are not missed, as has historically been the case.

Five of the 11 studies explained how they validated their results in alternative ways. For example, two forms of analysis informed "cluster profiles" on chosen metrics (Brown, Blackmon, and Shiflett 2017), there was comparison with past research (Rosenthal and Lobel 2020), and framing of results through the historical dynamics that have existed within the realm of privilege and power in society (Crooks, Singer, and Tluczek 2021).

We found that none of the studies documented that they sought out the knowledge or input of other Black laywomen or Black women scholars before they disseminated their work. Validating the work we do on Black women's reproductive and sexual health by engaging Black women beyond the study helps reduce the essentializing and romanticizing of Black women's stories. This is especially important, as researchers insert themselves in the research by determining which of the stories and quotes to include or exclude in their analysis. Recognizing the importance of understanding historical context and recommending the importance of using an intersectional lens are all promising practices in research. However, the work remains incomplete until the voices of those who stand to benefit the most are front and center.

Recommendations

To voice silences in intersectional research, researchers should consider the following:

- Seeking out the expertise and collaboration of Black women scholars on research teams or as a review panel for research findings.
- Seeking out Black women beyond the research who can validate interpretations of the findings (even if the researcher is a Black woman or the study team includes Black women, because there are varied intersectional experiences of Black women's sexuality and reproductive wellness).

STAGE 4. WORKING WITH "SILENCES" (RE-CONTEXTUALIZATION AND DISCUSSION)

The final stage is to work with the silences. Serrant (2020) admonishes us to translate marginalized perspectives into proposed policy, educational interventions, future research, and/or clinical practice in a way that will impact the life chances of Black women. For our intersectional research to have an impact on the realities that Black women experience, our findings must be interpreted for their benefit. This stage allows us to answer this question: Are my findings translated in real ways?

In this stage, we evaluated the ways in which authors wrote about the implications of their work. Most of the authors relied on several different methods for re-contextualizing and translating the experiences of study participants into tangible suggestions for future public health research, education, and practice. Of the 11 studies we reviewed, all of the authors reframed research implications, incorporated specific recommendations, critiqued existing structures, or identified room for improvement within a particular field.

Seeking to reframe Black women and girls' sexuality in the context of efforts to prevent HIV and other sexually transmitted infections, Opara et al. (2021) propose a new integrated intersectional framework that suggests four pillars for reevaluating research, education, and thought on Black women's and girls' sexuality. Similarly, Alson et al. (2021)

conclude their literature review on manifestations of structural racism in reproductive health with a focus on the importance of using an intersectional life-course perspective to examine social structures and barriers to improving Black women's reproductive health outcomes. While this framework is more broadly focused, it calls out systemic racism and patriarchy as threats to reproductive health equity. Jenkins Hall and Tanner (2016) suggest increasing the number of Black women and girls in intersectional public health research, particularly in disciplines dominated by white narratives. In this vein, Crooks, Singer, and Tluczek (2021) reframe their findings to inform nursing education to improve quality of care and clinical encounters for Black women. Other studies translated recommendations into community-level interventions.

It is important that study findings move beyond a set of recommendations alone. Serrant (2020) describes how intersectional research must recontextualize findings to benefit Black women in tangible and measurable ways. This is modeled particularly well in a study by Logan et al. (2021), who used focus groups to understand the role of socialization and marginalized identities in Black women's and girls' perception and experiences with sexual and reproductive health. The researchers used the study space to consult Black women on their perceptions of the effectiveness of proposed solutions and recommendations. This study normalizes Black women's expertise in ways that disrupt how the knowledge of Black women gets treated as supplementary to Westernized biomedical models of health.

Recommendations

To work in the silences in intersectional research, researchers should consider the following:

- Recontextualizing findings that center the experiences, values, and histories of Black women.
- Engaging Black women in the sense-making of data to propose holistic and relevant interventions.
- Identifying challenges with proposed policies and recommendations to increase the likelihood that proposed next steps are feasible.

CONCLUSION

Negating the silences in our intersectional research brings harm to the disciplines and fields that attempt to advance knowledge, science, and policies to protect Black women. We must be forthright with what brings us to our research and how we design, interpret, and discuss social identities, power, and inequity in our work. This context shapes how we conceptualize Black women and the histories and experiences brought to bear on our research process. The Silences Framework is helpful in bringing to the surface the often-neglected processes we tacitly undergo as we select and write about our research on Black women's health. In addition to valuing within-group differences and varied experiences with power and privilege, we also need more uniformity on how intersectional research is cataloged and carried out. Without this understanding of what makes one's research intersectional, we cannot translate what we learn from our research into our classrooms, clinical practices, or workplace cultures.

REFERENCES

Agénor M, Pérez AE, Wilhoit A, et al. Contraceptive care disparities among sexual orientation identity and racial/ethnic subgroups of US women: a national probability sample study. *J Womens Health (Larchmt)*. 2021;30(10):1406–1415. https://doi.org/10.1089/jwh.2020.8992

Alson JG, Robinson WR, Pittman L, Doll KM. Incorporating measures of structural racism into population studies of reproductive health in the United States: a narrative review. *Health Equity*. 2021;5(1):49–58. https://doi.org/10.1089/heq.2020.0081

Bagwell-Gray ME, Jen S, Schuetz N. How intimate partner violence and intersectional identities converge to influence women's sexual health across environmental contexts. *Soc Work*. 2020;65(4):349–357. https://doi.org/10.1093/sw/swaa031

Bowleg L. The problem with the phrase women and minorities: intersectionality—an important theoretical framework for public health. *Am J Public Health*. 2012;102(7):1267–1273. https://doi.org/10.2105/AJPH.2012.300750

Brown DL, Blackmon S, Shiflett A. Safer sexual practices among African American women: intersectional socialisation and sexual assertiveness. *Cult Health Sex*. 2017;20(6):673–689. https://doi.org/10.1080/13691058.2017.1370132

Burger K, Evans-Agnew R, Johnson S. Reproductive justice and Black lives: a concept analysis for public health nursing. *Public Health Nurs*. 2022;39(1):238–250. https://doi.org/10.1111/phn.12919

Cerdeña JP, Plaisime MV, Tsai D. From race-based to race-conscious medicine: how antiracist upbringings call us to act. *Lancet*. 2020;396(10257):1125–1128. https://doi.org/10.1016/S0140-6736(20)32076-6

Collins PH. *Black Feminist Thought*. New York, NY: Routledge; 2000.

Crear-Perry J, Maybank A, Keeys M, Mitchell N, Godbolt D. Moving towards anti-racist praxis in medicine. *Lancet*. 2020;396(10249):451–453. https://doi.org/10.1016/S0140-6736(20)31543-9

Crenshaw K. Demarginalizing the intersection of race and sex: a Black feminist critique of antidiscrimination doctrine, feminist theory and antiracist politics. *Univ Chic Leg Forum*. 1989;(1):139–167.

Crooks N, Singer R, Tluczek A. Black female sexuality: intersectional identities and historical contexts. *ANS Adv Nurs Sci*. 2021;44(1):52–65. https://doi.org/10.1097/ans.0000000000000332

Durkheim, E. *Division of Labor in Society*. New York, NY: Free Press; 2014.

Goes EF, de Souza Menezes GM, Chagas de Almeida MDC, et al. Barriers in accessing care for consequence of unsafe abortion by Black women: evidence of institutional racism in Brazil. *J Racial Ethn Health Disparities*. 2021;8(6):1385–1394. https://doi.org/10.1007/s40615-020-00900-w

Hill Collins P. *Black Sexual Politics: African Americans, Gender, and the New Racism.* New York, NY: Routledge; 2005.

Jackson FM, Rowley DL, Curry Owens T. Contextualized stress, global stress, and depression in well-educated, pregnant, African-American women. *Womens Health Issues.* 2012;22(3):e329–e336. https://doi.org/10.1016/j.whi.2012.01.003

Jenkins Hall W, Tanner AE. US Black college women's sexual health in hookup culture: intersections of race and gender. *Cult Health Sex.* 2016;18(11):1265–1278. https://doi.org/10.1080/13691058.2016.1183046

Logan RG, Vamos CA, Daley EM, Louis-Jacques A, Marhefka SL. Understanding young Black women's socialisation and perceptions of sexual and reproductive health. *Cult Health Sex.* 2021;24(12):1–15. https://doi.org/10.1080/13691058.2021.2014976

Opara I, Abrams JA, Cross K, Amutah-Onukagha N. Reframing sexual health for Black girls and women in HIV/STI prevention work: highlighting the role of identity and interpersonal relationships. *Int J Environ Res Public Health.* 2021;18(22):12088. https://doi.org/10.3390/ijerph182212088

Prather C, Fuller TR, Jeffries WL IV, et al. Racism, African American women, and their sexual and reproductive health: a review of historical and contemporary evidence and implications for health equity. *Health Equity.* 2018;2(1), 249–259. https://doi.org/10.1089/heq.2017.0045

Rosenthal L, Lobel M. Gendered racism and the sexual and reproductive health of Black and Latina women. *Ethn Health.* 2020;25(3):367–392. https://doi.org/10.1080/13557858.2018.1439896

Serrant L. Silenced knowing: an intersectional framework for exploring Black women's health and diasporic identities. *Front Sociol.* 2020;5:1. https://doi.org/10.3389/fsoc.2020.00001

30

Designing New Futures: Essential Wrap-Around Services for Reproductive Justice–Informed Scholars

Joia Crear-Perry, MD, Asha Hassan, MPH, Tonni Oberly, MPH,
Jaleah Rutledge, MA, Daphne Scott-Henderson, MS, RN,
Daniel Suárez-Baquero, PhD, MSN, RN, Najjuwah Walden, MSW,
and Monica R. McLemore, PhD, MPH, RN

The purpose of this chapter is to describe essential services built to support Black doctoral students to become reproductive justice–informed scholars. This chapter describes pathways between pipeline programs at primarily white institutions and essential services necessary for Black scholars to conduct reproductive justice research and to be successful and thrive. Voices from scholars participating in these programs are centered to provide important insights into how we best develop the next generation of knowledge producers who will unlock discoveries in health and human services to improve outcomes and resolve health inequities.

The chapter is divided into three sections. First, we describe two pipeline programs, National Birth Equity Collaborative (NBEC) and Abortion Care Training Incubator of Outstanding Nurse Scholars (ACTIONS), and we provide basic statistics for workforce projections in health care and human services provision. Second, scholars present their experiences, strategies, and tools learned from the frameworks embraced by the NBEC and ACTIONS programs to combat stereotype threat, imposter syndrome, racism, and microaggressions. Finally, the chapter ends with a discussion of reimagining programs to support scholars based on lessons learned from the NBEC and ACTIONS programs including the cohort model, intergenerational shared learning, access to nationally recognized scholars for mentorship and sponsorship, works in progress, and prioritization of wellness and self-actualization.

PIPELINE PROGRAMS FOR REPRODUCTIVE JUSTICE SCHOLARS

This chapter represents a collaborative writing effort between the leadership and scholars from NBEC and ACTIONS. Given the focus of both programs to support Black, Indigenous, other people of color (BIPOC; ACTIONS), and Black women and femmes

(NBEC), some background is provided about each program and how these programs fit into the larger landscape of pipeline programs geared toward diversifying the nursing, public health, and social science research workforces.

NBEC is one of the nation's leading experts and an advocate for change in the Black maternal health and infant mortality crises. As an organization focused on the sexual and reproductive health and well-being of Black women and birthing people worldwide, NBEC creates transnational solutions that optimize Black maternal, infant, sexual, and reproductive well-being. Established in 2015, NBEC was created to combat the increasing rate of infant mortality within the most marginalized populations—Black and Brown people. As an obstetrician/gynecologist, NBEC founder Dr. Joia Crear-Perry witnessed the disparities experienced by Black women and birthing people, as well as children dying during childbirth and the postnatal period. Recognizing that ensuring better care for Black babies had to start with better care for Black mamas, NBEC expanded its mission to focus more on mothers' experiences along with the baby, in hopes of creating safe and healthy conditions for both moms and their babies.

One major aspect of the work has been awareness of the crises and offering actionable solutions. With the launch of its training program, NBEC began training providers and birthing facilities on ways they could be more equitable in delivering care to Black and Brown birthing people. However, with every step forward, it became clear that to truly solve the Black maternal mortality crisis, this fight must be fought on several different fronts. It is through this expanded focus that NBEC has evolved to become one of the leading organizations within the maternal mortality crisis, using advocacy, collaboration, strategic communications, policy, research, training, and technical assistance to accomplish its mission.

Through these channels, NBEC hopes to not only help to significantly curb the maternal and infant mortality rate but to also shift the culture within public health, creating an all-around more equitable and respectful level of care for all women, birthing people, and their babies. NBEC is a proud member of Black Mamas Matter Alliance.

The ACTIONS program, currently housed at the University of California, San Francisco (UCSF) School of Nursing, is funded in three-year increments by an anonymous donor to train the next generation of nursing and public health leaders. The ACTIONS program provides funding for predoctoral and postdoctoral scholars at UCSF to design studies that prioritize reproductive justice as the primary approach to reproductive health services provision, including abortion, birth, contraception, healthy sexuality, parenting, and pleasure. This fellowship provides a unique opportunity to train the next generation of thought leaders and change agents in nursing, public health, and social science scholarship. The program participants have launched several research projects, written op-eds, co-authored an amicus brief, and actively participated in the California Future of Abortion Council. The ACTIONS program launched in 2018.

Former postdoctoral fellows are now pursuing academic careers and leading reproductive justice work at other institutions across the country.

RETROFIT, REFORM, AND REIMAGINE FRAMEWORK

The conceptual framework that informs the structure of this chapter is the retrofit, reform, reimagine (3R) framework (McLemore 2022). In our view, pipeline programs are at best a retrofit to the existing structures of academia. What makes NBEC and ACTIONS innovative is the NBEC program was purposively designed to be adjunctive to existing institutional support. The NBEC scholars are predoctoral scholars at accredited academic institutions in 18 unique departments working to obtain research degrees. Both the NBEC and ACTIONS programs use a cohort approach to allow scholars to have peer-to-peer opportunities for learning and partnership on projects. Scholars in both programs are institutionally bound and required to complete all competencies and coursework required by their academic institutions.

Capturing scholar experiences is a reformation using the 3R framework. We believe co-creating the programs to meet the needs of the scholars allows for specific content to be offered including dissertation workshops, restoration and reflection retreats, teach-ins with expert scholars who have expertise with populations of interest and those with methodological and/or theoretical expertise, and opportunities to interface with the work of other NBEC and ACTIONS scholars. Group interviews were used to obtain scholar experiences and are presented with methods consistent with qualitative research.

The programmatic supports of both NBEC and ACTIONS are considered a reimagining of academia—specifically, the process and the content necessary to become a scholar and to complete doctoral programs. Current academic curricula are inadequate to develop the innovative work of BIPOC, Black women, and femme scholars, particularly at primarily white institutions. Therefore, it is why NBEC and ACTIONS programs were founded—to develop the opportunities, coaching, mentorship, and sponsorship that are crucial for successful completion.

Retrofit: Brief History of Pipeline Programs

A substantial body of evidence exists that describes health disparities between populations. Yet this important work has not spawned effective, novel, or sustainable interventions designed to mitigate disparities and achieve health equity. Similarly, there have been pipeline programs (Sullivan 2004; Smith et al. 2009a; Smith et al. 2009b) that theoretically should result in improved health outcomes due to the mechanism of racial concordance—the notion that stress from racism and mistreatment would be reduced. However, there has been little movement in the diversification of the health professions (Zambrana 2018).

Programs funded by both the federal government and the private sector have had mixed results. Assessments of these programs have found that (1) people of color in the health professions are more likely to serve minority populations, (2) health care providers who are people of color are more likely to work with publicly insured and minority populations, and (3) programs that provide financial incentives to any health care provider who serves minority populations have not been more successful than programs that develop minority health care providers in ensuring adequate workforce serving in underresourced settings (Sullivan 2004; Smith et al. 2009a; Smith et al. 2009b).

As of 2018, only 65.6% of the US population was classified as white, however, 83.2% of licensed nurses and 90% of certified nurse-midwives are white. While the physician community is more diverse (49% white), only 4% of physicians are Black or African American, 4.4% Hispanic, and 0.4% American Indian or Alaska Native (Zangaro et al. 2018). While 93% of licensed nurses or certified nurse-midwives are women, only 34% of physicians are women (Association of American Colleges of Medicine 2014). While there are more Black or African American women physicians (54.7%) than men (45.3%), in all other racial and ethnic groups, there are more men than women for Asians (56.4% men), American Indians or Alaska Natives (58.1% men), Hispanics or Latinos (59.0% men), and whites (65.2% men; Association of American Colleges of Medicine 2014). For the purposes of this chapter, scholars of color, people of color, and communities of color refer to the underrepresented racial and ethnic categories specific to the health sciences from the National Science Foundation (National Science Foundation 2017) abbreviated as URM (i.e., American Indian or Alaska Native, Black or African American, Hispanic or Latino, Native Hawaiian or other Pacific Islander).

Globally, researchers recognize that the health and well-being of our modern world is tied to the health and well-being of women and girls (Davidson et al. 2011). If applied in the United States, these types of programs should enable women to fully participate as citizens in society and therefore improve their health and the health of their communities. However, when considering the unique challenges of the advancement of education for women and girls of color in the United States, it is necessary to understand the complex relationship of gendered racism (the intersection of racism and sexism experienced by URM women; Rosenthal and Lobel 2020) reproductive well-being, and life trajectory (Figure 30-1).

In the United States, across the reproductive spectrum (e.g., family planning, maternal fetal medicine, reproductive endocrinology and infertility, gynecologic oncology), Black and Brown women and girls have poorer outcomes than their white counterparts. For example, Black women are three to four times more likely to die in childbirth, are more likely to have advanced and aggressive disease when diagnosed with breast and gynecologic cancers, and are half as likely as white women to be able to access infertility and assisted reproductive technology (Eichelberger et al. 2016).

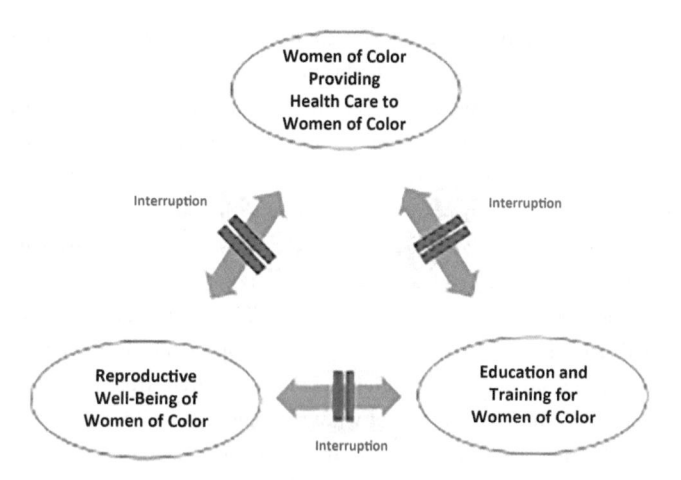

Figure 30-1. Potential Interruption of Life Trajectory for Women of Color

Exposure to gendered racism leads to poor reproductive well-being of women of color, which further narrows the pool of potential scholars—the exact people most likely to have the greatest influence over these outcomes. Gendered racism also serves as a predictable interruption in the life trajectory for women of color; specifically, decreased access to health insurance does not allow for full range contraception or pregnancy termination. Given these findings and the dearth of faculty and students of color, it is necessary to ensure that these individuals are supported for success and to be able to be to complete their academic programs and career goals. In the next section, we provide scholar experiences to provide support for our approach. In addition to including single vignettes from scholars, which were obtained between September 1 and November 30, 2021, we conducted a focus group on Zoom on October 1, 2021, and November 15, 2021, which was recorded and transcribed. All interviews were conducted in confidentiality, and the names of the interviewees are withheld by mutual agreement. We include portions of the transcript to support our thematic analyses.

Reform: Scholar Experiences

One scholar described their experiences in the ACTIONS program in the following vignette:

> When I was notified of my acceptance into the Abortion Care Training Incubator for Outstanding Nurse Scholars (ACTIONS) program as an incoming predoctoral student, I wasn't sure what to expect from the program. The ACTIONS team explained their program model and I received ample supplemental information before and after acceptance, but I never assume what a new experience would be like, and I was wary of setting my expectations too

high. I can say with certainty, now that I have completed my first year as a doctoral student at UCSF, that ACTIONS has been an integral factor in my academic success.

ACTIONS lives up to its name and is truly an incubator for ideas, creativity, and camaraderie. Although my PhD cohort is supportive, there is an undercurrent of competition that runs through the cohort. ACTIONS has provided me with an alternative academic social outlet wherein I can network and collaborate with graduate students—within and outside of the School of Nursing—who are genuinely encouraging and who are interested in the kinds of social justice-focused research that I am most passionate about. As a member of the lesbian, gay, bisexual, transgender, queer (LGBTQ+) community, I frequently seek welcoming and affirming spaces, and ACTIONS is that space for me at UCSF. During my first year as a doctoral student, I applied for and received a grant from the UCSF School of Nursing chapter of Sigma Theta Tau International to conduct a pilot research study. I was informed that this grant rarely goes to early career students.

As an ACTIONS scholar, I feel empowered, and I am encouraged to be vigilant and proactive when opportunities arise that align with, or could potentially support, my research interests, research projects, and/or my academic or professional growth. As a full-time student who also works full-time, I don't depend on my ACTIONS stipend for my costs of daily living. Nevertheless, I greatly appreciate the financial support. Of course, the stipend helps with funding crucial components of research projects, but the financial support also gives credence to the message that ACTIONS believes in my abilities as a scholar and as a social justice warrior-in-training and is doing everything possible to remove obstacles to my success. Lastly, a benefit of ACTIONS that is priceless: the program encourages us to be outspoken scholars and fearless research scientists, but to never forget to be compassionate and ethical human beings.

Theme 1: Filling Programmatic Gaps

This quote exemplifies what we heard from many scholars in that NBEC and ACTIONS filled essential gaps in their formal programs:

> In my department at my university, I did not have anybody whose research interests directly aligned with mine, so I was super excited to apply for the fellowship program because I felt that it would give me an opportunity to do work on what I was really interested in with populations that I'm interested in working with. That's not something that I really had the opportunity to do within my program, like I could have done it, but then the pandemic happened, so I really wasn't able to leverage the community in the ways that I would have wanted to, because people were worried about so many other things. They were not thinking about me trying to push a research agenda forward, no matter how community-based it was. They had my real-life problems that were happening right then and there around COVID-19. And, so, when I saw the fellowship opportunity, I was like, oh wow, this will really give me an opportunity to do work that I really want to do and I'll probably get a different set of skills that I would not have necessarily gained by only working with the faculty mentorship and people that were available to me at my institution.

Theme 2: Belonging and Building Community

Another student remarked on the space that is intentionally curated to support the students in different ways than their academic homes:

> It would be really interesting to see our committee members in that engagement in this space; yeah, that would be really, really interesting and probably very helpful for them to understand more about where we're coming from, or how we communicate with each other and how we operate in this space and how it is different and beneficial to us as graduate students in the program. So, I would say that's really great insight. And just to build off of what was just said, I'm just thinking about more of a focus on us hitting our milestones to finish our degrees. So, wherever people are in their program, making sure that we're on whatever flexible timeline (acknowledging that timelines change) but are we meeting milestones and are we progressing could be helpful. I think if we started doing that, with our individual development plans but just more tracking of actually finishing these degrees, I think it could be useful.

Another student was adamant about why they applied and stated that she wanted to build on the previous statement:

> Yes, so I had an advisor who I had worked with for about a year, and I gravitated to her, because she was the only Black and female faculty on the public health sciences side, but her research areas of interest and my research area of interest were very different. She was an environmental epidemiologist. I was studying social epidemiology at the time, and she wanted to make sure that I was in a community of scholars, of academics, of faculty members who could support my area of interest and also critique it. Because, often times what happens, especially at my school, is that you might have students who have areas of interest that are different from their committee members and so there's no one able to really challenge or critique or ensure that you're doing accurate and rigorous research, and so she sent the information over to me and I decided to apply because I felt like it would be a place where I could study the experiences of Black women without having to explain why the experiences of Black women were important to study. So, I had hoped that that would be the outcome and that's absolutely been my experience but I think the second reason I also applied was absolutely for financial support, because my area of interest isn't on the grant funding radar right now; there aren't people who are interested in studying the effects of lifestyles on reproductive health across the life course, you know, there's not a lot of research on this.

Another scholar said,

> What both of you are saying resonates to me. The academic support to be challenged in my research was also important to me. The funding was crucial. My program is funded, but you know grad school funding is only like $20,000 a year and that's really not enough, and so I was working full time while being a part-time student, instead of being a full-time student. So, I wasn't really getting the full experience of being a full-time student. I wasn't able to engage with my cohort in the same way. And in both my academic setting and my professional setting I was the only Black person so, even though I was in the maternal-child health

space, I was the only Black person, and others didn't really get it. It was just a really traumatic environment so being able to apply to a space where I knew that, like our colleague said, I wasn't going to have to explain myself or why it mattered but to actually just go ahead and go deeper was really, really helpful.

Another ACTIONS scholar said,

The experience of mentoring depends so much more on the mentor rather than the mentee. Even the components of the program or the resources that you have available are nothing if you don't have a mentor that is committed with your success, committed with the completion of your goals. One can have all the resources one needs but, without a committed mentor, that is nothing. I think that's something that is important to have, I don't know if it could be possible, to have a training or something for white mentors, because they are replicating the behaviors that we are trying to avoid from academia and actually that was one of the reasons why I came to ACTIONS, because I thought, the director of the program is a Black woman who has strong opinions and she does not give a shit of what anybody thinks about it. So I said, I'm going to go there; I want to be like her.

However, the ACTIONS program is at UCSF, and UCSF is a primarily white institution, so it has white professors who are maintaining and replicating behaviors that are harmful for people of color and we have contact with them. Another ideas is to have maybe a mechanism in which we can address or report this harm, because we are not feeling safe or comfortable when these faculty members are in the same room; for example, I personally stopped having meetings with one of these faculty members because I really felt harmed by them, so I decided to stop having meetings with this person because it's really harmful, because this person not only discourage me about my research, but also about me as a person. So, I think that that is something important because, in these programs, we are looking for a safe space in which we can build community.

Theme 3: Demystifying the Doctoral Process

One NBEC scholar made a statement that perfectly captures the third theme of demystifying the doctoral process:

The first thing that came to mind is this additional dissertation proposal support because I felt like the dissertation retreats, I am still really reaping the benefit of those last couple of days that we've been together. But, at the same time, I feel like after the retreat, you know I went back to my institution and didn't receive the same level of feedback, didn't receive the same level of support, and, so, if there was any way that that could be continuous, I don't know if that looks like having a weekly or bi-weekly sessions to be able to work on our proposal or just having additional workshops or guest speakers talking about opportunity to do research, but I feel like there's a lot more that I need to understand about doing equitable and birth justice, enabling research, and all of it couldn't be contained within the retreat, I felt like there was so much more that I needed in a lot more that we had time to give, given the fact that the fellowship is two years.

Another added,

> One thing that I'm starting to think about, especially now that graduation is quickly approaching, is opportunities in terms of job support or maybe some type of job club or something. I know that we are all applying for different things, and so I appreciate that, but I think it will be really helpful to have some type of, I don't know, program or workshop that's really built to help us think about next steps in terms of our careers. Because, and I know we kind of talked about postdoc opportunities and stuff like that, but something that's a bit more formal that can really set us up to walk directly into something after we finish would be really, really helpful and I don't think I've experienced that yet.

Several scholars discussed international models of education and training. One in particular spoke of Latin America, where there is something that is called *semillero* (seedbed/hotbed)—that is, space in which you plant the seeds for them to grow and you care for the seeds to become big plants:

> In the *semillero*, what we do is to communicate with undergrad students and the students of all the levels in the school. This is a space in which we can share not only a research project but also initiatives and ideas, and find ways and places in which we can find support for us in all different levels of education. So, in that way, we are growing together with the future scholars, clinicians, or those who will be in different settings. Something similar happens in ACTIONS and NBEC; they are *semilleros*, and we have that seed of reproductive justice, health equity, of anti-racism in us. Also, to continue with the idea is to bring other ways of knowing and ways of living, bring those to our discussions, research and meeting, not only to have the Eurocentric focus in academia, but also other knowledges that are so valuable, especially when we are talking about midwifery and Black maternal health. It is important to start acknowledging these other ways of knowing at the same level as the Eurocentric traditional way, because in a certain point, only the knowledge that is built inside the academia is valuable and recognized, but I learned ways of knowing [i.e., from *parteras, curanderas*, and granny midwives] that are also important and have not been recognized. Moreover, they have been oppressed by formal structures of academia, so it's important to recognize them, embrace them, and invite them to or groups and to our programs.

Theme 4: Deeper Need for Community Engagement and Embedded Research

When thinking about our work and building both competence and confidence, the scholars also reflected on the theoretical underpinnings and conceptual frameworks of their research. One scholar said,

> One thing that comes to my mind, I love all of those suggestions [work using Black feminist perspective from a reproductive justice perspective and from a birth justice perspective] that have been made, is also maybe building a better connection with community, whether

it's community-based organizations or directly with community members. I know at NBEC, we talk about being community-centered in the research, but I feel like there could be more done there, whether it's maybe scholars are somehow linked up with a local community-based organization and you do some research for them, or with them, or I don't know. I'm just thinking that there might be a way to plug scholars in to their communities as researchers in some way.

Another scholar added an important point specific to intergenerational opportunities for learning:

I don't know the name of the program, I think Robert Wood Johnson has some type of program with community leaders [Culture of Health Leaders]; I believe it is a fellowship-type thing. I think that would be something that NBEC could implement to leverage community more in the work we do, especially as a part of the scholars program. And I also would have loved something like this program in undergrad as I was just kind of dipping my toe into the water and trying to understand what all of this was. I don't know that I would have done, like, a different path, if I had been exposed earlier, but I definitely think it would have helped me become more sure of my research interests and what it was that I wanted to do if I had had an opportunity like this in my junior or senior year of undergrad. So, I think, maybe an undergrad internship program or summer program would be really, really good if we can even like pair them with scholars.

Theme 5: Readiness for Postdoctoral Experiences

Another student remarked on the support and preparation they received with becoming reproductive justice scholars:

I found in the ACTIONS program an open space where I can freely share my ideas with other BIPOC scholars and experts, continue our research paths, and quench our thirst for reproductive and social justice. In the ACTIONS program, I learned that the most important feature to combat stereotype threat, imposter syndrome, racism, and microaggressions is to have a faculty mentor committed to see in the mentee a human being embedded in an intersection of characteristics, someone who recognizes those wounds and scars that academy has left in us just because of what we are.

During my postdoctoral path and considering that ACTIONS is still a part of a primarily white institution, I must acknowledge all the good and kindness I received in the program, but also the harm produced from white faculty members who replicate behaviors I have gone through across other US academic institutions—namely, giving unrequested opinions, breaking students' confidence, putting barriers to develop one's ideas, among others. However, thanks to the support received from my BIPOC mentor in the ACTIONS program—a Black woman who has undergone the same experiences on her own skin, and who is highly passioned for guiding students—I received the essential tools to stand and speak up.

In the ACTIONS program I found a shelter for my own self becoming and a place full of resources to develop my research program. Indeed, the main characteristic that makes

ACTIONS the greatest program from reproductive justice scholars in the world, is the people that move you to believe in yourself because here you feel at home. When I think of ACTIONS and my mentor, it comes to my mind the memory of my grandmother teaching a young 5-year-old me how to cook to share with all the family; the smell of the coffee floods the kitchen and a warm feeling comes from the inside; this is the best way I can describe the program, it is about reproductive justice, but it is about love and caring as well.

Together, all of us, pre- and postdoc fellows, mentors, project directors, interns, graduate student researchers, and collaborators, combine our strengths to fight racism through our collective research projects, communications, policy briefs, podcast, videos, and social media presence that prioritize reproductive justice as the primary approach to reproductive health services provision. We create a safe environment in which you are not threatened by others judging you based on who you are, including your race, gender, culture, ethnicity, or other forms of identity. In ACTIONS, besides learning how to apply reproductive justice theoretical framework, practice, and strategy, this program promotes the 3Rs model developed by its creator, Dr. Monica R. McLemore. In this model, we retrofit, reform, and reimagine a different future based on social justice and our own paths as future scholars.

In ACTIONS, I have learned courage to take the chance and go beyond. Now that I start my transition to become a faculty mentor, I clearly know the kind of professor, mentor, and scholar I aspire to be. I am committed to antiracism, diversity, equity, and inclusion to confront biases and racism at the individual, institutional, and systemic levels. When I arrived in ACTIONS, I heard with disbelief how they positively described my work and myself, mainly because during the recent years I was labeled as a failure for going against the canons of my school. Today, looking back, I take ACTIONS because I cannot bear that more people must live the experiences I lived. Particularly, in academia and in nursing science, where from the very beginning, the ideas and world views of a predominant privileged group have mandated "what [nursing] is, and what it is not."

Reimagining: Programmatic Supports

Many scholars discussed the protective supports within NBEC and ACTIONS as a result of being with other scholars of color when they are "onlys" at their home academic institutions. One summed it up this way:

> And it's just so healthy for my development and my growth as a scholar. And I went to an HBCU [historically Black college or university], right, so I've been around Black academics, I know that they exist, but the value in having that community of other Black women doctoral students as you go through this process is really affirming and comfortable and, like, obviously, I knew that we would have people, but I really did not think that I would have the community that I have in the scholars program. That's not something I really expected, and I think that has honestly been one of the greatest benefits of the programs and making sure that I just kind of stay on track, like me and the other scholars will hold each other accountable to doing what we need to do and, yeah, I think that has made a really big difference in my matriculation.

One scholar also clearly articulated the toll that doctoral studies can take on individuals and put this into a larger context, linking what we study to our own personal experiences and trauma:

> I also feel like, as an NBEC scholar, we really get to imagine what it looks like for Black women and Black birthing people to be well and to be healthy, because at my institution whenever I first came in, you know, with social determinants of health, it was packed. It was like everybody was talking about it. You know, everybody was conducting research and looking to know whether or not, you know, Black people had worse outcomes. And to discover that was almost, you know, a glorification, you know, of their research. But at the same time, I feel like for Black people and additional people of color who have to be told over and over and over again that we're more at risk for this and more at risk for that, it can be traumatizing, and it's also not explanatory. Like you telling me that I'm more likely to experience this, this, and this. Because I'm Black doesn't tell me what I get to do about it; it doesn't tell me how I can prevent those outcomes; it doesn't tell me, you know, what about my experience of being Black makes me vulnerable. And we know that in the background those conversations don't exist. But I have never had a conversation in a year that I've been a birth equity research scholar where someone has said, you know, in conclusion, Black women are more at risk. That is not the conclusion. That may not even be the starting point. Here we really get the opportunity to understand why these vulnerabilities exist, whether it's on the individual or the cellular or the systemic level, and then we also get encouraged to imagine what it looks like in a world where those things don't happen for Black women, okay, and then, how do we enable Black women to get there.

DISCUSSION

In our application of the 3R approach to diversification of the workforce, pipeline programs, and support for scholars, we highlight five recommendations that are supported by the five themes identified in our interviews and focus groups (Box 30-1). First, both NBEC and ACTIONS programs use cohort models where multiple individuals are onboarded in a shared experience to build community and connection. This approach is purposively employed to remove the stigma of being an only and the ease of which scholars are hypervisible and vulnerable.

Box 30-1. Identified Themes of Scholars' Experiences

Theme 1: Filling programmatic gaps
Theme 2: Belonging and building community
Theme 3: Demystifying the doctoral process
Theme 4: Deeper need for community engagement and embedded research
Theme 5: Readiness for postdoctoral experiences

Next, we deploy opportunities for intergenerational shared learning; however, this looks different in each program. Within the NBEC program, scholars have access to other scholars within the organization as well as Black women researchers and leaders of community-based organizations as NBEC currently only accepts predoctoral students. The ACTIONS program operationalizes intergenerational learning by including ACTIONS alumni and pre- and postdoctoral scholars in addition to faculty to support the research projects, seminars, and symposia. Both programs grant access to nationally recognized scholars for mentorship and sponsorship with a focus on reproductive health, rights, and justice-informed individuals. Specific to these activities, the programs employ teach-ins, which are opportunities to share works in progress and other networking opportunities for scholars to emerge and present their work.

Finally, both the NBEC and ACTIONS fellowships focus on the prioritization of wellness and self-actualization for the scholars such that the process of their development is aligned with the content they are studying, learning, and using in their work. We believe these are the essential components to diversifying the workforce while ensuring a focus on health equity and justice.

REFERENCES

Association of American Colleges of Medicine. Current status of the US physician workforce. 2014. Available at: http://www.aamcdiversityfactsandfigures.org/section-ii-current-status-of-us-physician-workforce/index.html

Davidson PM, McGrath SJ, Meleis AI, et al. The health of women and girls determines the health and well-being of our modern world: a white paper from the International Council on Women's Health Issues. *Health Care Women Int*. 2011;32(10):870–886. https://doi.org/10.1080/07399332.2011.603872

Eichelberger KY, Doll K, Ekpo GE, Zerden ML. Black lives matter: claiming a space for evidence-based outrage in obstetrics and gynecology. *Am J Public Health*. 2016;106(10):1771–1772. https://doi.org/10.2105/AJPH.2016.303313.

McLemore MR. Using retrofit, reform, and reimagine to advance toward health equity. *J Perinat Neonatal Nurs*. 2022;36(2):99–102. https://doi.org/10.1097/JPN.0000000000000639

National Science Foundation. Women, minorities, and persons with disabilities in science and engineering. 2017. Available at: https://www.nsf.gov/statistics/2017/nsf17310

Rosenthal L, Lobel M. Gendered racism and the sexual and reproductive health of Black and Latina women. *Ethn Health*. 2020;25(3):367–392. https://doi.org/10.1080/13557858.2018.1439896

Smith SG, Nsiah-Kumi PA, Jones PR, Pamies RJ. Pipeline programs in the health professions, part 1: preserving diversity and reducing health disparities. *J Natl Med Assoc*. 2009a;101(9):836–840, 845–851. https://doi.org/10.1016/s0027-9684(15)31030-0

Smith SG, Nsiah-Kumi PA, Jones PR, Pamies RJ. Pipeline programs in the health professions, part 2: the impact of recent legal challenges to affirmative action. *J Natl Med Assoc*. 2009b;101(9):852–863. https://doi.org/10.1016/s0027-9684(15)31031-2

Sullivan L. Missing persons: minorities in the health professions, a report of the Sullivan Commission on Diversity in the Healthcare Workforce. 2004. https://doi.org/10.13016/cwij-acxl

Zambrana RE. *Toxic Ivory Towers: The Consequences of Work Stress on Underrepresented Minority Faculty.* New Brunswick, NJ: Rutgers University Press; 2018.

Zangaro GA, Streeter R, Li T. Trends in racial and ethnic demographics of the nursing workforce: 2000 to 2015. *Nurs Outlook.* 2018;66(4):365–371. https://doi.org/10.1016/j.outlook.2018.05.001

31

We're at a Turning Point: How Investments in Black Women–Focused Organizations and Leaders in Philanthropy Are Impacting Black Women's Reproductive Health and Sexuality

Regina Davis Moss, PhD, MPH

There is increasing recognition throughout the philanthropic sector that advancing reproductive justice and birth equity is critical to protecting the health and well-being of Black women. Yet, investments in efforts supporting Black women–focused and Black women–led organizations have continually been underfunded. In 2018, only $15 million of almost $428 billion in philanthropic giving (less than 1%) in the United States supported Black women and girls (Couvson and McHarris 2022). According to an Echoing Green and The Bridgespan Group (2020) report on racial inequities in philanthropic funding, the revenues of Black-led organizations are, on average, 24% smaller than those of their white-led counterparts. Moreover, organizations led by Black women consistently receive less funding than those led by Black men as well as those led by white women.

Philanthropic efforts that lack an intersectional analysis and understanding of culturally relevant strategies or those that over-rely on specific forms of evaluation and deprioritize the missions of organizations working closest with the community are several factors that contribute to inequitable investments (Dorsey et al. 2020). When organizations do receive funding, it is often highly restricted or does not allow for the ability to build infrastructure, further fueling barriers.

There is a growing movement of philanthropic leaders across the country working to dismantle barriers in securing funding and center Black women's health-focused funds. This chapter presents the results of a key informant study that asked some of these leaders about their first-hand knowledge and experiences. The goal was to deepen the understanding of how philanthropy is impacting change in Black women's reproductive health and sexuality and included fundamental questions such as, "What are the overall funding practices of grant-making organizations?" and "What types of organizations and programs are receiving funding?" Their insights about solutions to overcome the funding gap, as well as directions for the future, were also sought. Special thanks to the leaders for sharing their time and stories. The sections that follow highlight the key findings.

METHODOLOGY

Key informant interviews were conducted between June and September 2022 with 13 leaders with extensive knowledge in grant-making, and particular experience funding Black women–led or Black women–focused reproductive health and sexuality programming. All interviewees identified as female, with 92% identifying as persons of color. Respondents represented 11 entities focused on philanthropy and investments in health-related projects, including national- and state-level organizations, large philanthropic funders, private companies, and philanthropy watchdog groups. Interviewees held various professional roles, including experience directing large funding organizations, leading programs focused on Black women's reproductive health and sexuality funding, and managing relationships between funder and grantee organizations. Respondents reported a range of 5 to 25 years of experience in grant-making and/or philanthropy, and many reported additional professional experience in the field of reproductive health and sexuality not related to grant-making. All interviews were conducted in confidentiality, and the names of the interviewees are withheld by mutual agreement.

Interview transcripts were reviewed and edited for accuracy using the appropriate recording. After all interview notes were finalized, the resulting data were coded and analyzed. Key themes and patterns of responses were then assigned to the appropriate interview objective and utilized to create a summary of common responses.

FINDINGS

Detailed findings are organized by interview objective and include general impressions of trends in respondent data. Specifically, this section presents

- Characteristics of funding organizations
- Characteristics of organizations receiving funding
- Funding practices
- History of funding programs and advancing the work
- Impact and future of funding focused on Black women's reproductive health and sexuality

General Impressions

- Funding programs or activities specifically focused on Black women's reproductive health and sexuality and/or Black women–led organizations is still an emerging area within philanthropy and grant-making. This area of funding has had a history of inequity. Organizations are often required to justify their decision to fund these types of programming. However, the environment is shifting as acceptance of the existence

of systematic racism increases and the importance of work focused on Black women's reproductive health and sexuality becomes more visible to professionals in the field and the public in general.
- Funding is often awarded to large, well-known organizations that have the capacity to search for, apply, and manage funding, as well as meet funding requirements. Funders should shift some of their focus to building the capacity of grantees and incorporate practices that lessen the burden on smaller organizations working closest to the issues being addressed. Funders also should approve the distribution of more unrestricted funds that allow smaller community organizations to continue their good work. This will increase positive outcomes and diversify funding.
- There is a positive trend in the funding of programs and activities focused on Black women's reproductive health, and there is a feeling that supporters of this type of funding should "seize the moment" to both increase awareness of inequities in funding and push the movement forward.

Characteristics of Funding Organizations

Respondents were asked to describe the general characteristics of organizations that fund programs or activities focused on Black women's reproductive health and sexuality. Organizations that fund these types of programs or activities were described as focused on equity, having people of color in decision-making positions, and willing to take risks. It was also mentioned that these organizations must substantiate their decision to direct funds to programming that supports Black women's reproductive health and sexuality by conducting their own research and collecting their own data:

> Organizations that are committed to equity…we are cognizant, and our grantees are cognizant of the racial disparity in outcomes and that they are focused on more systemic change and sustainable change…Organizations funding in this area are clear that the disparity that we are seeing is generally rooted in racism, and it's going to take efforts that are addressing the systemic racism to be truly effective.

> Candidly I would say it's the organizations that are interested in taking risks…organizations don't identify themselves as that, but usually that [funding programs or activities focused on Black women's reproductive health and sexuality] happens as a result of the leadership, or someone who had developed a taste for taking a risk.

> Most of them are Black women led…I used to do birth work. In doula trainings, I would ask, 'What makes you want to become a doula?' and the white women in the room would say, 'I want everyone to have the amazing experience that I had,' while the Black women in the room were all saying, 'I want to make sure no one has the experiences that I went through.' In philanthropy, I am seeing a lot of the same…The folks that are doing it right, have somebody at the table who has been a victim of the systems that folks are trying to fight…There

are foundations that aren't quite moving money yet, but they are moving their staff and their boards to understand how they contributed to the gap.

The number one thing we find is that we have Black women at the table leading discussions. The second thing is that we partner with other Black women in the field and partner with other Black women organizations...putting Black women in these leadership roles and having them fund other Black women organizations is key.

Organizations that fund this work have often done some pre-work to document the data around this issue, whether that is nationally or in a given space. Usually there is a case that has to be made by the organization to begin to fund it as a grant-maker.

Another common point made by respondents was that the characteristics of the organizations and the environment around funding programs or activities focused on Black women's reproductive health and sexuality is shifting and adapting to the current political and social climate:

It's shifting...it's become a more visible topic, and there are more people working in this space. There is a range, meaning there are people who have been in this space from the beginning who are thinking about reproductive justice and how to address not only maternal health and equity but also how that is inextricably linked to other inequities...and there are others that are newer in the space, that may think about maternal health, but not as equity. They focus on the gender piece, but haven't necessarily focused on the racial piece... or how do you ensure that you are partnering appropriately with people that have been doing this work for a long time. Now, with *Dobbs* and the reproductive health quagmire that we find ourselves in, there's a lot more interest in the space. Now there are conversations looking at how to reimagine capital, reimagine philanthropy, and help catalyze true change.

Within the last about 15 years there has been a shift...a major focus on our work, with literally hundreds of grants to local communities, to research, to midwifery, to the issue of breastfeeding and the whole continuum...recently [major funders] have decided to make maternal health part of their structural racism work...there have been a lot more nonprofits emerge that are focused on Black women's reproductive health. This is an emergent area.

Characteristics of Organizations Receiving Funding

Respondents were asked to describe the types of organizations that receive funding focused on Black women's reproductive health and sexuality. Respondents generally agreed that large, national organizations that have the infrastructure in place to handle the management of funds and the requirements that come along with funding are most likely to receive funding. They also mentioned that the organizations receiving funding often have an advocacy arm, are policy- or research-focused, and provide direct services:

There needs to be funding for general operating support, and unrestricted, and multi-year. Right now, it's going to Black women–led work; however, it's still the national-level conversation. It's the same conversation we were having around abortion access, meaning so much money is going to national organizations, and it's a state- and local-level issue. We have the data around Black maternal health. Why not invest in Black doulas in the state, in addition to the Black women–led organizations. There's enough money to go to everyone, but I think that philanthropy is still trying to figure out how they can continue to invest in the white women–led national efforts, and give a piece to Indigenous people, and a piece to Black folks that are doing the work.

Organizations that receive funding have a strong infrastructure in place to handle the funds. This is the more traditional nonprofits. The organizations that care and demonstrate advocacy for Black women's health tend to be smaller organizations who are created to deliver services in response to the inequity or are advocacy organizations that are fighting for policy change. These smaller organizations are less likely to get funding. The funding tends to follow the federal model, which means organizations well positioned to receive money are the organizations usually getting the funding.

As a national funder, I think a lot of the organizations that are receiving large investments are those typical institutional partners or organizations that have worked in those areas but have much more of a national influence. As a national funder, those are the ones that we are typically in conversations with, and in partnership with.

The ones that are receiving funding tend to be more policy- and research-focused, and the funders are more comfortable funding that work because they understand that approach… Organizations with a national footprint are being funded, because especially national funders want to see things that can scale. It's organizations led by people that have operated within health care systems as physicians or things like that, so there's that commonality of 'Oh, a Black doctor is running that org,' or 'This person has worked in government and public health,' so they are getting funded more than some of the groups on the ground, and certainly more than midwifery-led work. Organizations being funded must have an advocacy arm.

When asked how equitable the decision-making process is around funding Black women–led or Black-focused organizations, respondents generally agreed that this process is not equitable and that Black-led organizations often do not have the capacity to search for or apply for available funding. However, some mentioned that the decision-making process is trending toward becoming more equitable:

> I do not think it is equitable. Candidly, I don't think it is equitable on both sides. We don't fund Black-led organizations in the way that they need to be funded, but I also think Black-led organizations don't ask for their work. Meaning, I think Black-led organizations are doing the work and not looking at the actual cost of the project, so they are often bidding and pitching us projects at a lower rate. I don't think they are doing this intentionally, but

maybe because they haven't had time to assess the amount of people and time needed for the project, because they are busy on the ground doing the work. When you are on the ground doing the work, you don't have free-thinking time.

It's not quite equitable yet. People are trying, but the money hasn't moved yet. I think the scales might tip in the coming years. There are some heavy and important conversations happening in philanthropy right now that are led by Black women...this might shift how Black women–led reproductive and feminist work, in particular, are funded in the next couple of years. There's going to be a lot of money shifting now.

If you look like all the other large corporate-looking nonprofit organizations and you have been able to establish yourself, then you can get funding from me...Black women-led organizations...have systematically been less likely to secure the resources that they need. They don't have the development staff and the HR office and the programs team...I need to understand that to build equity, I need to be able to take risks in your funding...these Black-led organizations need us to fund deep and long to allow them to sustain their work.

Funding Practices

Respondents generally agreed that there is no standard of funding practices within funding organizations and that the process related to selecting programs to receive funding is specific to the funder. It was mentioned that funds are generally restricted to a narrow time period and can often only be used for programmatic work. In addition, it can be hard to access funds if an organization does not have an existing relationship with the funder. Participants also stated that there is often a disconnect between the decision-makers and the organizations receiving the funding:

It's kind of all over the map in how we fund those organizations...when you have boards and people making the decisions that still don't represent the population you're trying to fund. Many of the boards don't have significant representation of people of color. I am fortunate, because my leadership and program officers are Black women, and that is unheard of.

They are all over the place. It depends on the foundation or funding mechanism, the structure of the funding. They are very different because even people's interpretation of birth equity and reproductive health can be very different. When I say reproductive health, I'm talking about everything, but for others it's about abortion and contraception...a lot of the foundations, especially those that don't include abortion as part of their work or funding, they are funding very differently than the groups that have a more holistic approach.

Funding is usually constrained in the sense of you are trying to make major societal change. It's not a Band-Aid; it's real work...the funding tends to be time-limited for a one- or two-year grant. Those types of grants are not so helpful when you are trying to change conditions in communities...bottom line on the practices of funding is that they are too narrow in scope and too short.

There is no standardized process by which philanthropy decides who gets the funding. A big piece of that is who is applying. We have many organizations in the country that aren't applying, but not because they aren't interested...foundations are typically solicited proposals, and there aren't a huge number of RFPs [requests for proposals] or public call for grants around this space...philanthropy tends to work with the usual grantees around this space and not fund the new, up-and-coming organizations.

Other commonalities in funding practices were the tendency to fund via intermediaries and to fund programs that focus on birth outcomes rather than the overall health of the Black woman:

A lot of the organizations that we fund as a national funder are what we call intermediaries, even though they might not call themselves intermediaries...these are organizations that already have deep investments into the field...they have the network and connections and history and expertise and have earned the trust of those stakeholder organizations and partners. As a national funder, it is more difficult for us to know who those folks are. It is more difficult for us to get out a lot of smaller grants to those orgs, so we fund through intermediaries.

There is a whole slew of organizations that are led and staffed by people of color that make up a broader infrastructure that supports the work that is happening. That is how we show up as a national funder...we are now just beginning to understand what it takes for these intermediary-like organizations to do the work that they do and understanding that more of those organizations are important to sustain the field.

It's still very much about 'What is the clinical program that is connected to this hospital or government?' or 'How do we get Black women to participate in this and get what they need out of this particular program?' but not a general 'How do we support Black reproductive health and sexuality?' I don't think anyone would frame their funding around that.

Most funding of reproductive health, particularly of women of color, was still going around those issues of birth outcomes, particularly in birth mortality. This broader holistic understanding of reproductive health was in the context of social determinants and equity issues. That's been a more recent understanding, at the most within the last 20 years.

Some respondents commented that these funding practices were shifting in a positive direction:

The funding practices for larger national funders are in flux—in a good way. I am starting to see more of an emphasis on grant-making practices, which includes things like reducing the amount of program-related investments and giving more flexible funding and general operating support funding to help build the capacity of many of the organizations that we are looking to support. Giving more unrestricted funding and leaning into trusting in those that have been leading the work for some time and trusting that they will use the funds that make sense for their work...I also see a shift towards more participatory grant-making...allowing those that are most impacted to decide on where the funds will be allocated in whatever work that we are prioritizing. That is promising, all the way down to the technical and administrative burdens that we often place on potential grantees. We have been doing a lot to try to remove some of those obstacles as it relates to how to even apply for opportunities.

When asked to describe practices specific to funding Black women–led or Black women–focused organizations specific to Black women's reproductive health and sexuality, respondents stated that there were no defined practices in this area, but that funding Black women–led or Black women–focused organizations is becoming more intentional:

> I don't think there are standardized practices in the field of philanthropy that focus on Black-led organizations.

> It is becoming a little more intentional. I have had conversations with Black women-led organizations, and Black women that are organizing that are telling me they are having different experiences than they have had with their program officers in the past. Part of that is the moment we are in with the 2020 summer uprising, and COVID, and *Dobbs*. People are starting to get it.

> These organizations are not known to the grants committee or the board. We almost have to go in and prove the organizations' worthiness…to support organizations that have never gotten a $50,000 or even $10,000 grant. For some organizations, that grant is what they need to make them legitimate…they are working with and for their community, providing services and programs, so are already legitimate. But just getting one grant can open the door for other grants.

History of Funding and Advancing the Work

Respondents were asked to discuss the history of funding programs or activities focused on Black women's reproductive health and sexuality and what can be done to improve and advance these funding efforts. Respondents indicated that most of this funding grew from a focus on infant mortality or maternal health, not a holistic approach to Black women's reproductive health across the life stage. It was also generally agreed that the issue of systemic racism or racial justice was historically ignored in funding these efforts:

> I don't think it has largely focused on the holistic aspect of a woman's reproductive rights and justice. It definitely had not had a justice lens until recent years. Even now a justice lens is not easily implemented into an organization unless their top leadership is for this. I have researched organizations that have transformed their bodies of work and grant-making calls that include the word *justice*. Most of the Black women's reproductive justice work falls under advocacy, and not under direct health philanthropy programming.

> The global indicator for the well-being of a nation is infant mortality, and we have such horrible results in this country, as well as such gross disparity. The history of funding for

Black women's health grew out of that mindset. The elephant in the room was racism, but nobody has ever really dealt with that directly, although it may just now be the beginnings of dealing with that within the last decade...from a philanthropic standpoint, there's not enough innovation to lead to meaningful change in those outcomes, but that is changing now.

Overall, women's health and women's reproductive health funding has been in existence for about 50 years, but, in terms of a focus on Black women's health and maternal health, it has only been for the last two years.

At least there's now a conversation about it. The conversation has shifted because there have been some brave people in different movement areas that are not afraid to call out philanthropy. The more conversations we have...about outcomes for Black women in this country and as this enters the mainstream, foundations have to pay attention to it, especially those that have been funding maternal health work forever.

When asked what additional practices organizations should incorporate into funding efforts that address Black women's reproductive health and sexuality, respondents mentioned diversifying funding efforts, allowing more unrestricted funds, building sustainability, increasing the length of funding cycles, and lessening the burden of applying for and reporting on funding:

> Trust-based and accountability. Black women-led organizations are very small, but they do great work. We need to get to a place of not having a lot of reporting requirements for these small but mighty organizations.

> Thinking about their sustainability and recognizing that they may not want to be a huge corporation. An example is the idea of creating cooperatives to provide that back office, so they don't have to hire an office person or development person...help them to seize the moment. Right now, there is a lot of wind behind the work that is happening on improving birth outcomes for Black moms. There will be a new thing in town within a few years, but the problem won't go away. How do we assist these organizations in capitalizing on this moment?

> How do you not fund the usual suspects? Looking at who are you funding, what do they look like; are they the same ones you have been funding? Looking at how to diversify funding. It's more than just liking an organization's idea and wanting to fund them—it's really understanding the barriers in place...For some it's easier to pull off a grant application. A lot of it is about building relationships, which takes resources for the foundations to build new relationships. So, the how we provide grants, the who we provide grants to, the processes we have, and looking internally to understand where those processes create barriers.

> Collaborating with Black women, identifying Black women-led organizations. Removing bureaucratic policies that prevent these organizations from being able to apply for grants, or being able to participate...Shifting power, meaning a lot of organizations need to remove

themselves from being in the position of directing the work, and trust grantees to identify what the output of the work should be.

We need to support organizations who are moving forward with a full spectrum of care... The funding approach can't be 'I just want to do the birth justice piece because that's easy and I don't want to get into the abortion issue.' All of it is needed...Funders need to show up to support communities with a full spectrum of care and support people on the ground.

Change the bureaucracy of funding. The application process is insane for the tiny bit of money, with crazy timelines. It can be 12 to 18 months of going back and forth with the foundations before getting funded for only about $50,000 for their work. There are boards that often are filled with people that don't understand the issues but are making the decisions about the grants that move forward...Not sure philanthropic institutions understand or want to acknowledge that they are a significant part of the problem. They need to take bigger risks. People say, 'We need to see data on this,' but this has never been done before.

In philanthropy, there is a culture and a power dynamic that suggests that we are the experts, but we are not. The best thing we can do is work to earn the trust of organizations that have been doing this work for decades and be in true relationships and partnerships with them, show up as a true ally in the work, and let them define what that means.

If we are going to change health outcomes for women of color, we are going to have to change the social context in which they live...so many of the board members in the philanthropic sector come from the private sector who are driven by a whole different world view of effectiveness; they are driven by quarterly profits...If I am going to change the ethos of a community, it might take three years to see a real change...these are complex things that take time to build up a critical mass of both understanding and support for the intervention. But if I have a foundation that says I need to see that you reduced the mortality by 25% within the year of receiving this grant, then we have a mismatch (and we often do)...I can give you a count on how many meals were served or how many taxi rides we paid for to see the doctor, but that is not the same as a creating a trajectory for change within the community. That has to be dealt with.

Due to the nature of how philanthropy is set up...we get into that pattern of being used to funding organizations that have a lot of manpower to complete high-level reporting that leaves behind the smaller grassroots organizations that are directly serving communities, because they are forced to complete tasks that require a larger workforce...a lot of foundations and a lot of organizations have to evaluate who has had an easier time applying for grants.

Impact and Future of Funding Focused on Black Women's Reproductive Health and Sexuality

Respondents generally agreed that the impacts of funding that focuses on Black women's reproductive health and sexuality cannot currently be measured. Many expressed that we are amid the growth of this movement and that the impacts could be limitless if funders take advantage of this moment in history, continue to recognize the importance of this work, and allow funding practices to evolve to truly meet the needs of the community over an extended period of time:

> We don't yet know the true impact because we are in the midst of it. The hope is that we will dismantle some of the racist structures, and create an environment in which Black lives thrive, and their outcomes are better, and they will have access to what they need to have successful birth outcomes. Has that happened yet—'no'; we are still working on it—'yes.' I think more organizations are recognizing the importance of this work.
>
> The impact is endless. To me, the impact is Black liberation. When you fund it, Black folks feel supported and cared for when they are trying to receive reproductive health care. I have been telling funders that if you want to fund Black liberation, then fund Black reproductive health. The impact helps us get access to health care, allows us to choose when we have children, and [impact] if our babies and birthing people survive. If you fund Black repro health, you are funding Black children and Black joy.
>
> The fact that we have this emerging movement is a clear impact...The fact that you have so many programs and projects right now is a big impact. You have doula programs, and Baby-Friendly Hospitals, community-based breastfeeding programs, and women's empowerment programs—all of that didn't exist 20 years ago. The state of the field today is an indication of impact...We are not where we need to be because we don't have enough improvement in outcomes, but that's because we haven't done the hard work of eliminating racism and racist conditions.
>
> The impact is that we are starting to see the future but haven't quite reached the place where funding is abundant enough, because people want to see progress so quickly...I'm now getting to see other incredible Black women in other foundations doing this work, and we're doing it together. We're creating pathways for young Black women becoming midwives, and doulas, and running programs in their communities. There's a visibility of the issue and the visibility of Black women being at the helm of it. There are still a lot of orgs where there aren't Black women leading this work and this conversation at funding institutions, so the visibility of us is important, too, and it's much bigger than the strategy of the foundation.
>
> Right now, we don't know. It's ambitious to think we will know the impact within the next five years. We must be in this for at least 10 years...It's a long haul for epidemiologic data to move. I am hoping in 10 years we will have moved the needle, and we will have reformed pre-professional education, and pre-provider education, and we will have worked to transform systems of care to include support for licensed and unlicensed individuals in that space...Our model is built in white patriarchy. When you look at the medicalization of birth, it didn't start out this way. You have white men making the big decisions for women. It is really incredible when you sit back and look at it...It will take 10 years of funding and staying in this space to see the needle move.

> We are just starting to scratch the surface. When we look at federal funding and private funding, we've been able to fund a lot of Black women and Black leaders and allow their voices to be heard…we are in a very special era, where we can see the fruits of the funding, through elevation of these voices…in the future, if organizations can be more strategic and more aware of the possible barriers their processes can pose to Black women accessing these funds, we could see larger impacts.
>
> I think the field has finally validated Black-led women orgs. The problem is the validation doesn't yet translate to dollars.
>
> We are working on an intractable problem that has existed for decades, in terms of poor outcomes for Black birthing people related to pregnancy and childbirth. We are in this for the long haul. We are not looking to pivot out of here if it doesn't change in the next five years, because this is going to take a while, and we need to stay the course.

Respondents mentioned that the movement to fund Black women's reproductive health has been evolving over time but that we are currently in an important moment in history that is providing great opportunities to advance this work. There was an indication that funders should seize this opportunity and focus efforts on advancing efforts to fund programs focused on equity:

> We are at a turning point. We now have more women of color in leadership positions within philanthropy, so there is a different level of awareness and understanding, and that is one way that funding is evolving. They are funding Black women-led orgs now in ways that were unheard of 20 years ago. There's a deeper understanding now, that structural racism is an underlying problem, which is another evolution.
>
> The evolution I've seen in the last two years has been an increase in trust…We are building real trust, and we…know that the work that they are doing is good. We are seeing that this money is going to these Black women. More intentionality around elevating their voices. We are seeing direct mentoring. We want to have a maternal health summit and we want these Black women to speak.
>
> I have observed in the last couple of years a lot of funders coming to the birth justice table. I think broader health-funder philanthropy has struggled to figure out how to get into this space, but are moving there now.
>
> The year 2020. Direct identification of racial inequities exists, and, when it comes to reproductive health, we know that Black women have the worst outcomes. Calling that out, and having orgs putting that in their strategies, operationalizing it has helped. I keep hearing about 2020, which makes sense, but these things have been going on for hundreds of years. What was different about 2020? The pandemic. We didn't have time to be distracted. COVID was already disproportionally affecting Black people, and the triggers of the unjust deaths… In 2020, all of these burdens being placed on Black people, and Black women specifically. I would say it's the trifecta of all this information was coming out at the same time, when we were all on lockdown.

Respondents often mentioned capacity building, easing requirements, dismantling racist structures, and targeted funding when discussing the future of funding efforts that focus on Black women's reproductive health and sexuality:

> Addressing and dismantling the racist structures that have resulted in these poor outcomes. We have to be cognizant that, traditionally, we've blamed the victim. We've victimized them by saying their outcomes are attributable to something that they did or didn't do, but it actually is the result of the environment in which they have lived and tried to deliver babies, and what's happened to them.

> I think the future looks bright. The philanthropies that have the biggest footprints drive trends in the field. It is no small thing that the Robert Wood Johnson Foundation is shifting to structural racism as a primary focus. They have a maternal focus now, and the disparities and inequities in that space. They are determined as an organization to put money in the hands of the innovators on the ground in communities…Several years ago, as I walked into this hospital, there was a big banner that said, 'We are a Baby-Friendly Hospital'…those things we have fought for, for decades, were in place and happening in this hospital. I know that change can and does happen and, if you live long enough to see it, it's a blessing.

> Funding reproductive health also supports professional development, education, strengthening of communities, and reduction of violence, and so on. If we understand that, then the way that we support Black women-led organizations will change radically, because we understand it's linked to so many other things.

> It's going toward having more community-led and Black-led organizations. Getting the health care system to address the systemic racism in the American society. Even five years ago, you could not go into any health care settings and talk about racism, because the reaction would be, 'What, you're calling me a racist?' But now the reaction is, 'Yes, there is racism and bias'…We need to work together to make systemic changes instead of just a little bubble of changes.

> The other challenge is the need to be patient and to fund generously, and with funding general operating supports, so that these orgs both build capacity but also have the freedom to invest to innovate long term to get real results. And to navigate the system [system meaning the publication world, research world, and institutional world], the systems driven by the majority population of white women and white men. It takes a lot for women-led and Black women-led small community organizations to develop the partnerships and the collaboration and the credibility to navigate these complex systems.

> Many large funder organizations have practices, policies, and approaches that perpetuate structural racism and that hold onto white supremacy culture and make it difficult for people of color even in their own institutions. It then becomes a harmful and traumatizing experience. I think that is the biggest challenge that we have in front of us. Trying to push money into the field, at the same time trying to challenge and advance the institutional changes that need to be made.

CONCLUSION

The results of the study lend a rich sense of urgency to funding Black women–focused and Black women–led organizations, particularly those working to advance reproductive health and sexuality. There must be significant investment in Black women's and girls' leadership, advocacy, and well-being if we are to achieve population-level impact. Funders have an opportunity to proactively define their role as the momentum around racial justice and Black women's reproductive health continues. In the words of one respondent,

> A lot more organizations are wanting to fund Black-led teams and community-based work. Many are thinking about how we help support and grow so that these organizations can be self-sustaining, so they are not always operating on a shoestring and not sure where their next funding cycle is coming from...In the last five years, I went from knowing two possible co-funders who would fund in this space. Now we see a birth equity funders group, where we meet to talk the issues, and how we can better coordinate and address them. Now there's a group of about 25 or 30 funders nationwide. It's nice to see that a lot of them are people of color. A lot of philanthropies have hired staff that look like the communities they want to serve.

ACKNOWLEDGMENTS

Special acknowledgement of Dana J. Martin, MPH, of Shattuck & Associates Inc. for her analysis that made this chapter possible.

REFERENCES

Couvson M, McHarris T. Let Black women-led funds and Black girls lead the way: centering Black women-led funds to lead social justice efforts. Philanthropy News Digest. October 19, 2022. Available at: https://philanthropynewsdigest.org/features/commentary-and-opinion/let-black-women-led-funds-and-black-girls-lead-the-way-centering-black-women-led-funds-to-lead-social-justice-efforts

Dorsey C, Kim P, Daniels C, Sakaue L, Savage B. Overcoming the racial bias in philanthropic funding. *Stanford Social Innovation Review.* May 4, 2020. Available at: https://ssir.org/articles/entry/overcoming_the_racial_bias_in_philanthropic_funding

Echoing Green, The Bridgespan Group. Racial equity and philanthropy: disparities in funding for leaders of color leave impact on the table. May 4, 2020. Available at: https://www.bridgespan.org/insights/disparities-nonprofit-funding-for-leaders-of-color

Appendix IV: From the Archives

- Villarosa L, ed. *Body & Soul: The Black Women's Guide to Physical Health* and *Emotional Well-Being*. New York, NY: Harper Perennial, 1994.

Written by and for Black women and sponsored by the National Black Women's Health Project, this self-help guide draws on the expertise of Black female scientists, academics, health care practitioners, and writers to address some of the most pressing physical, emotional, and spiritual health issues and concerns of Black women.

- **Black Mamas Matter, Center for Reproductive Rights. Black Mamas Matter: advancing the human right to safe and respectful maternal health care. New York, NY: Center for Reproductive Rights; 2018. http://blackmamasmatter.org/wp-content/uploads/2018/05/USPA_BMMA_Toolkit_Booklet-Final-Update_Web-Pages-1.pdf**

This toolkit has helped lay the groundwork for policy change while highlighting Black Mamas' human right to safe and respectful care. It provides a comprehensive overview of information and resources on Black maternal health and identifies action policymakers can take to address maternal health within the human rights and reproductive justice frameworks.

Afterword

In *Black Women's Reproductive Health and Sexuality: A Holistic Public Health Approach*, the authors have done an extraordinary job of examining an aspect of Black women's health that has been historically fraught while being systematically denied. Much of what has been taught in the academy that is focused on as research and funded as interventions stems from efforts to describe or explain disparities in health outcomes and perpetuate harmful perceptions of Black women's sexuality. The result has been a deficit-driven system of research, policy, and medical care and to portray Black women as having no independent interpretation of their historical oppression. We are so much more.

This edited volume arose from the need for a comprehensive and intersectional approach to understanding Black women's reproductive health and sexuality that informs the next generation of scholars, practitioners, and policymakers. It also addresses a long unmet need to center Black women scholars and their work. Here, the authors have placed Black women's reproductive health and their sexuality firmly in the context of a public health issue. They are both studying and witnessing reproductive health praxis through the lens of Black women's lived experiences and, thus, their own. And, in doing so, they have provided essential guidance for needed changes in the design of public health research, the organization and delivery of care, the development of policies to both protect and advance the reproductive health of Black women, and, importantly, how these changes connect to the dissemination of authentic narratives of their sexuality.

To be sure, producing a book of this kind was no small endeavor. In conducting and writing about their research, the authors were confronted with their own experiences of having their expertise challenged or research second-guessed. During the course of writing these chapters, some of the authors faced bias and ignorance while receiving health care for themselves and family members. Their knowledge and expertise provided no protection from racism and low expectations. And then there was the reversal of the Supreme Court decision on *Roe v. Wade*. This unconscionable act placed into stark relief how deadly sexism-fueled policies can be.

The promise of this body of work is that, in presenting both a qualitative and a quantitative analysis of approaches to Black women's reproductive health and sexuality, our understanding of the underlying contributors to inequalities is clarified and, notably, contextualized so as not to blame Black women. For if Black women could actually change the research landscape, their health, economic outcomes, or bias in health care, one could argue, why have they not done it sooner? This is a question the authors have had to grapple with repeatedly. The assumption by many is that if Black women work harder, advocate more, or raise their voices louder, then barriers to quality care or even being seen as valuable human beings would fall. The responses to these assumptions can be found in the characterizations of gender, race, health, and data. Future research and pedagogy should be informed by the authors' use of language: for example, race is not a risk factor; racism is a risk factor.

In women's studies and public health coursework, legions of professors should frame their syllabi through the lens of historical oppression and contemporary perceptions of Black women as reproducing and sexual beings who have been vilified for being such. Furthermore, any discussion or future analysis of Black women's reproductive health and sexuality must take place, as many of the authors demonstrate, in the context of an evidence-based understanding of existing societal power structures. Only in examining the spaces Black women occupy in health, education, the economy, elected office, or the corporate ladder can we fully appreciate the structural changes required to improve birth outcomes, fund research relevant to the Black woman's experience, or ensure Black women have access to respectful, quality reproductive and sexual health care. With structural changes come changes in power.

Much of the work in *Black Women's Reproductive Health and Sexuality: A Holistic Public Health Approach* was funded through philanthropy of one sort or another. Many of the authors receive federal or foundation funding for their research. A great amount of academic research at many institutions is only through grant writing. Some of the authors are employed in the nonprofit industry. Grant writing is the heart and soul of keeping the lights on and salaries paid. As the authors provide analysis on systems and structures that limit Black women's access to reproductive health care or their ability to engage in healthy relationships, it is important to note the very bedrock of their work—philanthropy—and the role it has in shaping research, evidence, and best practices.

Black women in philanthropy who have the responsibility for grant-making often report limitations on their ability to fund what, in their opinions, are research and programs that deeply investigate the root causes of inequalities in Black women's health and wellness. They must conform to the strategic guidance of leadership, who are often the board of directors. While this is understandable, it has important implications for how research and data are interpreted, are presented, and become accepted as factual. What becomes evidence depends on who is asking the question, whom they are asking, and who is funding the research.

Black women who work in academe and the nonprofit industry often develop grant proposals that must be tailored to the strategic and, in some cases, political interest of the funder rather than those that directly address the issues of research or program interest. The work in this volume is remarkable in its depth and breadth and clearly demonstrates the determination, resilience, and persistence of the authors in obtaining sufficient funding to produce such a detailed and comprehensive exploration of Black women's reproductive health and sexuality. As one seasoned grant writer put it: when seeking funding from philanthropic organizations, one must either be best friends with the executive leadership or have a well-established legacy of support. Without power or access to power, everything else is begging.

By bringing together experts in public health, medicine, media, policy, and the social sciences, the editor of this book has helped Black women in the academy create partnerships and a community that center Black women and amplify their voices together with the importance of their scholarship. Moreover, as we consider the transforming demographic composition of the US population toward the point, 20 years from now, when the majority of adults will not be white, the ramifications of omitting Black women's scholarship cannot be overstated.

This volume forges an evolved path forward to policy, research, and practice grounded in an authentic reconstruction of historical events and their impact on Black women's reproductive health and sexuality. In the classroom, students and scholars of all backgrounds will appreciate the context and contribution of the lived experiences of Black women to their reproductive health. For example, there will be a more defined and nuanced comprehension of why the reversal of *Roe* will be so detrimental to Black women. Scholars will understand that Black maternal mortality and morbidity rates are agnostic of genetics and biology but, rather, are determined by what care is accessible and what attitudes and behaviors Black women encounter in the examination room or on the birthing chair.

The authors caution us about a potentially troubling picture of a future health care system that will be largely led by white men convinced their responsibility is to make health care and health policy decisions for a largely nonwhite female population. As power and decision-making are likely concentrated among a steadily smaller percentage of the population, scholars and practitioners focused on Black women's health must uncover ways to continue their scholarship and work to provide a consistent, evidence-based counternarrative to the devaluing of Black women.

This requires change. Change in systems. Change in policies. Change in behaviors of those whose hands are on the levers of power. The authors astutely point to the fact that maternal health and chronic disease outcomes for Black women have not improved for more than 40 years. Sadly, the gap between Black and white women is worse now than in the 1980s. All of this has occurred against a backdrop of more than $200 billion having been invested in community-based participatory and clinical research to alleviate health disparities and improve maternal, sexual, and reproductive health since 1985.

The editor and authors of *Black Women's Reproductive Health and Sexuality: A Holistic Public Health Approach* have given current researchers and practitioners as well as those in training or considering this work a gift. We now have a unique volume from which to articulate the facts of Black women's reproductive health and sexuality, provide a historical context to examine the most determinative elements of Black women's lived experiences, and expose the science-based methods required for innovation in supporting Black women's reproductive health and sexuality.

As a final word, the authors have a tremendous voice and much more to say. They know, to say something of consequence, there may be consequences, but to say nothing is to be inconsequential. *Black Women's Reproductive Health and Sexuality: A Holistic Public Health Approach* is anything but.

Linda Goler Bount, MPH

Contributors

EDITOR

Regina Davis Moss, PhD, MPH, is the president and CEO of In Our Own Voice: National Black Women's Reproductive Justice Agenda. She has more than 20 years of experience in the public, nonprofit, and political sectors and has dedicated her entire career to advancing complete physical, mental, and social well-being for women through research, programmatic initiatives, and the development of innovative strategies for informing health policies.

AUTHORS

Siwaar Abouhala is the founder and senior advisor of MARCH: Maternal Advocacy and Research for Community Health, the largest undergraduate-led maternal health organization in the United States. Siwaar currently works as a founding member and research assistant at the Maternal Outcomes for Translational Health Equity Research (MOTHER) Lab in the Research and Grants Committee and as a policy intern at the Center for Black Maternal Health and Reproductive Justice at Tufts University School of Medicine. She is also the founder and project coordinator of the Arab Maternal Health in Ohio Study, a three-year long project based at The Computational Epidemiology Lab in the College of Public Health, Ohio State University, a project which will fill major gaps as the first qualitative maternal health project among Arab birthing people in America.

Osub Ahmed, MPH, is a policy officer at the Robert Wood Johnson Foundation. She focuses on issues related to health and racial equity, coverage, and access, leveraging her expertise in the public health and health policy fields and experience working on reproductive and maternal health policy.

Kobi V. Ajayi, PhD, MPH, MBA, holds a PhD and MPH from Texas A&M University. Her research addresses the socioeconomic, sociocultural, and sociopolitical factors affecting health behaviors, access to care, and health outcomes among women across the life course. Ajayi's work comprises (1) behavioral science methods to generate, test, and evaluate hypotheses; and (2) applied research through community engagement, as implemented in her nonprofit organization based in Nigeria. She employs equity and social justice lenses in her research and practice to promote and protect women's health. Ajayi also received an MBA from Edinburgh Business School at Heriot-Watt University, United Kingdom.

Kamila A. Alexander, PhD, MPH, RN, is an associate professor at the Johns Hopkins School of Nursing. Her research examines the sociostructural determinants of trauma and violence on sexual, mental, and reproductive health outcomes among marginalized young people.

Aishwarya Amarnath is a student at Tufts University studying community health and sociology. She is a research assistant on the SHARE Study at Tufts.

Ndidiamaka Amutah-Onukagha, PhD, MPH, is the Julia A. Okoro professor of Black Maternal Health in the Department of Public Health and Community Medicine at Tufts University School of Medicine. She is the founder and director of the Center of Black Maternal Health and Reproductive Justice, and the Maternal Outcomes for Translational Health Equity Research (MOTHER) Lab.

Yoann Sophie Antoine, MPH, is a health equity strategist and consultant. Her experience as public health professional spans from environmental health to reproductive and mental well-being. She focuses on equitable access to care, social determinants of health, health policy, and population well-being.

Kimberly A. Baker, DrPH, MPH, is an assistant professor at the UTHealth Houston School of Public Health and cofounder of Full Circle Strategies and The Race Equity Leadership Collective in Houston, Texas.

Anna Barickman is a recent graduate of The George Washington University's Milken Institute School of Public Health. She is currently working in hospital administration and aims to translate her passion for women's health and health equity into creating and fostering diverse and inclusive health care settings.

Allyson S. Belton, MPH, is the director of education and training for the Satcher Health Leadership Institute at Morehouse School of Medicine. She has long maintained a heart for working with people and working within the public health sector to bring about better awareness towards optimal physical, mental, and emotional health.

Kristin Z. Black, PhD, MPH, is an assistant professor in the Department of Health Education and Promotion at East Carolina University. Black is committed to utilizing community-based participatory research, mixed methods, and racial equity approaches to understand and address the individual- and systems-level factors that may hinder or facilitate birthing people's journey through health care services.

Linda Goler Blount, MPH, is the president and CEO of the Black Women's Health Imperative, the only national organization focused on Black women's emotional, physical, and financial health. Since joining the organization in 2014, Blount has overseen the Imperative's strategy to increase research for Black women to prevent chronic disease and HIV, to ensure reproductive justice and healthy maternal outcomes, and to advocate for health-promoting policies.

Elizabeth Bolarinwa is recent graduate who majored in clinical laboratory sciences at Howard University. Outside of school, she works to progress health equity through community engagement and research.

Davondra I. Brown, MEd, is a New Orleans native with over 25 years of experience in sexual wellness education and health promotion services. Her expertise and entrepreneurial spirit infuses her various roles as a speaker, author, volunteer, business owner, mother, wife, and director. Her life's mission is to facilitate health education and promote relationship health, sexual wellness, and interpersonal communication, all through an equitable lens. Brown has earned her BA in philosophy, an MA in education, an advanced certificate of innovative technologies in health science education, and she is due to complete a doctorate of systemic studies in marriage and family therapy in 2024.

Haywood L. Brown, MD, is the senior associate vice president of faculty and academic affairs for University of South Florida Health, vice dean of faculty affairs and associate dean of diversity for the Morsani College of Medicine, and a professor of obstetrics and gynecology. Brown has served in numerous local and national leadership positions, including as the 68th president of the American College of Obstetricians and Gynecologists.

Keri Carvalho, PhD, MS, is a postdoctoral scholar, experimental psychologist, and public health researcher. Her research uses quantitative methods to examine the role of psychosocial stress (e.g., discrimination, financial strain, relationship strain) on health outcomes, with a particular focus on obesity. Other research includes the intersectionality of race and weight, as well as psychosocial factors that contribute to health and racial disparities.

Aja Clark, MPH, is a doctoral student in the Department of Population, Family, and Reproductive Health at the Johns Hopkins Bloomberg School of Public Health. She is interested in sexual and reproductive health education and experiences across the life course.

Camille A. Clare, MD, MPH, is a board-certified obstetrician and gynecologist. She is a certified physician executive as conferred by the Certifying Commission on Medical

Management. Clare is chair and tenured professor in the Department of Obstetrics and Gynecology of Downstate Health Sciences University (DHSU) College of Medicine and Professor of Health Policy and Management in DHSU School of Public Health.

Joia Crear-Perry, MD, is a physician, policy expert, thought leader, and advocate for transformational justice who identifies and challenges racism as a root cause of health inequities. She is a highly sought-after trainer and speaker who has been featured in national and international publications, including *Essence* and *Ms.* magazines. She has twice addressed the Office of the United Nations High Commissioner for Human Rights to urge a human rights framework to improve maternal mortality. A proud recipient of the Congressional Black Caucus Healthcare Heroes award, Crear-Perry currently serves on the Board of Trustees for Community Catalyst, the National Medical Association, and the New Orleans African American Museum. Crear-Perry completed her medical degree at Louisiana State University and her residency in obstetrics and gynecology at the Tulane University School of Medicine. She was also recognized as a fellow of the American College of Obstetricians and Gynecologists.

Shubhecchha Dhaurali is a recently graduated student that studied community health at Tufts University. As a maternal and reproductive health researcher at the Maternal Outcomes for Translational Health Equity Research (MOTHER) Lab and Center of Black Maternal Health and Reproductive Justice, Dhaurali focuses on topics like maternal health equity and reproductive justice. She aims to pursue an MD/PhD in maternal medicine and population health.

Brenice Duroseau, MSN, is a highly accomplished certified family nurse practitioner, with over a decade of comprehensive health care experience. She has established herself as a leader in her field, through her expertise and distinctions in infectious diseases, women's health, and community health. Currently, she is pursuing a PhD at Johns Hopkins University School of Nursing, where she is conducting research to enhance the sexual and reproductive health of Black women through community-informed interventions. In addition to her PhD studies, her research interests encompass a range of topics, including endemic and emerging infectious diseases, health communications and delivery, health equity, and community-informed interventions.

Yanica F. Faustin, PhD, MPH, is an assistant professor of public health at Elon University. Faustin's research investigates the diversity in Black diasporic birthing persons' infant and maternal health outcomes and structural barriers to health equity.

Akayla Galloway, JD, is a reproductive justice activist and Black feminist, using law and policy to advocate for the liberation of folx. She is the founder and CEO of The Social Justice Center, a social change organization dedicated to dismantling the regimes of oppression that impact Black women, girls, femmes, and gender-expansive folx at the intersection of their race, gender, class and sexuality.

Christy M. Gamble, JD, DrPH, MPH, is a senior vice president and the head of the Research and Policy Analysis Department at Forbes Tate Partners, a government and public affairs advocacy firm, where she works at the intersection of policy, research, and politics. She leverages her numerous years of research experience to develop creative and strategic policy solutions in ways that resonate with members of Congress, as well as industry, academia, and nonprofit organizations.

Dawn Godbolt, PhD, MS, is the director of health equity at Maven Clinic, the world's largest virtual clinic for women's and family health. Prior to joining Maven, Godbolt worked in the reproductive justice space and at the National Partnership for Women & Families where she integrated a reproductive justice framework into the maternal health portfolio. Godbolt was involved in the drafting and development of critical federal health legislation, including the Health Equity Accountability Acts of 2018 and 2020, the Black Maternal Health Momnibus Act of 2021, and the COVID-19 Safe Birthing Act.

Lisa Grace-Leitch, EdD, MPH, MA, is a professor and deputy chair of the Health Education Department at the City University of New York-Borough of Manhattan Community College. She teaches courses in women's health, gerontology, spirituality, community health education, public health, health communication, and the social and behavioral determinants of health.

Lesley L. Green-Rennis, EdD, MPH, is a tenured full professor and chair at the City University of New York-Borough of Manhattan Community College. Green-Rennis's expertise is in public health history, health disparities, and social determinants of health. Her research focuses on the use of contemplative pedagogy to enhance classroom teaching and learning, online pedagogy, the development of health professions career paths, and Black women's health.

Kanika A. Harris, PhD, MPH, is a mother of three, near-miss survivor, reproductive justice advocate, doula, and filmmaker. She currently serves as the senior director for maternal health for the Black Women's Health Imperative.

Nicole L. Harris, MA, is a doctoral student at the University of South Florida's College of Public Health. She studies the root causes of disrespect during prenatal care and how Black women resist and re-story narratives that fuel their mistreatment.

Asha Hassan, MPH, is a doctoral student in the Department of Health Policy and Management at the University of Minnesota School of Public Health. She studies the mechanisms linking structural racism and restrictions in bodily autonomy.

Kisha B. Holden, PhD, MSCR, is the Poussaint-Satcher endowed chair in mental health and associate director of the Satcher Health Leadership Institute at Morehouse School of Medicine (MSM). Holden is also a professor and director of research and scholarship for the Department of Psychiatry and Behavioral Sciences and professor in the Department of Community Health and Preventive Medicine at MSM. She is also an adjunct professor at Emory University's School of Medicine in the Department of Psychiatry and Behavioral Sciences.

Jon M. Hussey, PhD, MPH, is an assistant professor in the Department of Maternal and Child Health at the Gillings School of Global Public Health, University of North Carolina at Chapel Hill. He is a sociologist and demographer with a primary interest in the association between social stratification and health across the life course.

Kendra Ippel, MS, is the vice president of strategy and engagement at Commonsense Childbirth, a nonprofit dedicated to eradicating racial disparities in birth outcomes. She coordinates the training and consulting efforts to replicate The JJ Way model in clinical and nonclinical settings.

Tia Jackson-Bey, MD, MPH, is a reproductive endocrinologist and infertility specialist at Reproductive Medicine Associates of New York and assistant professor of obstetrics, gynecology and reproductive science at the Icahn School of Medicine at Mount Sinai. Jackson-Bey is passionate about reproductive justice and ensuring access to fertility care for all. She works with various organizations and medical societies, including the diversity, equity, and inclusion committee of the American Society for Reproductive Medicine, to enhance fertility options for underrepresented minorities and reduce health disparities.

Sascha James-Conterelli, DNP, is an assistant professor of nursing and midwifery at Yale University School of Nursing. She is a proud Afro-Caribbean woman dedicated to achieving health equity for Black and Brown people globally.

Michelle S. Jerry is a graduating biology student at Tufts University. Her academic interests also include community health, sociology, and women's, gender, and sexuality studies. Jerry is particularly fascinated by the intersection of health care and access, with a specific focus on understanding the social determinants that impact women and racial minorities.

Kenya Johnson, PhD, MSW, is the co-owner of Full Circle Strategies, where she focuses on antiracist organizational change research and training. She is also a founding board member to the Race Equity Leadership and Research Collective. She works in solidarity with those committed to building and sustaining spaces that center equity, liberation, and justice.

Jennie Joseph, LM, fights for perinatal health and equity for all childbearing people. A British-trained midwife, Joseph is one of the world's most respected midwives and authorities on improving birth outcomes and was a TIME Magazine Woman of the Year in 2022. Joseph is the founder and executive director of Commonsense Childbirth and the creator of The JJ Way, a common sense maternity model that saves lives.

Mother Mother Binahkaye Joy is a spatial architect, dancing mother, spiritual midwife, sacred nourishment practitioner, and ringshout synergist. She is the generative pulse of the Fertility Abundance Garden, a congregation for creators and a sanctuary for mothers. Through her core enterprise, Mother Space Luminaries, Joy cultivates soft learning portals that amplify and expand the reach of maternal intelligence.

Anna Kheyfets is a fourth-year MD/MPH candidate at Tufts University School of Medicine pursuing obstetrics and gynecology. She focuses her research on equity-focused quality improvement, immigrant health, and combating structural racism to improve health outcomes.

Marwah Kiani is a recent graduate of Tufts University with a BA in Community Health. She is currently a clinical research coordinator at the Mount Sinai Adolescent Health Center and is hoping to eventually go to medical school. She hopes to pursue an MD/MPH and further center equity and justice within her practice.

Nekisha Killings, MPH, is a board-certified lactation consultant and perinatal equity strategist who consults birth worker organizations on applying cultural humility in the care setting. Killings is on a mission to normalize brown breasts in health care provider education, thereby expanding provider acumen and improving care experiences for people of color. In 2022, Killings was awarded the inaugural Black Breastfeeding Week Birth Award for Tech Innovation for founding The Melanated Mammary Atlas, a digital resource showcasing conditions of the breast/chest on skin of color.

Lorraine J. Lacroix-Williamson, MPH, is a pleasure activist, health advocate, and social epidemiologist. She is a doctoral candidate in the Department of Health Sciences at Northeastern University's Bouvé College of Health Science. She investigates how sociocultural factors influence Black women's sexuality to mitigate sexual and reproductive health inequities.

Blessing Chidiuto Lawrence, MPH, is an epidemiologist by training, founding member of the Tufts Maternal Outcomes for Translational Health Equity Research (MOTHER) Lab, and medical student at The State University of New York Upstate Medical University. She has experience working in health care settings, nonprofit, and state agencies. Her work focuses on improving systems of care, maternal and child health outcomes, and promoting effective contextualization and interpretation of scientific data.

Ashleigh LoVette, PhD, MA, is an assistant professor of health behavior and health promotion at the Ohio State University. Prior to this role, she completed a T32 postdoctoral fellowship focused on addressing violence and trauma at the Johns Hopkins University School of Nursing. LoVette uses community-engaged, strengths-based, and trauma-informed approaches to promote the sexual health of Black girls and young women in the United States and abroad.

Inas K. Mahdi, MPH, is currently a fourth-year doctoral student at the Johns Hopkins Bloomberg School of Public Health within the health equity and social justice program. She focuses on interventions that use Black women's theoretical frameworks to mitigate the impact of racial and sexual violence on Black birthing people. Mahdi is particularly interested in research related to anti-Black racism, human rights, sexual and obstetric violence, and trauma-responsive care.

Monica R. McLemore, PhD, MPH, RN, is a tenured professor in the Child, Family, and Population Health Department and the interim director for the Center for Antiracism in Nursing at the University of Washington School of Nursing.

Gloria Shine McNamara, PhD, MS, is a professor at the City University of New York (Borough of Manhattan Community College campus) in the Health Education Department. Her research focuses on health behaviors, specifically diet and exercise, as well as pedagogical practices in educating health care professionals.

Bailey Moore is an undergraduate public health major with a minor in human services and social justice and micro–minor in health equity on the premedical track at The George Washington University, graduating in the spring of 2024. She is an aspiring obstetrician-gynecologist and is passionate about Black maternal/reproductive health and justice, health equity, informed health education, and decolonizing what is known about Black birth and birth work in America.

DaKysha Moore, PhD, MHS, MS, is an associate professor in the speech program at North Carolina A&T State University. Her research area is health communication. Specifically, she focuses on health disparities, mainly in the African American community, within the context of HIV/AIDS, sickle cell disease, and women's health issues.

Jerrine R. Morris, MD, MPH, is a reproductive endocrinologist and infertility specialist at Shady Grove Fertility in Baltimore, Maryland. She has research interests in polycystic ovary syndrome, health disparities, and third-party reproduction. She is passionate about expanding access for equitable and effective infertility treatment.

Vanessa Nicholson, DrPH, MPH, is an assistant professor at Tufts University School of Medicine within the Department of Public Health and Community Medicine. As a health equity research scientist, she has coauthored the original unit lead positions within Tufts

University's Center for Black Maternal Health and Reproductive Justice. She also is credited with being the chief report editor and lead technical writer for the Report of the Special Commission on Racial Inequities in Maternal Health for the Commonwealth of Massachusetts.

Tonni Oberly, MPH, is a doctoral candidate in city and regional planning at The Ohio State University. Oberly's research investigates the intersections of place, racism, and health outcomes.

Folashade Omole, MD, is a professor of family medicine and a licensed acupuncturist. She is the Sarah and William Hambrecht Endowed Chair of the Department of Family Medicine at Morehouse School of Medicine. Omole has served as a principal investigator (PI)/co-PI of several grants and has authored and coauthored several manuscripts. She is known for her commitment to educating the next generation of health care providers and has received several awards, including being inducted into the Alpha Omega Alpha Honor Medical Society and receiving the Georgia Academy Family Physician (GAFP) Educator of the Year award. In 2015 and 2019 she was also named the Georgia Family Physician of the Year and awarded the Community and Volunteer Services Awards respectively; the highest awards bestowed on a GAFP member that recognize excellence in peer leadership in professional affairs and outstanding contributions to family medicine and the community. In 2018, she was recognized as an Inspiration Physician by the Women Physicians of the American Medical Association.

Elijah O. Onsomu, PhD, MPH, MS, is an associate professor of nursing at Winston-Salem State University. He is a health services researcher that uses various methodological and data analytical approaches in health services research and public health. He has written extensively in the areas of maternal and child health, domestic violence, HIV/AIDS, and high-risk sexual behaviors.

Stacey C. Penny, MSW, MPH, is a builder, collaborator, and maternal and child health expert committed to creating systems-level changes to reduce health inequities and improve pregnancy and birth outcomes for women of color.

Torie Comeaux Plowden, MD, MPH, is double board-certified in obstetrics/gynecology and reproductive endocrinology and infertility. She has clinical interests in fibroids, sexual wellness, and infertility and also conducts clinical research. She is a leader in diversity, equity, and inclusion efforts in her field and is also heavily involved in community service.

Sharon Rachel, MA, MPH, is principal faculty in the Department of Physician Assistant Studies at Morehouse School of Medicine and a PhD student in the School of History and Sociology at the Georgia Institute of Technology. Her research focuses on intersectional and climate-related determinants of health disparities.

Tiffany L. Reddick, MEd, LPC, is an Atlanta-based licensed counselor, healing arts practitioner, and consultant specializing in holistic mental health and wellness. She is the founder of SavvyLife Group, which offers personal and professional development services and also runs Flourish Therapy Bar, an online therapy practice centering neurodivergent Black women.

Rhonda Reid, MD, is a resident physician in the Department of Psychiatry and Behavioral Sciences at Morehouse School of Medicine. Her clinical and academic interests include addressing the mental health of African American women and girls and implementing collaborative care models to reduce mental health disparities.

Jaleah Rutledge, MA, is a birth equity research scholar for the National Birth Equity Collaborative and PhD candidate in ecological-community psychology at Michigan State University. Her research focuses on strengths-based approaches for the promotion and protection of Black women's sexual and reproductive health.

Daphne Scott-Henderson MS, RN, is an informatics nurse and doctoral nursing student at the University of California, San Francisco. Her research interests include sexual and reproductive health care disparities of Black LGBTQ+ persons.

Maria J. Small, MD, MPH, is a maternal-fetal medicine specialist and associate professor of obstetrics and gynecology at the Duke University School of Medicine. Her clinical, scholarly, and community engagement work focuses on reducing severe maternal morbidity and mortality. Other areas of focus include maternal hypertensive disease and cardiac disease.

Shawna G. Shipley-Gates, MA, MPH, is a doctoral candidate in the Women, Gender, and Sexuality Studies Department at the University of Kansas. She explores Black feminist digital erotic resistance as a form of resistance against sexual oppression and its impact on the sexual health behaviors of Black women.

Candace Stewart, MPH, is the program manager for the Maternal Outcomes for Translational Health Equity Research (MOTHER) Lab housed within the Center for Black Maternal Health and Reproductive Justice at Tufts University School of Medicine. She is a child health policy advocate and a law student at Northeastern University School of Law.

Daniel Suárez-Baquero, PhD, MSN, RN, is a Colombian assistant professor at the School of Nursing at the University of Washington and a former postdoctoral fellow at Abortion Care Training Incubator for Outstanding Nurse Scholars (ACTIONS) at the University of California San Francisco. His research and practice concern qualitative research methods, reproductive justice, Latine reproductive health experiences, and community/cultural memory of ethnic minoritized women.

Zainab Sulaiman, MSc, is a reproductive justice and mental health advocate, feminist, and pan-Africanist. She is a sexual and reproductive health researcher, educator, and communications expert passionate about health equity, reproductive and gender justice, and access to knowledge, information, and services to produce sustainable communities.

Aurora Sullivan, MPH, is an adjunct professor of Public Health at Stetson University in Deland, Florida. Her professional work and interests lie in equity with a focus on the social determinants of health. Sullivan received her MA in public health and her BA in religious studies, allowing her to bring a deep intersection of health, humanities, and culture to her work.

Jamila K. Taylor, PhD, MPA, is president and CEO of the National WIC Association, the nonprofit education arm and advocacy voice of the special supplemental nutrition program for Women, Infants, and Children (WIC) program. She is a long-time advocate, researcher, writer, and policy professional with expertise in health policy and equity, reproductive justice, and maternal and child health. The proud two-time HBCU graduate has published widely and has been featured in top media outlets including the Washington Post, NPR, The Hill, Politico, CSPAN, Fox News, and more.

Shemeka Thorpe, PhD, is a sexuality researcher and educator. She is an assistant professor of health promotion at the University of Kentucky. Her research interest is the sexual well-being of Black women, focusing primarily on barriers to sexual pleasure.

Claudia Tillman, PhD, MA, is a sociologist, communicator, facilitator, and coconspirator for health equity. She currently directs communication at Commonsense Childbirth.

Ashley Townes, PhD, MPH, is an epidemiologist based in Atlanta, Georgia. She has 15 years of work experience in a variety of academic and public health entities. Her research focuses on Black women's sexual experiences and their access to sexuality-related information and health services.

Ruth Vigue, MS, is a graduate student at Boston University Chobanian & Avedisian School of Medicine studying medical science.

Hena Wadhwa, PhD, MS, MA, is a women's and reproductive health activist and scholar in South Asian American women's mental health. She has completed an MA in curriculum and teaching inclusive education (general and special education) from Columbia University-Teachers College, an MS in sociology, and a PhD in sociology with a concentration in demography from Florida State University. Wadhwa serves on a FemTech board and is determined to bring forward the voices of women of color in literature and research.

Najjuwah Walden, MSW, is a doctoral student in the public health sciences program at Washington University in St. Louis where she studies the nutritional epidemiology of postpartum depression. Influenced by the connection between diet and psychoneuroimmunology, her global research explores how popular diets, including traditional confinement and Western diet, impact people's ability to maintain psychoneuroimmunological resilience and prevent biological mechanisms of mood shifts. Walden joined the National Birth Equity Collaborative as a research scholar to deepen her exposure to traditional postpartum practices across the African diaspora and develop dissemination methods to implement in home-based settings.

Angela Wangari Walter, PhD, MPH, MSW, is an associate professor of public health at the Zuckerberg College of Health Sciences, the University of Massachusetts Lowell. She is also a faculty member in the health promotion and resiliency intervention research program at the Mongan Institute, Massachusetts General Hospital. Her intervention research focuses on advancing equity in behavioral health prevention and treatment.

Maranda C. Ward, EdD, MPH, is an award-winning diversity, equity, inclusion, and justice scholar, public health practitioner, and community engaged researcher who serves as an assistant professor and director of equity in The George Washington University School of Medicine and Health Sciences. Her scholarship focuses on preparing the health workforce to meet the challenges of health and racial equity.

Deanna J. Wathington, MD, MPH, is a public health practitioner and family physician whose work and scholarly efforts have centered on health equity, clinical-community linkages, maternal and child health, equitable community development, community health initiatives, and expanding diversity within the health professions. She currently serves as the clinical director at REACHUP, executive director of the Consortium of African American Public Health Programs, and as an affiliate professor in the University of South Florida College of Public Health.

Phoebe Wescott, MPH, is a senior birth equity analyst at the National Birth Equity Collaborative. She focuses on maternal health and health equity priorities through cofacilitating antiracism training and providing organizational assessments for health departments and hospital systems.

Wendy C. Wilcox, MD, MPH, MBA, is the chief women's health officer for New York City Health and Hospitals. She focuses on population-based efforts to improve quality and safety in women's health, as well as improving maternal health and equity for Black and Brown birthing people.

Gail Elizabeth Wyatt, PhD, MA, is a distinguished professor and is a Dena Bat Yaacov Endowed Chair of Psychiatry and Biobehavioral Sciences at the Jane and Terry Semel

Institute of Neuroscience and Behavior at the David Geffen School of Medicine, University of California, Los Angeles (UCLA). She directs the Center for Culture, Trauma and Mental Health Disparities, The Sexual Health Program, and codirects National Institutes of Health–funded domestic and international training programs on the effects of health disparities, substance use, sexual and physical health risks, and trauma on mental health. She celebrates 50 years at UCLA.

Rauta Aver Yakubu, MPH, MHA, is a doctoral candidate at Saint Louis University's College for Public Health and Social Justice, as well as a research assistant in the Maternal Outcomes for Translational Health Equity Research (MOTHER) Lab at Tufts University School of Medicine. Yakubu has 10 years of experience working in perinatal health equity.

Telesha B. Zabie, MD, MBA, is a graduate from Windsor University School of Medicine with a primary focus on maternal black health. She is a lead research assistant for the SHARE Study (Stopping the Spread of HIV/AIDS through Relationship Engagement). She focuses on Black maternal health, birth equity, and uplifting Black autonomy.

Index

Page numbers in *italics* indicate figures.

A

abortion care, 17, 20–21, 23, 113
Abortion Care Training Incubator of Outstanding Nurse Scholars (ACTIONS), 379–391
abstinence-only-based sex education, 316–317, 325–326
abuse
 physical, 128
 psychological, 128
 sexual, 124, 304, 360–362
ACA (Affordable Care Act), 31, 53–54, 139, 220
access to accurate sexual wellness education, 349–351
access to birth control, 137–139, *139*, 141–143
access to care, 9, 31–33, 113, 237
 maternity care deserts, 111–112
 in rural counties, 51
access to social support, 235–236
ACEs (adverse childhood experiences), 338
ACNM (American College of Nurse Midwives), 167, 171
ACOG (American College of Obstetricians and Gynecologists), 164, 194, 285, 317
ACTIONS (Abortion Care Training Incubator of Outstanding Nurse Scholars), 379–391
Adams, Alma S., 113–116, 150–151, 316
Adams-Santos, Dominique, 92–93
adolescent girls
 identity, 336–338
 Kellye's story, 335–337
 media and, 82
 physical development, 336–337
 puberty, 336–337
 recommendations for, 306–307
 reproductive health, 337
 sex education for, 314–315
 sexual orientation, 337–338
 wellness, 301–309
adolescent pregnancy, 98, 317, 337–338
adultification, 21–22, 301, 335–337
adverse childhood experiences (ACEs), 338
Affordable Care Act (ACA), 31, 53–54, 139, 220
African American women
 breastfeeding, 218
 exoticization of, 81
 fertility preservation, 230
 gendered racism against, 49
 heart health, 249–250
 matriarchs, 78
 older, 251
 preterm births, 187–188
 transgender, 292
 See also Black women
African diaspora, 166, 203–206
African women, 3–4, 203–208. *See also* Black women
Afrocentricity, 353–354
afterlife of slavery, 362
age compression, 312
age-related brain disorders, 251
aging
 biologic age (BA), 168
 in HIV care, 281–282, 285
 premature, 47–48. *See also* weathering
agricultural economy, 3–4
Aina, Angela D., 150
Akil, Mara Brock, 98
Akil, Salim, 98
Alabama, 123, 140
allostatic load, 46–47
allostatic overload, 47
alternative medicine, 65–67
Alzheimer's disease, 250–251
AMA (American Medical Association), 4, 7, 167, 317
American Association of Sexuality Educators, Counselors, and Therapists, 350
American College of Nurse Midwives (ACNM), 167, 171
American College of Obstetricians and Gynecologists (ACOG), 164, 194, 285, 317
American Indian or Alaska Native women, 161, 382
American Medical Association (AMA), 4, 7, 167, 317
American Nursing Association, 167
American Sexual Health Association, 87
Anarcha (enslaved woman), 4–5
anatomical images, 328
Ancient Song Doula Services, 198
anesthesia, 4–5
anti-inflammatory agents, 256
Anti-Racist Public Health Praxis, 320
antioxidants, 256
archetypes. *See* stereotypes
Arkansas, 317
ART (assisted reproductive technology), 231–232, 237–238
arthritis, 341

articulation, politics of, 93
Asian American women, 100
Asian women, 45, 128, 250, 312, 382
Aspen Institute, 146
asset-based programs, 306, 328
assisted reproductive technology (ART), 231–232, 237–238
Associated Press, 7–8
Association of Women's Health Obstetric and Neonatal Nurses, 9, 194
asthma, 29
"at risk" (term), 302
Atlanta, Georgia, 53
Aunt Jemima, 77
authenticity, 331
autonomy, 352–354, 356

B

Baartman, Saartjie (Sara or Sarah), 6–7, 122
baby bonds, 53
Baby Friendly Hospital Initiative (BFHI), 218–219, 403
Bailey, Moya, 91, 93, 95, 312
Baker, Josephine, 76
Baldwin, Tammy, 115
Ballet After Dark, 284
Barickman, Anna, 368
Bateson, Gregory, 352
Beard, Mary, 170–171
beauty ideals, 265
behavior, sexual, 263, 266–270
Being Mary Jane (BET), 97–102
"A Belle in Brooklyn" blog (Lucas), 94–95
belonging, 385
best practices for research, 71
"best-practices" training, 189
beta-carotene, 256
Bethune, Mary McLeod, 137, *138*
Betsy (enslaved woman), 4–5
Beyoncé, 94–95
BFE (Black feminist epistemology), 352
BFHI (Baby Friendly Hospital Initiative), 218–219, 403
bias
 adultification, 21–22, 301, 335–337
 co-therapy case study, 355
 explicit, 182, 218, 236, 312
 identification of, 351–352
 implicit, 52, 182, 218, 236, 312
 resolution of, 351–352
 Sexual Attitude Reassessment workshops, 351–352
Biden, Joe, 151
biologic age (BA), 168
BIPOC (Black, Indigenous, other people of color), 10
birth control, 18, 136–138
 access to, 137–139, *139*, 141–143
 forced, 137
 oral contraceptives, 6
Birth Control Federation of America, 137, *138*
Birth Detroit, 198
birth justice, 110–111
birth movement, 195

Black, Indigenous, other people of color (BIPOC), 10
Black birth workers, 115, 220
Black Breastfeeding Week, 219
Black church, 105, 266, 298, 303
Black Codes, 5, 122
Black feminist epistemology (BFE), 352
Black girls
 adolescents, 82, 301–309, 341
 adultification of, 21–22, 301, 335–337
 "at risk," 302
 comprehensive sexuality education (CSE) for, 327–328
 education of, 302–303
 incarceration of, 125
 Kellye's story, 335–336
 as kin-keepers, 126
 mental health, 341
 oversexualization of, 303–304
 philanthropic support, 393
 reproductive and sexual health, 311–317
 school suspensions, 125
 school-to-prison pipeline, 125
 sex education for, 314–315, 319–320
 sexual violence against, 359–360
 strengths-based methods for, 306–307
 wellness, 301–309
Black infants, 34, 203–213
Black lady stereotype, 80
Black liberation, 403
Black Lives Matter (BLM) movement, 91, 126
Black Mamas Matter Alliance (BMMA), 148–150, 219, 372
Black Maternal Health Caucus, 113, 151, 153
Black Maternal Health Federal Policy Collective, 151
Black Maternal Health Momnibus Act (Momnibus), 9, 33, 145–156, *147*, 169
 House of Representatives version, 152
 key concepts, 113–117
 Senate version, 152–153
Black Maternal Health Week, 150, 153–154
Black Mothers' Breastfeeding Association, 219
Black nativity, 205–206
Black perinatal birth workers, 111–112
Black physicians, 237
Black Radical Teaching, 320
Black Sexual Politics (Collins), 372
Black Systems of Care, 320
Black women
 Alzheimer's disease, 251
 best practices for research, 71
 birth control, 136–138
 breastfeeding, 215–225
 chronic health conditions, 28–29
 chronic stress, 46–55
 college-age and adult, 266–268
 comfort with providers, 237
 comprehensive sexuality education (CSE) for, 327–328
 doulas, 64–65
 ectopic pregnancy, 232
 educators, 328

emerging sexuality, 265–266
endometriosis, 233–234
engaging, 374
enslavement of, 3–5, 10–11, 15–17, 122, 136, 166–167, 194, 215–216, 360
exploitation of, 3–13, 28
family-building considerations, 234–240
feminist digital erotic resistance, 87–96
fertility awareness, 227
fertility issues, 97, 230–234, 240
fertility misconceptions, 235
fertility treatment, 227–228, 230–231
forced sterilization of, 112
foreign-born, 203–210, 218
funding focused on, 402–405
heads of households, 33
health inequities, 62
health outcomes, 46–48, 382
heart health, 249–250
historical perspective on, 3–13
HIV burden, 275–276, 283–284, 291
HIV testing, 228
immigrant, 205–209, 218
incarceration of, 19–20
infertility, 99–100, 227, 230–235, 240
interview #1, 292–295
interview #2, 295–299
intimate partner violence (IPV), 127–128
Kellye's story, 339
leadership, 149–152, 154
legal subjugation of, 15–25
LGBTQ+ women, 291–300
low birth weight babies, 186–187, *187*
maternal health, 34–35, 145–147, 203–213
maternal morbidity, 34
maternal mortality, 3, 33–34, 45–46, 62, 145, *146*, 161, 165, 168, 172, 179, 361
media portrayals of, 81–82, 90, 98
menopausal, 247–261
mental health, 34–35, 335–345
midwives, 170
multiple identities of, 368–369
older, 251–252, 269–270
pansexual, 292–295
perinatal and postpartum health, 33–35
philanthropic support, 393
physicians, 382
polycystic ovary syndrome (PCOS), 234
postmenopausal, 269–270
pregnancy-related maternal mortality ratio (PRMR), 162
preterm births, 186–188, *187*, 203–208
professionals, 231
reproductive health, 27–43, 109–120, 311–317, 402–405
research on, 370
responses to sexual trauma, 126–127
self-help guide for, 407
severe maternal morbidity (SMM), 62
sex education programs targeted to, 319–320
sex-positive research for, 329–330
sex workers, 128–130
sexual abuse of, 360–362
sexual health, 311–317
sexual minorities, 238, 270
sexual oppression, 89–91
sexual pleasure, 280–281
sexual violence against, 121–125, 128–130, 359–362
sexuality, 27–43, 75–85, 335–345, 402–405
sexually transmitted infections (STIs), 228, 311–312
stereotypes of, 75–78, 82–83, 303–304
sterilization of, 17–18
strong Black woman (SBW), 34–35, 75, 78–79, 264–265
third-party reproduction (TPR), 239–240
transgender, 20, 128–130, 275–276, 292
uterine fibroids, 62, 231–232
victimhood, 21–22, 304, 360–362
violence against, 20, 312
weathering, 168
young women, 301–309
Black Women for Wellness (BWW), 319–320
Black women living with HIV (BWLH), 275–276, 281–284
Black women–led or Black focused organizations, 393, 397–398, 402–406
Black Women's Health Imperative (BWHI), 199
Black Women's Health Study (BWHS), 253
#BlackBreastsMatter, 223
Blue Cross Blue Shield, 36
Blumenthal, Richard, 114
BMMA (Black Mamas Matter Alliance), 148–150, 219, 372
bodily changes, 340–341
body surveillance, 336
Booker, Cory A., 117, 152, 154, 316
Bosom Buddy Program, 221
brain health, 250–251
branding, 92
breastfeeding, 215, 223
    community-based programs, 403
    community services and resources, 217–223
    current states, 217
    historical context, 215–217
    strategies to support, 219
Breckenridge, Mary, 170–171
Brown, Cyntoia, 127
Brown, William Wells, 216
Brown women, 32–33, 370, 382
Build Back Better Act, 153
Burke, Tarana, 121, 125
Burwell v. Hobby Lobby, 139
Business Case for Breastfeeding program, 220
BWHI (Black Women's Health Imperative), 199
BWHS (Black Women's Health Study), 253
BWLH (Black women living with HIV), 275–276
BWW (Black Women for Wellness), 319–320

C

calcium, 256
California, 112, 152, 315

California Future of Abortion Council, 380
Call to Action to Support Breastfeeding (US Surgeon General), 219
Canada, 129, 161
cancer, 31
carbohydrates, 256
CARDIA (Coronary Artery Risk Development in Young Adults) study, 168
cardiovascular disease (CVD), 28–29, 172–173, 249–250
Caribbean Black women, 203–208
caricatures. *See* stereotypes
Cartwright, Samuel, 167
case study, 355–356
Casey, Robert P., Jr., 115
CDC (Centers for Disease Control and Prevention), 9, 27–30, 117, 163
cell senescence, 48
Center for American Progress, 149
Center for Reproductive Rights, 149–150
Center for Social Inclusion, 219
Centering Racial Justice in Sex Education: Strategies for Engaging Professionals and Young People (SEC), 330–331
Centers for Disease Control and Prevention (CDC), 9, 27–30, 117, 163
Centers for Medicare and Medicaid Services (CMS), 115, 154
certified nurse-midwives, 382
cervical cancer, 31
cesarean section, 167, 199
Chatman, Donald, 234
chestfeeding, 215–225
Chicago, Illinois public school system, 313
Chicago Family Case Management, 221
childbirth, 11, 216
children, 338. *See also* Black girls
Children's Health Insurance Program (CHIP), 115
Chinese American women, 100
Chisolm, Shirley, 135
chlamydia, 30, 311
chronic health conditions, 28–29, 293–294
chronic stress, 46–55, 247–261
CHWs (community health workers), 185
Cite Black Women Critical Praxis, 331
Civil Rights Act, 7
Civil Rights Era, 7–8, 20, 123
Civil Rights Movement, 8, 123, 137
classism, 182, 326
#Clemency4CyntoiaBrown movement, 127
climate change, 117
clitoris, 347
cluster profiles, 373
CMS (Centers for Medicare and Medicaid Services), 115, 154
co-therapy case study, 355–356
cohort models, 390
Colen, Shellee, 236
collaboration, 36, 61, 64–65
college-age women, 266–268
Collins, Patricia Hill, 88, 90, 105, 319, 352, 372

colonialism, 303, 355
Combahee River Collective Statement, 372
coming-out stories, 92–93
Committee for Equal Justice, 123
Commonsense Childbirth (CSC), 180–181, 186–190, *187, 189*
Community Action Network (Healthy Start), 36
community-based doulas, 194, 197–200
community-based organizations, 115–116, 219
community-based sexuality education, 318–320
community building, 385–386
community-centered peer-to-peer breastfeeding trainings, 219
community collaboration, 64–65
community engagement, 331, 387–388
community health workers (CHWs), 185
community inclusion, 331
community partnerships and collaborations, 36
community services and resources, 217–223
Competitive SRAE program, 316
complementary and alternative medicine (CAM), 65–67
comprehensive sexuality education (CSE), 303–305, 312–315, 326–328
  calls for, 318, 320
  culturally aware comprehensive assessment and intervention, 352
  recommendations for, 326
congestive heart failure (CHF), 293–294
Connecticut, 53
consent, 304–305
content experts, 372
contextualization, 369–371, 374–375
contraception, 6, 18. *See also* birth control
contraception deserts, 140
Coronary Artery Risk Development in Young Adults (CARDIA) study, 168
counseling
  empowerment, 52–53
  fertility, 229
  peer counselors, 221
counter-narratives, 372
COVID-19 pandemic, 9, 117, 139–140, 145, 184, 188, 219, 400
Cox, Laverne, 299
crack cocaine, 81
Crear-Perry, Joia, 380
Crenshaw, Kimberlé Williams, 157, 368
criminal justice system (CJS), 124
critical race theory, 372
cross-disciplinary collaboration(s), 61, 64–65
CSC (Commonsense Childbirth), 180–181, 186–190, *187, 189*
CSE. *See* comprehensive sexuality education
Cult of True Womanhood, 80
cultural awareness, 352, 355
cultural factors, 179–180, 264–266
cultural humility, 331
culturally appropriate services, 218
culturally centered sexual wellness education, 351–356

culturally relevant sexuality education, 330–332
culture, hookup, 266–267
culture of silence, 265

D

data collection
   sex research data, 329
   standardized processes, 116–117
data justice, 209–210
data limitations, 209–210, 329
Data to Save Moms Act, 116
Davids, Sharice, 116
decision-making
   in funding Black women–led or Black focused organizations, 397–398
   sexual, 263, 266–270
dementia, 251, 341
denial of victimhood, 21–22
Depo-Provera, 18
depression, postpartum, 339
development, 353
diabetes, 28–29
dietary supplements, 257
diets, healthy, 256
digital alchemy, 92
digital erotic resistance, 92–95
digital media, 90–91, 349
digital storytelling, 94
discrimination
   adultification bias, 21–22, 301, 335–337
   gender, 137
   racial, 203–213, 216. *See also* racism
   racial-gendered, 326
discussion, 374–375
District of Colombia, 53, 94, 218, 314
Dobbs v. Jackson Women's Health Organization, 23, 113, 400
doctoral process, 386–387
Douglas, Kelly Brown, 105
doulas, 193–197, 403
   Black women, 64–65
   community-based, 194, 197–200
   future directions, 200
   Medicaid reimbursement for, 200
   radical, 194, 197
   recommendations for, 54
Doulas of North America (DONA), 195
drapetomania, 167
drug abuse, 81–82
Du Bois, W.E.B., 80
Duckworth, Tammy, 117
Duncan, Ruby, 135
dysaesthesia aethiopica, 167

E

Early Intervention, 221
early sex-positive research, 329–330
Easy Access Clinics, 184–186, 188, *189*, 190
economic factors

   burden of maternal mortality, 163
   determinants of chronic stress, 51
   maternity leave, 169
   out-of-pocket spending, 66–67
   recommendations for, 53–54
   socioeconomic status (SES), 20, 267
   See also funding
ectopic pregnancy, 232–233
education
   of Black girls, 302–303
   co-therapy case study, 355–356
   community-based sexuality education, 318–320
   comprehensive sexuality education (CSE), 303–305, 312–315, 318, 326–328
   culturally affirming sexuality education, 325–333
   culturally centered sexual wellness education, 351–356
   formal sex education, 315
   HIV education, 314
   Indigenous wellness indicators, 353
   Personal Responsibility Education Program (PREP), 315–316
   public schools, 124–125, 313
   Real Education and Access for Health Youth Act (REAHYA), 316
   sexual and reproductive health education, 314–315
   Sexual Attitude Reassessment workshops, 351–352
   sexual-risk-avoidance education (SRAE), 316–317
educators, 328
elders, 353
elevation, 354–356
embarrassment, 100
embedded research, 387–388
empowerment, 181, 354–356
empowerment counseling, 52–53
Ending the HIV Epidemic in the US initiative, 282
endometrial cancer, 31
endometriosis, 233–234, 294–295
engagement, 331, 374, 387–388
Enovid, 6
environmental factors, 50–51, 53, 179–180
epistemology, Black feminist, 352
The Equality Act, 130
equitable outcomes at scale, 188–190, *189*
equity-based resilience approach, 283–284
eroticism, 76, 87–90, 92–95, 355
estradiol (E2), 248
estriol (E3), 248
estrogen, 248, 250
estrogen deficiency, 255
estrone (E1), 248
ethnic disparities, 203–204
eugenicist movement, 6–7
eugenics, 6–7, 17, 313
eugenics movement, 5–6, 20, 123, 137
eugenics programs, 112
Eurocentrism, 219, 265, 387
evidence-based medicine, 186–188, *187*
evidence-based programs, 61–69, 315–316, 326

exclusive sexual relationships (ESR), 269
exercise, 256–257, 295–296
experimentation, 4–6, 166–167, 217, 361
expertise, 355
explicit bias, 182, 218, 236, 312
exploitation, 3–13, 15–25

F

Facebook, 91–92
faith, 80–81
Family, Youth, and Services Bureau, 315–316
family building, 234–240
Family Connects Chicago, 221
Family Focus, 221
fathers, 173, 222–223, 296
Federal Comstock Act, 137
federally funded evidence-based programs, 315–316
Felix, Allyson, 153–154
feminism
    Black feminist digital erotic resistance, 87–96
    Black feminist epistemology (BFE), 352
    "Knob-Slobbing Feminism" (Jones), 93
    "Live and Love With HIV" project (Carter), 94
Ferebee, Dorothy Boulding, 137, *138*
fertility awareness, 227
fertility counseling, 229
fertility issues, 97, 101–102, 230–234, 237–238.
    See also infertility
fertility preservation, 229–230
fertility treatment, 227–230, 235–239
fetishization, 303–304
fibroids, uterine, 30–31, 62, 66, 231–232, 294–295
fight-or-flight response, 253
financial stress, 20, 139, 163, 169
Finland, 171
Florida, 140, 186–188, *187*
folk medicine, 66
Food and Drug Administration (FDA), 18, 31
food choices, 256, 295–296
food deserts, 51, 172–173
food-grade supplements, 257
food swamps, 51
forced sterilization, 217
formula feeding, 216–218
framing language, 372–373
France, 161
free body movement, 353
freedom, reproductive, 18, 135–144
Friere's Theory of Freeing, 355
funding
    for Black women–led or Black focused organizations, 397–398, 402–406
    for breastfeeding, 217–223
    characteristics of organizations that provide, 395–396
    characteristics of organizations that receive, 396–398
    decision-making around, 397–398
    future directions, 402–405
    history of, 400–402
    philanthropic practices, 398–400

future directions, 210–211
    for research, 209–210, 370
    for sex-positive research, 330

G

gangs, 216
gender-affirming care, 19–20
gender-based violence, 128–130, 360–361, 369
gender discrimination, 137
gender identity, 337–338
gender reassignment surgery, 297
gender roles, 369
gendered racism, 49, 71, 369, 383
Genesis, 170
genetic testing, 239
genitourinary syndrome of menopause (GSM), 251
Georgia, 5, 140
Germany, 171
gestational diabetes, 28–29
Get Smart B4U Get Sexy, 319, 327
Gey, George, 8
Gillibrand, Kirsten E., 114–115
girl phase, 265
girls. *See* Black girls
goddess rituals, 354–355
Gonaquasub group, 122
gonorrhea, 311–312
granny midwives, 216
Group Insight, 223
group practice, 354
grown phase, 265
growth, personal, 354
GSM (genitourinary syndrome of menopause), 251
Guttmacher Institute, 27

H

Haitian immigrants, 209
Hamer, Fannie Lou, 217
Hamilton, Darrick, 53
Hammonds, Evelynn, 92
Harambee Village Doulas, 198
harm-reduction efforts, 93–95
Harris, Kamala, 150–151, 153–154
Hartman, Sadiya, 362
Harvard Public Health Magazine, 33
hate crime laws, 130
HCWs. *See* health care workers
HDL (high-density lipoproteins), 250
healing, 284, 353
healing justice, 354
health care
    calls for more responsive care, 362–364
    inhumane practices, 19–20
    integrated care, 169–170
    interview #1, 292–295
    interview #2, 295–299
    race-conscious approach to, 10
    racialization in, 360–361
    traditional delivery, 65–67

unequal, 20–21
well-woman visits, 291
health care policy, 113–117
health care system, 111–112, 115–116, 236
health care workers (HCWs), 163, 237, 382
    Black birth workers, 111–112, 115
    community health workers (CHWs), 185
    explicit and implicit biases, 218
    maternal fetal medicine (MFM) providers, 172
    perinatal workforce, 111–112, 115, 185
    physicians, 237, 382
    support for menopausal Black women, 255
    workforce development, 183–184
health disparities, 252–253
health equity, 62–63
health inequities, 62
health insurance, 220, 236–237
health literacy, 291
HealthConnect One, 198–199, 219
Healthy Families Illinois, 221
Healthy Start, 36, 221–222
heart health, 249–250
HeLa cells, 8
herbal medicine, 66
heterosexism, 89
Higginbotham, Evelyn, 79
high-density lipoproteins (HDL), 250
Hirono, Mazie, 316
Hispanic women, 31
    fertility treatment, 227–228, 230–231
    heart health, 250
    intimate partner violence (IPV), 128
    low birth weight babies, 186–187, *187*
    maternal mortality, 33, 45, 145, 179
    physicians, 382
    preterm births, 186–187, *187*, 188
historical context
    of birth control, 136–137
    of Black breastfeeding and chestfeeding, 215–217
    Civil Rights Era, 7–8, 20, 123
    of comprehensive sexuality education (CSE), 312–313
    of exploitation, 3–13
    Jim Crow Era, 5–7, 22, 112, 122, 167, 216
    for justice-oriented frameworks, 110–111
    of midwifery, 170–171, 180
    of pipeline programs, 381–383
    Progressive Era, 313
    for reframing narratives about sexuality, 75–85
    of reproductive oppression through policymaking, 112–113
    of sexual violence, 121–125
    of trauma, 370
    why we need doulas, 193–197
Historically Black Colleges and Universities (HBCUs), 142, 152, 199
HIV/AIDS, 62, 317
    Black women living with HIV (BWLH), 275–276
    comprehensive HIV care, 281–283
    Ending the HIV Epidemic in the US initiative, 282
    equity-based resilience approach to, 283–284
    healing-focused interventions for, 284
    holistic approach to, 277–278, 284–285
    knowledge gaps related to, 270
    life course approach to, 278
    "Live and Love With HIV" project (Carter), 94
    in older adulthood, 341
    people living with HIV (PLWH), 281–282
    prevention of, 278–281, 305
    resilience to, 283–284
    Sistas, Informing, Healing, Living, and Empowering/Sisters Informing Sisters About Topics on AIDS (SIHLE/SISTA) interventions, 306
    stigma related to, 277, 284–285
    strengths-based approaches to, 277–278, 283–284
    "Undetectable equals Untransmittable (U=U)" campaign, 282–283, 285
HIV/AIDS testing, 94–95, 228
HIV education, 314
holistic approach
    barriers to care, 66–67
    to HIV/AIDS, 277–278, 284–285
    to maternal mortality, 168–173
    to medicine, 65–67
    multisolution, 168–173
    out-of-pocket spending for, 66–67
    recommendations for, 148
    systems-thinking, 64
Home Owners' Loan Corporation, 112, 167–168
home remedies, 66
home visiting services, 221
homelessness, 129–130
homicide, pregnancy-related, 49–50
homophobia, 89, 91
hoochie, 90
hooks, bell, 88–89, 352
hookups, 266–267
hormone-replacement therapy, 257, 297–298
hormone therapy (HT), 257, 297
hot flashes, 250–251
Hotep Twitter, 91
Hottentot Venus, 122
human papillomavirus (HPV), 67, 228, 291
human trafficking, 304
humility, cultural, 331
Hyde Amendment, 17, 113
hypermasculinity, 267, 298–299
hypersexualized imagery, 89–90, 92, 98, 263, 303–304, 349, 355
hypertension, 28–29, 249, 293–294
hypothalamic-pituitary-adrenal (HPA) axis, 253
hysterectomy, 20, 31, 112, 294

I

ICD-10 (*International Classification of Diseases*, Tenth Revision), 163
ideals, beauty, 265
identity, 336, 353, 368–369
Illinois Momnibus legislation, 152
immigrants, 129, 170–171, 205–209, 218

IMPACT (3-2-1 Integrated Model for Parents and Children Together), 170
IMPACT to Save Moms Act, 115
implicit bias, 182, 218, 236, 312
implicit bias training, 52
"In Her Hands" program, 53
in vitro fertilization (IVF), 66, 98–100, 237–238
incarceration, 19–20, 117, 125, 131, 296
inclusion, 331
Indian Health Service (IHS), 18
Indiana Black Breastfeeding Coalition, 221
Indigenous women, 112, 353
infant feeding, 216–217, 223. *See also* breastfeeding; chestfeeding
infant health, 203–213
infant mortality, 34
infertility, 30–31, 66, 240
    Being Mary Jane portrayal of, 99–102
    causes of, 230–234
    definition of, 97, 227, 230
    stigma associated with, 100, 235
    tubal factor, 232–233
Inflation Reduction Act, 153
inhumane medical practices, 19–20
innovation, 116
Instagram, 92, 335–336
institutional racism, 370
institutionalized racism, 48–49
integrated care, 169–170
    comprehensive HIV care, 281–283
    for HIV prevention, 278–281
integrative medicine, 65
intergenerational learning, 391
intergenerational opportunities, 388
internalized oppression, 142
internalized racism, 49, 142
International Classification of Diseases, Tenth Revision (ICD-10), 163
intersectional research, 367–377
    recommendations for, 371, 373, 374, 375
    Silences Framework, 367, 369–375
intersectionality, 157, 367–368
interview #1, 292–295
interview #2, 295–299
intimate candor, 93
intimate partner violence (IPV), 50, 130–131, 276, 279, 369
    definition of, 121, 127
    interventions to reduce, 52–53
    research on, 372
    risk factors for, 127–128
intrauterine devices (IUDs), 6, 229
IPV. *See* intimate partner violence
iron deficiency, 294
Irving, Shalon, 150–151
isolation, 101

J

Jackson, Hogue, Phillips Contextualized Stress Measure, 54

Jane Crow, 32–33
Japan, 171
Jeferson, Thomas, 303
Jezebel stereotype, 75–76, 90, 100, 264, 312
Jim Crow Era, 5–7, 22, 112, 122, 167, 216
JJ Way, 181, 186–187, *187, 189*
JJ Way Framework, 180
Johns Hopkins Hospital, 8
Johns Hopkins University, 8
Johnson, Eddie Bernice, 116
Jones, Camara P., 48–49
Jones, Feminista, 91, 93
Joseph, Jennie, 181, 184
Joy, Mother Mother Binahkaye, 193
Just Be, Inc., 125
justice
    birth, 110–111
    criminal, 124
    data, 209–210
    racial, 327, 330–331
    reproductive, 15–25, 110, 125, 279–280, 359–366
Justice for Incarcerated Moms Act, 117
justice-oriented frameworks, 109–120

K

Kaine, Tim, 117
W.K. Kellogg Foundation, 222
Kelly, Robert (R. Kelly), 21–22
Kellye's story, 335–345
Kentucky, 140
Kenya, 94
Khoikhoi people, 122
Kinsey, Alfred, 329
Kira Johnson Act, 114–116, 148
"Knob-Slobbing Feminism" (Jones), 93
knowledge, shared, 181
knowledge gaps, 227–228, 270
    about HIV/AIDS, 276, 282–283
    about transitioning, 297
    fertility misconceptions, 235
    health-related misconceptions, 291
    sex-related misinformation, 350
knowledge keepers, 353
Kool G Rap, 93
#KSFem, 93

L

Lacks, Henrietta, 8
lactation programs, 221
lactation support persons, 220
Lancet, 171
Las Vegas Strip, 135
Latin America, 387
Latinx women, 203, 292, 312, 338, 382
law enforcement, 124–125
LDL (low-density lipoproteins), 250
leaders, 154
    coalition building, 149–152

interview findings, 394–405
in philanthropy, 393–406
learning
  intergenerational, 391
  Professional Learning Standards for Sex Education (SEC), 330–331
Lee, Barbara, 316
legal subjugation, 15–25
legislation, 169
  hate crime laws, 130
  new maternal health bills, 152–154
  police brutality laws, 131
  status of the mother laws, 4
  See also specific acts, bills
Leonard, Toni Bond, 372
lesbian, gay, bisexual, transgender, queer or questioning, intersex, asexual, and other gender minority (LGBTQIA+) folx, 19–20
lesbian, gay, bisexual, transgender, queer (LGBTQ+) women, 89, 91, 130
  fertility considerations, 237–238
  interview #1, 292–295
  interview #2, 295–299
  scholar experiences, 384
  sex education for, 327
  sexual minority youth (SMY), 337–338
  sexuality and sexual and reproductive health of, 291–300
liberation, 139–141, 403
liberation health framework, *139*, 141–143
liberation psychology, 354
liberty, lack of, 15–17
life course approach, 278
Life of Hope, 210
lifespan approach, 335–345
lifestyle programs, 256–257
Lipscomb, Breana, 150
literature review, 27–43
Little Sisters of the Poor v. Pennsylvania, 139
"Live and Love With HIV" project (Carter), 94
location, 371–373
longevity, 281–282
Lorde, Audre, 15, 88
Louisiana, 317
Louisiana Pregnancy Risk Assessment Monitoring System, 218
low birth weight babies, 186–187, *187*, 199
low-density lipoproteins (LDL), 250
Lucas, Demetria, 94–95
Lucy (enslaved woman), 4–5

M

macular degeneration, 293–294
Mama Glow, 198
Mamatoto Village, 198
mammy stereotype, 75–77, 312
March of Dimes, 36, 194
Markey, Edward J., 117
Maryland, 166
Massachusetts, 53, 99

Maternal CARE Act, 153
maternal care coordinators, 169
maternal fetal medicine (MFM) providers, 172
maternal health, 109
  across the Black diaspora, 203–213
  Black Maternal Health Momnibus Act (Momnibus), 9, 33, 113–117, 145–156, *147*, 169
  equitable, 116
  holistic approach to, 168–173
  key recommendations for, 172
  legislative investments, 153
  mental health, 34–35
  multisolution approach to, 168–173
  new legislation, 152–154
  partner-related recommendations for, 52–53
  racial disparities, 145–147
  racism and, 204–205
  social recommendations for, 52
  stress and, 204–205
  telehealth, 116
  toolkit for, 407
  ways to reduce inequities in, 114–115
  White House Maternal Health Day of Action Summit, 153
Maternal Health Pandemic Response Act, 117
maternal home, 169–170
maternal morbidity, 34, 62
maternal mortality, 3, 33–34, 45–46, 62, 179, 361
  acknowledgment of impact of loss, 162–163
  causal factors, 165–168
  definition of, 163–164
  economic burden of, 163
  pregnancy-related ratio, 161–162
maternal mortality review committees (MMRCs), 163–164
Maternal Vaccination Act, 117
maternity care, 9, 51, 115
maternity care deserts, 111–112
maternity leave, 169
maternity wards, 53
materno-toxic zones, 180–182
matriarch stereotype, 75, 78, 100, 102
McBath, Lucy, 114
McLemore, Monica R., 389
media portrayals, 81–82
  digital media, 90–91, 349
  hypersexualized imagery, 89–90, 92, 98, 263, 303–304, 349, 355
  of trans women, 299
  See also stereotypes
Medicaid, 21, 113, 115, 147
  coverage for doula work, 200
  equitable, 183–184
  expansion of, 9, 31, 139, 154
Medical College of Georgia, 5
medical experiments, 4–6, 166–167, 217, 361
medical illustrations, 328
medical racism, 154
Medicare, 21
medicine. *See* health care

Meigs, Joseph, 233
menarche, 336
Menendez, Robert, 116
menopause, 247–248, 341
    genitourinary syndrome of menopause (GSM), 251
    health disparities in Black women during, 252–253
    lifestyle programs for, 256–257
    stress–menopause cycle, 253–254, *254*
    support for women in, 255–257
    weight gain during, 249
mental health
    interview #2, 296
    Kellye's story, 335–345
    lifespan approach to, 335–345
    maternal, 34–35
    midlife, 339–340
mental health professionals, 339
Merck for Mothers, 33
metabolic syndrome, 234
#MeToo movement, 121, 125–127
micro-communities, 331
midlife, 339–340
"The Midwife Problem," 170
midwifery, 179–180
    enslaved midwives, 194
    granny midwives, 216
    history of, 170–171, 180
    JJ Way, 181
    model of care, 180–181
    recommendations for, 54
mind-body therapy, 66
minorities, sexual, 270
misogynoir, 21–22, 89, 91, 137, 304, 312
misogyny, 91
Mississippi, 140, 317
Mississippi appendectomies, 17, 217
mixed-methods approach, 207–208
MMRCs (maternal mortality review committees), 163–164
Momnibus Act. *See* Black Maternal Health Momnibus Act
Moms Matter Act, 114–115
Montgomery bus boycott (1955), 123
Montgomery Improvement Association, 123
Moore, Bailey, 368
Moore, Gwen, 115
Moore, India, 299
motherhood, 339
Moynihan, Patrick, 78
mulattos, tragic, 75, 77
multigenerational living, 195–196
multiple identities, 368–369
multiple sclerosis, 296
murder, 49–50, 128
myths
    fertility misconceptions, 235
    health-related misconceptions, 291
    impact on reproductive health and sexuality, 82–83

media stereotypes, 21–22
See also stereotypes

N

narratives
    coming-out stories, 92–93
    counter-narratives, 372
    digital storytelling, 94
    intimate candor, 93
    "Live and Love With HIV" project (Carter), 94
    reframing, 75–85
    self-naming in, 92
Nash, Jennifer, 88
National American Woman Suffrage Association, 22
National Association for the Advancement of Colored People (NAACP), 80, 123
National Association of Colored Women, 80
National Birth Equity Collaborative (NBEC), 379–381, 386–391
National Black Women's Health Project, 407
National Center for Complementary and Integrative Health (NCCIH), 65
National Council of Negro Women (NCNW), 137, *138*, 158
National Institutes of Health (NIH), 117
National Medical Association Breastfeeding Alliance, 222
National Perinatal Task Force, 180
National Provider Identifier (NPI), 183
National Research Act, 8–9
National Vital Statistics System (NVSS), 163
Native Americans, 166
nativity, Black, 203–213
naturopathy, 66–67
NBEC (National Birth Equity Collaborative), 379–381, 386–391
neonatology, 11
New Jersey, 53, 315
New York City, New York, 207–208
New York City Department of Health and Mental Hygiene (NYC DOHMH), 164
New York City Health + Hospitals, 170
New York Common Council, 166
New York State, 161, 164–166
New York State Department of Health (NYS DOH), 164
New York State Taskforce on Maternal Mortality and Disparate Racial Outcomes, 165
New York Times, 33
New Zealand, 161
newborns, 11
Nigeria, 94
Nixon, Richard, 8
"No Eggspectations" (*Being Mary Jane*, BET), 98–100
Noble, Safiya Umoja, 90
nonprofit organizations, Black women–led or Black focused, 393–406
Norplant, 18
North Carolina, 140, 152

NOURISH (New Opportunities to Uncover Our Resources, Intuition, Spirit, and Healing), 199
NPI (National Provider Identifier), 183
nurse-midwifery, 170–171
nurses, 382
NVSS (National Vital Statistics System), 163

O

Obama, Barack, 139
obesity, 28, 249
obstetric care, 171–173, 179–180
obstetric racism, 28
obstetric violence, 360–361
obstetrician-gynecologists, 231
obstetrics and gynecology, 166–167, 170
Office of Population Affairs, 315–316
Ohanian, Alexis, 154
older women, 251–252, 269–270
   bodily changes, 340–341
   with HIV, 281–282
   Kellye's story, 340
Older Women Embracing Life, 282
online support groups, 219
opioid use disorder, 81
oppression
   internalized, 142
   reproductive, 112–113
   sexual, 89–91
   tools against, 304–305
oral contraceptives, 6. *See also* birth control
Oraquick, 94–95
organizations, Black women–focused, 393–406
outrage, 186–188
ovarian reserves, 230–231
overweight, 249, 335–336

P

Pacific Islander women, 128
Pan-Africanism, 91
pansexual Black women, 292–295
Papanicolaou (Pap) testing, 31, 291
parent-child communication programs, 319
parents, nongestational, 222–223
Paris Museum of Mankind, 7
Parks, Rosa, 123
partner-related factors
   determinants of chronic stress, 49–50
   intimate partner violence (IPV), 50–53, 121, 127–131, 276, 279, 369, 372
   recommendations for, 52–53
partner support, 173, 236
partnerships, community, 36
partus sequitur ventrem, 112
paternalism, 326
Patient Protection and Affordable Care Act, 8–9
Patterson, Helen (character), 98, 100
Patterson, Niecy (character), 97–98, 100–101
Paul, Mary Jane (character), 97–102

PCC. *See* preconception care
PCOS (polycystic ovary syndrome), 234, 337
peer counselors, 221
peer support groups, 221
peer-to-peer breastfeeding trainings, 219
pelvic inflammatory disease (PID), 234
people living with HIV (PLWH), 281–282
perimenopause, 247–248
perinatal birth workers, 111–112, 115
perinatal care, 9, 179–180, 187, 362–365
perinatal health, 33–35, 63
Perinatal Quality Collaboratives, 36
Perinatal Safe Spots, 181, 185–186, 188–189, *189*, 190
perinatal workforce, 185
Perinatal Workforce Act, 115, 148–149
peripartum care, 49
Perry, Chris, 325–326
person-centered approach, 61
personal growth, 354
Personal Responsibility Education Program (PREP), 315–316
personally mediated racism, 48–49, 52
philanthropy
   decision-making process, 397–398
   funding for Black women–led or Black focused organizations, 397–398, 402–406
   funding organizations, 395–396
   funding practices, 398–400
   future directions, 402–405
   general findings, 394–395
   giving in the US, 393
   history of, 400–402
   impact of, 402–405
   organizations receiving funding, 396–398
physical abuse, 128
physical activity, 256–257, 295–296
physical development, 336–337
physical examination, 347
physicians, 237, 382
phytoestrogens, 256
pipeline programs
   history of, 381–383
   for reproductive justice scholars, 379–381
   See also specific programs by name
Planned Parenthood Federation of America, 6, 137
pleasure, 280–281
PLWH (people living with HIV), 281–282
PMDD (premenstrual dysphoric disorder), 337
PMSS (Pregnancy Mortality Surveillance System), 163
police brutality laws, 131
policy
   health care, 113–117
   justice-oriented frameworks applied to, 113–117
   priorities for, 149
   racist, 167–168
   reproductive justice framework applied to, 147–149
   reproductive oppression through, 112–113
politics, 22–23
   of articulation, 93
   of respectability, 79–80, 90
   of silence, 80

polycystic ovary syndrome (PCOS), 234, 337
pornography, 90
positive representation, 328
positivity
　sex-positive discourse, 263, 280
　sex-positive research, 329–330
　sex-positive sexuality education, 330–332, 348
post-traumatic stress disorder (PTSD), 128
postdoctoral studies
　pipeline programs for reproductive justice scholars, 379–381
　readiness for, 388–389
postmenopausal women, 269–270
postpartum depression, 339
postpartum health, 33–35
poverty, 20–21, 129–130, 297
Praxis Project, 62–63, 67
pre-exposure prophylaxis (PrEP), 279, 303, 305
Precious (2009), 97–98
preconception care (PCC), 29–30
preconception health (PCH), 29–30
pregnancy, 339
　adolescent, 98, 317, 337–338
　ectopic, 232–233
　mortality during, 163–164
　as sexual trauma reactivation period, 361–362
pregnancy-associated but not related death, 164
pregnancy-associated deaths, 163–165
Pregnancy Mortality Surveillance System (PMSS), 163
pregnancy-related deaths, 164–165, 172
pregnancy-related homicide, 49–50
pregnancy-related maternal mortality ratio (PRMR), 161–162
premature aging, 47–48
premenstrual dysphoric disorder (PMDD), 337
PREP (Personal Responsibility Education Program), 315–316
PrEP (pre-exposure prophylaxis), 279, 303, 305
prescription drug abuse, 81–82
Presidential Proclamation in recognition of Black Maternal Health Week, 154
Pressley, Ayanna, 117
preterm births, 186–188, *187*, 199, 203–208
Prevention Access Campaign, 282
Prevost, François Marie, 167
pro-choice movements, 23
Professional Learning Standards for Sex Education (SEC), 330–331
programmatic gaps, 384
programmatic supports, 389–390
programming, educational, 317
Progressive Era, 313
Project Dads in Nutrition Education, 222
promising approaches, 9–10
property taxes, 167–168
Protecting Moms and Babies Against Climate Change Act, 117
Protecting Moms Who Served Act, 117
protein, 256
psychological abuse, 128
puberty, 336–337

public health
　midwifery care and, 179–180
　sexual health education campaigns, 302–303
　strategies to address sexual violence, 130–131
　strategies to reducing maternal mortality, 161–177
Public Health Law Section 2509, 165
Public Health Service Act, 8
public school system, 124–125, 313
Puerto Rican women, 269
Puerto Rico, 6

Q

quality assurance, 183
quality improvement, 116, 183
quality of life, 281–282
quality of services, 183

R

race, 369
race-based medicine, 10
race-based sexual stereotypes (RBSS), 264
race-conscious approach, 10
racial discrimination, 203–213, 216. See also racism
racial disparities
　in infertility diagnosis and treatment outcomes, 231–232
　JJ Way and, 186–188, *187*
　in maternal health, 145–147
　in preterm births, 203–204
　in sexual health, 311–312
racial-gendered discrimination, 326
racial justice, 327, 330–331
Racial Justice and Equity Task Team (SEC), 330
racial sexual violence, 128–130
racial stress, 203–206
racialization, 360–361
racism, 9–11, 109, 182, 312, 326, 369
　and African American health, 167–168
　chronic exposure to, 48–49
　gendered, 49, 71, 369, 382–383
　in health care system, 111–112
　institutional, 370
　institutionalized, 48–49
　internalized, 49, 142
　and maternal health, 204–205
　medical, 154
　obstetric, 28, 360–361
　personally mediated, 48–49, 52
　in policymaking, 112
　role in reproductive and sexual health, 27–28
　and sexual health, 266
　structural, 146, 166
　systemic, 32, 114, 167–168, 216
radical doulas, 194, 197
radical self-love, 307
rape, 15–17, 312
rape culture, 303
RBSS (race-based sexual stereotypes), 264

re-contextualization, 374–375
Reaching Our Brothers Everywhere (ROBE), 222
Reaching Our Sisters Everywhere, 219, 222
Real Education and Access for Health Youth Act (REAHYA), 316
reality theme, 99
Reconstruction, 5
redlining, 29, 53, 112, 167–168
reference groups, 370
reflexive practice, 371
reform, 383–389
reframing narratives, 75–85
Relf, Mrs., 18
Relf sisters (Katie, Mary Alice, Minnie), 18
religion, 266, 298
reparations, 9–10
representation, 331
reproduction
  stratified, 236
  third-party, 239–240
reproductive coercion, 4, 121, 128, 166–167, 268
reproductive freedom, 18, *139*, 141–143
reproductive health, 337
  Being Mary Jane messages, 97–102
  of Black LGBTQ+ women, 291–300
  of Black women, 27–43, 62, 109–120, 402–405
  funding, 402–405
  justice-oriented frameworks for, 110–111
  myths and stereotypes, 82–83
reproductive health care, 20–21, 29–33, 140
reproductive health education, 314–315
"Reproductive Injustice: Gender and Racial Discrimination in US Health Care" (Center for Reproductive Rights), 150
reproductive justice, 15–25, 110, 279–280, 363–364
  pipeline programs for, 379–381
  programmatic supports for, 389–390
  scholar experiences, 383–389, *390*
reproductive justice framework, 125, 147–149, 157
Reproductive Justice Movement, 110
reproductive oppression, 112–113
research
  best practices for, 71
  broadening evidence and representation in, 67
  embedded, 387–388
  future directions, 209–210, 370
  intersectional, 367–377
  literature review, 27–43
  mixed-methods approach, 207–208
  pipeline programs for reproductive justice scholars, 379–381
  recommendations for, 54, 371, 373, 374, 375
  reference groups for, 370
  scholar experiences, 383–389
  sex, 329–330
  sex-positive, 329–330
  on STIs, 370
  wrap-around services for reproductive justice–informed scholars, 379–392
resilience, 283–284, 353

Resiliency in Sexuality Education Model, 331
resistance, digital erotic, 92–95
respectability, politics of, 79–80, 90
respectful maternity care (RMC), 9
respiratory health, 29
restoration, 353
resurrectionists, 5
retreats, 354–355
retrofit, reform, reimagine (3R) framework, 381–390
rhetoric, self-naming, 92
risky behaviors, 316
rituals, 354–355
RMC. *See* respectful maternity care
roadmap to equity, 182–184
Robert Wood Johnson Foundation, 405
Roberts, Dorothy, 157
Rochester, Lisa Blunt, 114–115
Roe v. Wade, 23, 32, 110, 113, 139–140
Roll Call, 158
Ross, Loretta, 372
rural health care, 51

S

Safe Motherhood Initiatives (SMIs), 164
safety
  for Black trans women, 297
  HIV/AIDS, 278–279
  perinatal, 179–191
  roadmap to equity, 182–183
  school, 124–125
safety trials, 6
salpingectomy, 232–233
salpingostomy, 232–233
Sanger, Margaret, 6–7, 137
Sapphire stereotype, 75, 77–78, 100, 312
SBW (strong Black woman) stereotype, 34–35, 75, 78–79, 264–265
Scandal (ABC), 98
scholar experiences, 383–389
school-based sex education, 317–318
school safety, 124–125
SDOH (social determinants of health), 168
Section 1115 waivers, 154
segregation, 112
self-awareness, 352–354, 356
self-care, 307
self-determination, 353
self-esteem, 265, 335–336, 353
self-help guide, 407
self-love, radical, 307
self-naming, 92
semillero (seedbed/hotbed), 387
senescence, cell, 48
severe maternal morbidity (SMM), 62
Sewell, Terri A., 117
sex education
  abstinence-only-based, 316–317, 325–326
  accurate, 349–351
  available curricula, 331–332

Centering Racial Justice in Sex Education: Strategies for Engaging Professionals and Young People (SEC), 330–331
co-therapy case study, 355–356
community-based, 318–320
comprehensive sexuality education (CSE), 303–305, 312–315, 318, 320, 326–328
culturally centered, 351–356
culturally relevant, 330–332
federally funded evidence-based programs, 315–316
formal, 315
lack of, 349–351
positive, 348
Professional Learning Standards for Sex Education (SEC), 330–331
public campaigns, 302–303
Resiliency in Sexuality Education Model, 331
school-based, 317–318
sex-positive, 330–332
Solidarity Statement for Racial Justice in Sexuality Education (The Women of Color Sexual Health Network), 327
suggestions for, 331–332
Sex Education Collaborative (SEC), 330–331
sex-positive and culturally relevant sexuality education, 330–332
sex-positive discourse, 263, 280
sex-positive research, 329–330
sex research, 329–330
sex trafficking, 304
sex workers, 128–131
sexism, 182, 312, 326
sexology, 350
sexual abuse, 304, 360–362
sexual abuse survivors, 124, 364–365
sexual agency, 263–270
sexual and reproductive health, 27, 62
sexual and reproductive health education, 314–315
sexual assault strategies, 305–306
Sexual Attitude Reassessment workshops, 351–352
sexual behavior, 263, 266–270
sexual health, 251–252, 266–271, 350, 369
  of Black LGBTQ+ women, 291–300
  definition of, 87, 280
  digital erotic resistance and, 93–95
  harm-reduction efforts for, 93–95
  indicators of readiness, 305
  inequities, 62
  role of racism in, 27–28
  rooted in eroticism, 88–89
sexual health campaigns, 302–303
sexual health care, 29–33
sexual minorities, 270
sexual minority youth (SMY), 337–338
sexual mores and taboos, 264–265
sexual oppression, 89–91
sexual orientation, 337–338
sexual pleasure, 280–281
sexual risk, 282

sexual-risk-avoidance education (SRAE), 316–317
sexual satisfaction, 263–270
sexual self-concept, 369
sexual stereotypes, race-based, 264
sexual violence
  against Black girls and women, 312, 359–362
  continuum of, 121
  history of, 121–125
  #MeToo movement, 121, 125–126
  public health strategies to address, 130–131
  racial and gender-based, 128–130
  responses to, 126–127
  against sex workers, 128–130
  social context of, 360–362
  state-sanctioned, 17
  trans panic defense of, 130
sexual well-being, 263–271
sexual wellness, culturally centered, 351–356
sexuality
  of Black LGBTQ+ women, 291–300
  of Black women, 27–43, 75–85, 335–345, 348–349, 402–405
  emerging, 265–266
  funding, 402–405
  lifespan approach to, 335–345
  midlife, 339–340
  older adulthood, 341
  oversexualization of Black girls, 303–304
  reframing narratives of, 75–85
sexualization, 123–124
sexually transmitted diseases (STDs), 312–313
sexually transmitted infections (STIs), 30, 311–312
  acquisition of, 228
  in adolescents, 317
  knowledge gaps related to, 270
  in midlife, 340
  in older adulthood, 341
  prevention of, 313, 326
  research on, 370
  screening for, 32
  in women of later reproductive age, 269
  in young people, 303
shame, 100, 348–349
Sheppard–Towner Act, 7, 180
SIHLE/SISTA (Sistas, Informing, Healing, Living, and Empowering/Sisters Informing Sisters About Topics on AIDS) interventions, 306
silence(s)
  culture of, 265
  hearing, 371–373
  politics of, 80
  voicing, 373–374
  working in, 369–371
  working with, 374–375
Silences Framework, 367, 369
  stage 1, 369–371
  stage 2, 371–373
  stage 3, 373–374
  stage 4, 374–375
silent generation, 281
Sims, James Marion, 4–5, 10, 166–167, 217

INDEX | 441

Sistas, Informing, Healing, Living, and Empowering/Sisters Informing Sisters About Topics on AIDS (SIHLE/SISTA) interventions, 306
SisterSong Women of Color Reproductive Justice Collective, 9–10, 149–150, 372
skin colors, 328
"Skye's the Limit" (Telusma), 94
slavery, 15–17, 112, 215–216, 360
　afterlife of, 362
　birth control methods, 136
　breeding plantations, 166–167
　history of, 3–5, 10–11, 122, 194
Small, Maria, 162
SMIs (Safe Motherhood Initiatives), 164
Smith, Barbara, 90
Smith, Tina, 116
SMM (severe maternal morbidity), 62
SMY (sexual minority youth), 337–338
social cognitive theory, 349
social conditioning, 348–349
Social Determinants for Moms Act, 114
social determinants of health (SDOH), 168
　determinants of chronic stress, 48–49
　determinants of health equity, 62–63, 67
　determinants of perinatal health, 63
social hygiene movement, 313
social media, 81, 223
social recommendations, 52
social safety net, 115–116
Social Security, 21
social support
　access to, 235–236
　resources for breastfeeding, 217–223
social workers, 169
Society for Adolescent Health and Medicine, 317
Society for the Scientific Study of Sexuality, 350
sociocultural context, 264–266
socioeconomic status (SES), 20, 267
Solidarity Statement for Racial Justice in Sexuality Education (The Women of Color Sexual Health Network), 327
South Africa, 94
South Carolina, 140
Southern Poverty Law Center, 18
Special Supplemental Nutrition Program for Women, Infants, and Children (WIC), 114, 152, 170, 218, 221, 223
specialty obstetric care, 171–173
spirituality, 80–81, 266
SRAE (sexual-risk-avoidance education), 316–317
Stallings, L.H., 92
standardized data collection, 116–117
state-sanctioned violence, 17, 19
Steele, Catherine Knight, 92
Stephens, Dionne, 123–124
stereotype threat, 82–83
stereotypes, 21–22, 100–102, 235, 326, 360–361
　Black lady, 80
　impact on reproductive health and sexuality, 82–83
　interview #2, 296

Jezebel, 75–76, 90, 100, 264, 312
mammy, 75–77, 312
matriarch, 75, 78, 100, 102
race-based sexual stereotypes (RBSS), 264
Sapphire, 75, 77–78, 100, 312
strong Black woman (SBW), 34–35, 75, 78–79, 264–265
tragic mulatto, 75, 77
welfare mother, 75, 78, 102
sterilization, 137
　compulsory, 17–18
　forced, 112, 217
　Mississippi appendectomies, 17, 217
　tubal, 18, 228–229
stigma
　associated with infertility and fertility treatment, 100, 235
　HIV-related, 277, 284–285
　interview #2, 296
storytelling, 94. See also narratives
stratified reproduction, 236
strengths-based approaches, 277–278, 283, 306–307
stress
　chronic, 46–55, 247–261
　definition of, 46
　determinants of, 48–54
　financial, 20, 139, 163, 169
　impact on health outcomes, 46–48
　impact on menopausal Black women, 247–261
　Jackson, Hogue, Phillips Contextualized Stress Measure, 54
　racial, 203–206
stress management, 257
stress-menopause cycle, 253–254, 254
strong Black woman (SBW) stereotype, 34–35, 75, 78–79, 264–265
Study of Women's Health Across the Nation (SWAN), 252
sub-Saharan African Black women, 206
subcultures, 331
subfertility, 230–234
substance abuse, 81–82
Substance Abuse and Mental Health Services Administration (SAMHSA), 114–115
substance use interventions, 305–306
sucklers gangs, 216
suicide, 129–130
Supplemental Nutrition Assistance Program (SNAP), 114, 170
support groups, 219, 221
sustainability, 353
SWAN (Study of Women's Health Across the Nation), 252
sympathetic nervous system (SNS), 253
systemic racism, 32, 114
systems thinking, 64

T

taboos, 264–265
tailored approaches, 210

"The Talented Tenth," 80
#TalkLikeSex, 93
targeted universalism, 52
Taylor, Recy, 123
Tech to Save Moms Act, 116
Teen Pregnancy Prevention (TPP), 315–316
tele-lactation services, 220
telehealth, 53, 116, 188
Telusma, Blue, 94
Ten Steps to Successful Breastfeeding (BFHI), 219
Tennessee, 140
terminology, 15, 92, 302
testosterone blockers, 297
thelarche, 336
theory of targeted universalism, 52
third-party reproduction (TPR), 239–240
3-2-1 Integrated Model for Parents and Children Together (IMPACT), 170
3R (retrofit, reform, reimagine) framework, 381–390
Title V, 316
Title X National Family Planning Program (Title X), 8, 113, 140, 147
    funding, 140
TPP (Teen Pregnancy Prevention), 315–316
TPR (third-party reproduction), 239–240
traditional Chinese medicine, 66
traditional health care delivery, 65–67
tragic mulatto stereotype, 75, 77
trans panic defense, 130
transgender women
    health care of, 292
    HIV prevalence, 275
    HIV risk, 276
    interview #2, 295–299
    sexual violence against, 128–130
    violence against, 20, 298–299
trauma, historical, 370
trauma-informed care, 363, *364*
trauma responses, 126–127
trauma-responsive care, 363–364
Trump, Donald, 139
Trump administration, 19–20, 140
trust, 353
tubal factor infertility, 232–233
tubal ligation, 229
tubal sterilization, 228–229
tube tying, 18
Tumblr, 92
Tuskegee Syphilis Study (Tuskegee Study of Untreated Syphilis in the Negro Male), 7–8, 10, 122, 146, 217
Twitter, 93, 121, 125–126, 299
two-generation care, 170

U

underrepresented racial minority (URM) women, 382–383, *383*
Underwood, Lauren, 113, 117, 150–151, 153
"Undetectable equals Untransmittable (U=U)" campaign, 282–283, 285
Union, Gabrielle, 98

United Kingdom, 171
United Nations Committee on the Elimination of Racial Discrimination, 150
United States
    Africans, 3–4
    agricultural economy, 3–4
    Biden-Harris administration, 153–154
    Black women, 3–13, 27–43, 62, 203–210
    breastfeeding, 217
    carceral system, 19–20
    Civil Rights Era, 7–8, 20
    compulsory sterilization, 17–18
    contraception deserts, 140
    COVID-19 pandemic, 9
    criminal justice system, 124
    Ending the HIV Epidemic in the US initiative, 282
    exploitation, 3–13
    health care system, 65, 111–112
    historical perspective, 3–13
    Hyde Amendment, 17, 113
    immigrants, 205–210
    Jim Crow Era, 5–7, 22, 112, 122, 167, 216
    "Live and Love With HIV" project (Carter), 94
    maternal health crisis, 109
    maternal mortality, 3, 145–146, 161, 179, 361
    materno-toxic zones, 180, 182
    midwifery care, 171
    philanthropic giving, 393
    political process, 22–23
    population, 382
    post–Civil Rights era, 8–9
    pregnancy-related deaths, 172
    Presidential Proclamation in recognition of Black Maternal Health Week, 154
    preterm births, 186–188, *187*, 203–206
    Progressive Era, 313
    public school system, 124–125, 313
    racism, 146–147
    Reconstruction, 5
    reproductive oppression through policymaking, 112–113
    sex education, 312–313, 315
    sexual and reproductive health education, 314–315
    slavery, 3–5, 112, 166
    Southeast, 9
    state-sanctioned sexual violence, 17
    Trump administration, 19–20, 140
United States Supreme Court, 110, 113. *See also specific cases*
universal birth control access, 139–141
universalism, targeted, 52
University of California, San Francisco (UCSF), 380, 386
Urban League, 80
US Department of Health and Human Services (HHS), 114–117, 148–149, 154
    maternal mortality, 145, *146*
    Office of Women's Health, 220
    Title X National Family Planning Program (Title X), 140

US Department of Housing and Urban Development, 114
US Department of Transportation, 114
US Public Health Service (PHS), 7–8, 10, 122
US Surgeon General, 219
US Vital Records system, 210
uterine cancer, 31
uterine fibroids, 30–31, 62, 66, 231–232, 294–295
U=U ("Undetectable equals Untransmittable)" campaign, 282–283, 285

V

vaccines, 67, 117
van Blarcom, Carolyn Conant, 170–171
vasomotor symptoms, 252
verbalization, 373–374
Veterans Affairs, 117
victimhood
  of Black women, 304, 360–362
  denial of, 21–22
Victorian family ideals, 313
violence
  against Black transgender women, 20, 298–299
  against Black women and girls, 312, 359–362
  gender-based, 360–361
  intimate partner violence (IPV), 50–53, 121, 127–131, 276, 279, 369, 372
  obstetric, 360–361
  sexual, 17, 121–126, 131, 359–362
  state-sanctioned, 17, 19
  trans panic defense of, 130
Violence Against Women Act, 130–131
Virginia, 4, 166
vitamin C, 256
vitamin D, 256
vitamin E, 256
Voting Rights Act, 22
vulvovaginal symptoms, 251

W

Wald, Lillian, 170–171
Walker, Alice, 105
Walker, James, 216
War on Drugs, 81, 216
Ward, Maranda C., 367–368
Warnock, Raphael G., 114–116
Warren, Elizabeth, 117
Washington, Booker T., 80
The Washington Post, 158, 167
"We Remember," 110
wealth disparities, 53
weathering, 29, 46–48, 71, 168, 206
web shows, 94
Webster v. Reproductive Health Services, 110
weight gain, 249
welfare mother stereotype, 75, 78, 102
welfare queens, 18

well-woman visits, 291, 347
wellness
  access to accurate sexual wellness education, 349–351
  of Black adolescent girls and young women, 301–309
  culturally centered, 351–356
  Indigenous indicators, 353
  interview #2, 296
  sexual, 263–271, 351–356
Western medicine, 65
White House Maternal Health Day of Action Summit, 153–154
white infants, 34
white supremacy, 137–138, 219
white women
  ectopic pregnancy, 232
  endometriosis, 233
  fertility preservation, 230
  fertility treatment, 231
  heart health, 250
  intimate partner violence (IPV), 128
  low birth weight babies, 186–187, *187*
  maternal mortality, 33, 45, 62, 145, *146*, 161, 168, 172, 179
  pregnancy-related maternal mortality ratio (PRMR), 162
  preterm births, 186–187, *187*, 188
  as reference group, 370
  reproductive coercion, 128
  severe maternal morbidity (SMM), 62
  sexual health, 312
  uterine fibroids, 62, 231–232
whiteness, 166, 370
whole-body autonomy and self-awareness, 352–354
whole person-centered approach, 61
WIC (Special Supplemental Nutrition Program for Women, Infants, and Children), 114, 152, 170, 218, 221, 223
Wilcox, Wendy C., 162
Williams, Serena, 154
woman phase, 265
womanism, 105
Women of African Descent for Reproductive Justice, 158, *158*
Women of Color Sexual Health Network, 327
women who have sex with women (WSW), 270
women who have sex with women and men (WSWM), 270
women's circles, 354
women's empowerment programs, 403
women's health, 4. *See also* African American women; Black women; Brown women; white women
Women's Rights Movement, 110
work gangs, 216
workforce development, 183–184
World Health Organization (WHO), 9, 87, 163, 280, 350
wrap-around services, 379–392

WSW (women who have sex with women), 270
WSWM (women who have sex with women and men), 270
Wyatt, Gail, 105–106

X

X, Malcolm, 36

Y

young women
  gender identity, 337–338
  Indigenous wellness indicators, 353
  Kellye's story, 337
  reproductive health, 337
  sexual behavior, 266–267
  sexual minority youth (SMY), 337–338
  sexual orientation, 337–338
  strengths-based methods for, 306–307
  wellness, 301–309
YouTube, 92–93

Z

zero-tolerance policy, 124–125